W9-ADD-485

DEATH BY MIGRATION

DEATH BY MIGRATION

EUROPE'S ENCOUNTER WITH THE TROPICAL WORLD IN THE NINETEENTH CENTURY

PHILIP D. CURTIN
The Johns Hopkins University

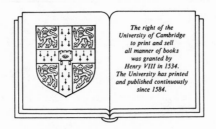

The right of the
University of Cambridge
to print and sell
all manner of books
was granted by
Henry VIII in 1534.
The University has printed
and published continuously
since 1584.

CAMBRIDGE UNIVERSITY PRESS

Cambridge

New York   Port Chester   Melbourne   Sydney

Published by the Press Syndicate of the University of Cambridge
The Pitt Building, Trumpington Street, Cambridge CB2 IRP
40 West 20th Street, New York, NY 10011, USA
10 Stamford Road, Oakleigh, Melbourne 3166, Australia

© Cambridge University Press 1989

First published 1989

Printed in the United States of America

Library of Congress Cataloging-in-Publication Data
Curtin, Philip D.
Death by migration : Europe's encounter with the tropical world in
the nineteenth century / Philip D. Curtin.
p. cm.
Bibliography: p.
ISBN 0-521-37162-7. – ISBN 0-521-38922-4 (pbk.)
1. Tropical medicine – History. 2. Soldiers – India – Mortality.
3. Soldiers – Algeria – Mortality. 4. Soldiers – West Indies –
Mortality. 5. Medicine, Military – History. I. Title.
RC961.C87   1989
614.4'0913–dc20   89-31414

British Library Cataloguing in Publication Data
Curtin, Philip D. (Philip De Armond)
Death by migration : Europe's encounter with
the tropical world in the nineteenth century.
1. Tropical regions. Europeans. Diseases,
1815–1914
I. Title
616.9'88'3

ISBN 0-521-37162-7 hard covers
ISBN 0-521-38922-4 paperback

CONTENTS

v

TABLES, FIGURES, AND MAPS

Tables

vii

Appendix Tables

Health Indicators – Great Britain

Health Indicators – The British West Indies

Miscellaneous

Figures

Maps

PREFACE

From the beginning of European trade and conquest overseas, Europeans knew that strange "climates" could have fatal effects. Later, they came to understand that it was disease, not climate, that killed, but the fact remained that every trading voyage, every military expedition beyond Europe, had its price in European lives lost. For European soldiers in the tropics at the beginning of the nineteenth century, this added cost in deaths from disease – the "relocation cost" – meant a death rate at least twice that of soldiers who stayed home, and possibly much higher.

This book is a quantitative study of the relocation costs among European soldiers in the tropics between about 1815 and 1914, but it has broader implications. For Europe itself, this was the crucial century of the "mortality revolution," with its profound influence on European and world demographic history. For the history of medicine, this was the transitional century between the kind of medicine that had been practiced in Europe since classical times and the kind of scientific medicine that would be spawned by the germ theory of disease. For Europe's global political and military relations, this marked the final period for the European conquest. For all these reasons, the relocation costs of this period have great bearing on human history.

In the longest run of time, human culture and human relationships to disease have passed through three phases. In the earliest, before the agricultural revolution of 10,000 B.C. – plus or minus a few millennia – human beings lived in small communities, as hunters, fishers, and gatherers. As they spread out from their presumed place of origin somewhere in eastern Africa, their ways of life changed and became increasingly varied. The major languages came into existence, along with ancestor ways of life that continue deep in the backgrounds of present human communities. Geographically, these early people occupied all of the major continents, including the Americas and Australia.

That earliest phase was by far the longest in human history, and it began a process of mutual adjustment between people and disease that has gone on ever since. In the 1940s and later, biological scientists began to see the relationships between diseases and people as part of a broader ecological system in which many different forms of life are interrelated. The ecological point of view suggests that, as human communities in semi-isolation spread, humans and their parasites engaged in a continuous process of adaptation and readaptation. Parasites evolved to take better advantage of their hosts; hosts responded with adjustments in their immune system, which sometimes promoted evolutionary change that resulted in genetic immunities. Most immunities, however, are acquired. The diseases of childhood are precisely that because they are broadly endemic in our society. Most people are infected in childhood and thus acquire the antibodies needed to protect them from further infection as adults.[1]

The process of adjustment between parasites and people is subtle, changing, and still not fully understood. In the preagricultural world, human communities were small and isolated. We can guess that they had comparatively few diseases, which had adapted and readapted to that particular community over a very long period of time. The human community in turn acquired a set of immunities that were limited but suited to their particular disease environment.

Then, with the development of agriculture, population density increased, which in turn led to widespread urbanization and intercommunication. Trade expanded across the Afro-Eurasian landmass, and by sea along its fringes. The intercommunicating zone for commerce became an intercommunicating zone for the spread of ideas and religions – and of diseases. As a result, the isolated disease environments were invaded by the diseases of their neighbors and underwent the painful process of acquiring immunities. The initial cost of entering the intercommunicating zone was a series of virgin-field epidemics with high death rates and probably a population decline until the necessary immunities were in place. The long-term cost was to live with a wider variety of parasites than the scattered hunting communities had had to put up with.

In the nineteenth century came the third phase, coinciding with the commencement of the industrial age. This period is comparatively short, barely two centuries, and the history of modern science is the account of its triumphs. With the rapid growth of science and technology, beginning in the late eighteenth century, Western countries learned how to produce more goods with less labor than any previous human society had used. Technical triumphs were not limited to manufacture and distribution. The new technology included means to intervene more effectively than ever before in the human battle against disease. People succeeded in reducing the threat of some diseases, like

[1] For a synthesis of this point of view, see Macfarlane Burnet and David O. White, *Natural History of Infectious Disease*, 4th ed. (Cambridge, 1972).

typhoid fever, and in destroying a few, like smallpox; but since that time they have also had to contend with new challengers, like AIDS.

We know much less about the middle period, between the agricultural and industrial revolutions. Medicine was comparatively ineffective in controlling parasites, though it laid the basis for modern medicine. In the history of disease, we are broadly acquainted with the impact of an unfamiliar disease on a nonimmune population, like that of the Black Death in Medieval Europe, the die-off of the American Indians from the sixteenth century into the nineteenth, or that of the Australian aborigines and the Pacific islanders in the late eighteenth and nineteenth.[2] We thus have some idea of the impact of alien diseases on isolated populations at the moment they entered the intercommunicating zone with its more diverse range of diseases.

Another important factor to consider is the European death rate as the Europeans moved overseas. We have some knowledge about this for particular areas, and the phenomenon is known generally, if not in detail.[3] For a better understanding of this process – of what happens when people leave their childhood disease environment – we need more than the impressionistic observations and scattered figures that make up most of the historical record. Ideally, we need experimental evidence. If several thousand human subjects could be recruited in a particular region of Europe, one part sent to live overseas while another stayed at home, and the health of both groups kept under careful medical observation over a period of years, with particular attention to the cause of death, we would have some hard evidence. The group at home could serve as a control from which to measure the changing health of the group overseas. The experiment should also exclude the application of modern medicine, and it should be repeated at intervals of ten years or so.

Needless to say, no such experiment is possible today. Aside from the cost, the loss of life would make it unthinkable. Yet the experiment was actually performed in the nineteenth century, not once but over and over again. European governments recruited men for military service, sent some overseas and kept others at home. They made careful records of the health of both groups – the most careful records of this kind available for any human group of equivalent size anywhere in the world before this century – and they published these records in

[2] Alfred W. Crosby, Jr., *Ecological Imperialism: The Biological Expansion of Europe, 900–1900* (New York, 1986); *The Columbian Exchange: Biological and Cultural Consequences of 1492* (New York, 1972); P. M. Ashburn, *The Ranks of Death: A Medical History of the Conquest of America* (New York, 1947); William H. McNeill, *Plagues and Peoples* (New York, 1976).
[3] K. G. Davies, "The Living and the Dead: White Mortality in West Africa, 1684–1732," in Stanley L. Engerman and Eugene D. Genovese, *Race and Slavery in the Western Hemisphere: Quantitative Studies* (Princeton, 1975), pp. 83–98; P. D. Curtin, "The White Man's Grave: Image and Reality, 1780–1850," *Journal of British Studies*, 1:94–110 (1961); "Epidemiology and the Slave Trade," PSQ, 83:191–216 (1968).

printed annual reports on the health of the army. These reports are especially comprehensive from the 1860s onward, but they exist for periods as far back as 1816 and occasionally date back into the eighteenth century. For much of the nineteenth-century tropical world, military health records are the earliest, and sometimes the only, quantifiable guide to the history of disease.

The nineteenth century was also the prime century of the mortality revolution in Europe itself. As the first century of the industrial age, it was a period of transition, among other things from a world in which birth rates and death rates were typically 30 or more per thousand, to one in which both were a small fraction of that number. For men of military age, even in Europe, death rates per thousand dropped by more than 80 percent in the course of that century. The improvement was still more striking for Europeans overseas.

Although this study focuses on the problem of relocation costs and death in the tropical world, the data have important implications for Europe as well. The control group of soldiers is not necessarily typical of European populations – even of populations in the twenty to forty age range – but the military doctors produced more careful and consistent data on cause of death than any contemporaneous civilian records did. These data add something to what was previously known about the transition in demographic history from the mainly agrarian to the industrial period in world history.

The first objective is to establish the principal patterns of European military death from disease in the tropical world, then to discover why they changed. The book contains two parts. The first deals with the period up to the 1860s, a period of relative stability in a mainly preindustrial world. The second deals with the 1870s to the beginning of the First World War, the transitional decades when scientific medicine became a major influence. Each part begins with a chapter measuring disease among the military at home and abroad. Chapters 2 and 5 examine major trends of European thought about tropical hygiene, while Chapters 3 and 6 take up the applications of that thought in the field situation.

The military medical data are rich and various. By the early twentieth century, they covered scores of different overseas territories and half a dozen European and North American armies. This study is limited, however, to the French and British armies, with special attention to three colonial settings – the British West Indies, Algeria, and the Madras Presidency of British India. The three sample territories represent different overseas environments. The British West Indies represents the New World, humid tropics, where malaria and yellow fever were especially serious. Algeria represents a Mediterranean climate similar to that of southern France, not strictly speaking tropical but epidemiologically different. South India is an example of monsoon

Asia, where the principal killing diseases were again different. Algeria and India provide the best samples because Europeans were there longer and in larger numbers than anywhere else. Other important disease environments are omitted. Tropical Africa was the most dangerous place in the world for Europeans, but the number of European troops there was not large enough to be used comparatively over a long period of time. Other sample areas might have been chosen in Asia – such as the Dutch East Indies, mainland Southeast Asia, the China coast, and other parts of British India – but, at this stage, it seemed preferable to work with the sample area that provided data for the largest number of troops over the longest period of time, with the least distortion from frequent campaigns.

These military records as a whole open several lines of investigation, of which the present study is only one. They report on the health of non-European as well as European recruits into Western armies. In a second projected study I plan to compare the mortality experience of "native" troops with those of Europeans serving in the same place. This topic has important implications for comparative immunology and for European colonial and military policy.[4] A third project will trace the patterns of disease and death among non-Europeans who were moved from their home environment as soldiers in European armies, including the nineteenth century West Africans who served in the French, British, and Dutch armies in places as various as the Caribbean, East Africa, Ceylon, Indonesia, and Morocco.[5]

The nineteenth century was the central period of European imperialism in the tropics, made possible by the achievements of industrial technology. One of those achievements was scientific medicine. Between the early nineteenth century and the eve of the First World War, the typical death rate of European soldiers in the tropics dropped by 90 percent. In due course, I hope to explore some of the policy implications of this decline in the cost of empire.

Every book leaves a trail of debt the author has accumulated that can never be repaid. The specialized collections in the field of military history at the National Library of Medicine in Bethesda are certainly the richest in the world, going back to the period when that library was the Library of the Surgeon-General of the United States Army. I am especially grateful to its staff, especially to the Division of Medical History, and in particular to Mrs. Dorothy Hanks for her uncanny skill in being able to lay her hands on uncatalogued works in the collection. The

---

[4] See, as a pilot study, P. D. Curtin, "Differential Military Mortality in the Nineteenth Century: European Medicine and Non-European Soldiers" (unpublished paper presented at the International Economic History Association, Bern, Switzerland, August 1986).

[5] Philip D. Curtin, "African Health at Home and Abroad," *Social Science History*, 10:369–398 (1986), is a pilot study for that project.

Interlibrary Loan staff at the Milton E. Eisenhower Memorial Library at The Johns Hopkins University in Baltimore also responded far beyond the call of duty to requests for aid.

The other inevitable debt is to those who have been kind enough to read manuscripts under construction and to reply with criticisms and suggestions. For this chore, I am especially beholden to my friends and colleagues James Cassedy, Anne G. Curtin, Robert S. Desowitz, Caroline C. Hannaway, Rachel Laudan, Harry M. Marks, and Charles Rosenberg.

ABBREVIATIONS

AHMC	*Annales d'hygiène et de médecine coloniale*
AHPML	*Annales d'hygiène publique et de médecine légale*
AHR	*American Historical Review*
AMN	*Archives de médecine navale*
AMPM	*Archives de la médecine et pharmacie militaire*
AMSR	British Army Medical Service Reports (later Army Medical Department)
BHM	*Bulletin of the History of Medicine*
DESM	*Dictionaire encyclopédique des sciences médicales* (Paris, 1861)
GMA	*Gazette médicale d'Algérie*
ICHD	International Congress of Hygiene and Demography
JAH	*Journal of African History*
JBS	*Journal of British Studies*
JIH	*Journal of Interdisciplinary History*
JRAMC	*Journal of the Royal Army Medical Corps*
JSSL	*Journal of the Statistical Society of London*
JTMH	*Journal of Tropical Medicine and Hygiene*
MH	*Medical History*
MS	*The Military Surgeon*
MTG	*Medical Times and Gazette*
PP	Great Britain, Parliamentary Sessional Papers
PSQ	*Political Science Quarterly*
RC	*Revue coloniale*
RGCMSM	*Revista general de ciencias médicas y de sanidad militar*
RHPS	*Revue d'hygiène et de police sanitaire*
RMMM	*Receuil de mémoires de médecine militaire*
RTC	*Revue des troupes coloniales*
WHO	World Health Organization

CHAPTER 1

THE MORTALITY REVOLUTION AND THE TROPICAL WORLD: RELOCATION COSTS IN THE EARLY NINETEENTH CENTURY

Between the seventeenth century and the middle of the twentieth, the Western world passed through a profound demographic change. Earlier patterns of high mortality and high fertility gave way to comparatively lower birth and death rates, like those that prevail today. The crucial change is generally (but not universally) interpreted as a "mortality revolution" – a one-time and dramatic change in death rates that opened the possibility for lower birth rates as well. By the mid twentieth century, the mortality revolution had reached most world societies. Not all of them chose lower fertility, but those that failed to do so experienced runaway population growth, sometimes as high as 4 percent per year.

In the nineteenth century, death rates not only dropped in Europe; they dropped even more dramatically among Europeans who went overseas. The change profoundly altered Europe's epidemiological relationship to the rest of the world. In the eighteenth century and before, death rates of Europeans moving into the tropical world at least doubled and could increase several fold – even for men in the prime of life.[1] When these death rates began to drop, Europeans were free to move into the tropical world at far less risk than ever before.

The Statistical Base

Military doctors have given us our best records of death and disease among mobile populations – and death from disease was far more serious in the nineteenth century than death in battle. Military doctors often treated men recruited in one part of the world and serving in another. From the early nineteenth century, they became especially concerned about recording what they observed. The statistical movement in British and French intellectual life was just then seeking quantitative measures of social phenomena that could be used to guide

---

[1] Philip D. Curtin, "Epidemiology and the Slave Trade," *Political Science Quarterly*, 83:191–216 (1968).

1

public policy in a number of areas, one of which was the health of the army, especially of the army serving overseas. Rising humanitarian sentiments from the late eighteenth century on brought increased sympathy for the common soldier, and practical considerations began to be important; the death of soldiers overseas was a burden to the taxpayer.

Although Britain did not begin to register births and deaths until the late 1830s, military records make it possible to reconstruct some annual mortality rates of British troops serving in India as far back as 1793.[2] These records reflect an even earlier concern for the health of British troops in the West Indies. Medical men and commentators of the early nineteenth century still recalled disease catastrophes of nearly a century earlier.[3] During the English attack on Cartagena on the Caribbean coast of South America in 1742, the English force spent only two months laying siege to the city, but its losses from disease alone were two-thirds to three-quarters of its more than 12,000 men – a big army for the Americas at that time. Even if they had lost only half the force, the annualized loss would come to 3,000 per thousand men.

Losses on a similar scale followed the English attack on Havana in 1762, the English intervention in Saint Domingue in 1793–98, and the French effort to reconquer that colony from rebellious slaves in 1802. In all these cases, fresh, nonimmune troops from the north met epidemic yellow fever. Even in normal times, the high death rate of troops on garrison service was cause for alarm.[4]

Wellington's losses in the peninsular campaign against Napoleonic France was another recent memory of high mortality. Sir James Mac-Grigor had been chief medical officer during that campaign. He then became director general of the Army Medical Department in the 1830s, where he was instrumental in ordering a retrospective statistical survey based on army medical reports back to 1816.[5]

[2] "Report of a Committee of the Statistical Society of London, Appointed to Collect and Enquire into Vital Statistics, upon the Sickness and Mortality among the European and Native Troops Serving in the Madras Presidency, from the Year 1793 to 1838," JSSL, 3:113–43 (1840).

[3] Moreau de Jonnès, Essai sur l'hygiène militaire des Antilles (Paris, 1817); John R. McNeill, "The Ecological Basis of Warfare in the Caribbean, 1700–1804," in Adapting to Conditions: War and Society in the Eighteenth Century, ed. Maarten Utlee (Tuscaloosa, 1986), pp. 16–42.

[4] F. Guerra, "The Influence of Disease on Race, Logistics and Colonization in the Antilles," Journal of Tropical Medicine and Hygiene, 49:23–35 (1966); David Geggus, Slavery, War, and Revolution: The British Occupation of Saint Domingue 1793–1798 (Oxford, 1982), pp. 347–72; Nicolas Pierre Gilbert, Histoire médicale de l'armée française à Saint-Domingue, en l'an dix: ou mémoire sur la fièvre jaune, avec un aperçu de topographie médicale de cette colonie (Paris, 1803).

[5] James MacGrigor, "Sketch of the Medical History of the British Armies in the Peninsula of Spain and Portugal during the Late Campaigns," Medical-Chirurgical Transactions, 6:381–489. For the statistical movement, see Theodore M. Porter, The Rise of Statistical Thinking (Princeton, 1986), esp. pp. 23–38; Michael J. Cullen, The Statistical Movement in Early Victorian Britain (New York, 1975), esp. pp. 45–52; see also Neil Cantlie, A History

In 1835, a medical crisis at an army hospital in the Bahamas added to the sense of urgency and led to the appointment of a special board of inquiry. Its chairman was Henry Marshall, an army doctor who had served in Ceylon and India and had already published statistical studies of army health. He, in turn, recruited Capt. Alexander M. Tulloch, a former foot officer with a legal background. Marshall was responsible for the overall design of the research that followed, and, when he retired in 1836, T. Graham Balfour took his place. Tulloch did most of the writing and supervised the assemblage of data, while Balfour kept the ensuing series of reports in line with medical knowledge. Together, the three men became the founders of systematic military medical statistics.

The first product of their research appeared in 1838 – the book-length "Statistical Report on Sickness, Invaliding, and Mortality among Troops in the West Indies."[6] Over the next four years the team followed up with equally impressive reports on England, North America, and the Mediterranean (1839); on Africa and the African islands (1840); and on Ceylon and Burma (1842). Each of these covered the two decades between 1817 and 1836 as nearly as possible.[7] Even before the last report had appeared, the British Navy began to produce its own medical statistics, and the United States government ordered a compendium of reports on its own army's health over the period 1819–39.[8] Tulloch and his colleagues began work on a second series covering the decade, 1837–46, but only one full report appeared – on troops in Britain, North America, and the Mediterranean.[9] The Crimean War diverted attention from leisurely retrospective views of army health to the dramatic toll of military deaths from disease in Turkey and the Crimea.

By the end of the 1850s, it was again possible to resume regular reporting – now in the form of annual reports by the Army Medical Department, published as a separate volume each year and also republished in the Parliamentary Sessional Papers. In 1859, the first of the new series summarized the unpublished data for 1837–46 in aggre-

of the Army Medical Department, 2 vols. (London and Edinburgh, 1974), 1:404–41. For its implications for the history of medicine, see James H. Cassedy, American Medicine and Statistical Thinking, 1800–1860 (Cambridge, 1984) and Medicine and American Growth 1800–1860 (Madison, 1986).

6 British Parliamentary Papers (cited hereafter as PP), 1837–8, xl (138).
7 In each case, Alexander M. Tulloch was listed as author, PP, 1839, xvi [C.166]; PP, 1840, xxx [C.228]; PP, 1842, xxvii [C.358].
8 "Statistical Reports on the Health of the Navy 1830–6, PP, 1840, xxx (163); PP, 1841, Sess. 2, vi (53); United States Army, Statistical Report on the Sickness and Mortality in the Army of the United States, from January 1819 to January 1839 (Washington, 1839).
9 Great Britain, Army Medical Department [Alexander M. Tulloch and T. Graham Balfour], Statistical Reports on the Sickness, Mortality, and Invaliding among the Troops in the United Kingdom, the Mediterranean, and British America (also published in Parliamentary Papers, 1853).

gated form, but the decade 1847–58 is still missing from the series. Parliamentary investigations took up the sorry sanitary record of armies in the Crimean War and the loss to disease among troops sent to suppress the Sepoy Mutiny in India in 1857. The government appointed a royal commission to survey the health of the troops in India and prescribe remedies.

When the Royal Commission on India reported in 1863, it found that the recent death rates of British military in India represented the trailing edge of a prolonged plateau of relatively high mortality stretching back still further into the past.[10] Most authorities date the beginnings of the mortality revolution as far back as the late seventeenth or early eighteenth century, and this was no doubt true for civilian populations.[11] The Indian commissioners, however, assessed the plateau rates for enlisted men in India over the whole period from 1800 to 1856 at about 69 per thousand; those for officers were 38 per thousand, and those for European civil servants about 20 per thousand.[12] The low rate for civilians highlights one of the fundamental facts of military medical experience; troops in barracks are much healthier than troops on campaign, even disregarding losses from combat, and military campaigns had been an ever-present reality in India before the 1860s.[13]

That same Royal Commission worked out the cost of Indian operations in pounds, shillings, and pence. It cost £100 to recruit a soldier and maintain him in India. With an army of 70,000 Europeans, 4,830 would die each year, and 5,880 hospital beds would be full at any given moment. Britain was therefore losing £588,000 annually from sickness alone. A similar force might have cost £200,000 in European conditions; the extra £388,000 was a surcharge for tropical service.[14]

---

[10] Great Britain, Royal Commission on the Sanitary State of the Army in India, *Report of the Commissioners Appointed to Inquire into the Sanitary State of the Army in India.... 2 vols. (London, 1863), 1:xi. A one-volume version consisting of the commissioners' report and a précis of evidence is printed in PP, 1863, xix [C.3184], but on different size sheets and with different pagination. See also William W. Hodges, "On Mortality Arising from Military Operations," JSSL, 19:219–71 (1856); John Pringle, *Observations on the Diseases of the Army*, 7th ed. (London, 1775), pp. 54, 60; Committee on the Preparation of Army Medical Statistics, PP, 1861, xxxvi (366), p. 44

[11] James C. Riley, "Insects and European Mortality Decline," AHR, 91:833 (1986).

[12] India Royal Commission, *Report*, p. xix. The data for officers and civilians, however, were not calculated over the same period or on the same basis as those for enlisted men, so that they are not strictly comparable. Officers and civilians, for example, had great freedom of choice to be "invalided" home in case of illness. Judging from later evidence, the commissioners' figures were probably too high for enlisted men and perhaps too low for officers. At later periods, death rates for officers and other ranks did not differ very much, and the health of officers was not necessarily better.

[13] This principle was well understood by the early statisticians; see, for example, Statistical Society of London, "Report of the Committee of the Statistical Society of London, Appointed to Enquire into Vital Statistics, upon the Sickness and Mortality among the European and Native Troops Serving in Madras Presidency, from the Year 1793 to 1838," JSSL, 3:113–43 (1840).

[14] India Royal Commission, *Report*, p. xvii ff.

Equivalent calculations had been published in France. Shortly after 1830, when the French conquest of Algeria began, French authorities became alarmed over the high death rate from disease among its troops in North Africa. In 1847, Jean Boudin, an army doctor who had served in Algeria, pointed to a recent death rate of 64 per thousand for Algerian service, or, with a total force of 100,000 in round numbers, an annual loss of 6,400 men – seven times the death rate in France for men of military age.[15] But the French had already begun to improve their performance, and the death rates dropped steadily from the mid-1830s. The French death rate from disease in the Crimean War, however, was even higher than the British, and the lesson was taken as seriously in France as in Britain. The French credited the British with superiority in military medicine and tried hard to catch up.[16] By 1866, they had succeeded so well in Algeria that the British War Office sent commissioners to investigate, hoping to use the lessons of French experience in India.[17]

The British Royal Commissioners of 1863 set their own goals for the future. They calculated that the "natural" death rate for men of military age in Britain was around 10 per thousand. Twenty per thousand seemed a reasonable short-run goal for India, to be achieved solely by applying known sanitary measures. In the longer run, they hoped to achieve what they called the "natural" rate of "no more than 10 per thousand per year."[18] As it turned out, the British Army in India met the first goal within the decade; it met the second, 10 per thousand, in 1907.

By the 1870s, most European armies and navies published annual reports on the health of the services. Dutch reports are especially important because of their sample size and length of continuous publication. Their forces in the East Indies were the largest in tropical Asia, after India itself, and some data are available as far back as the Dutch reoccupation of the islands at the end of the Napoleonic Wars. At least from 1848, these reports appeared in the annual *Kolonial Verslag*, matching those for the domestic army.[19] Spanish and Portuguese series also began to appear from the 1870s.[20]

Partial French returns had appeared here and there during the first

---

[15] Jean C. M. F. J. Boudin, "Études sur la mortalité et sur l'acclimatement de la population française en Algérie," AHPML, 37:358–9 (1847).

[16] Alphonse Laveran, *Traité des maladies et épidémies des armées* (Paris, 1875), p. xx.

[17] PP, 1867, xv [Cd.19447], *Report of the Causes of Reduced Mortality in the French Army Serving in Algeria*.

[18] India Royal Commission, *Report*, p. lxxxi.

[19] Netherlands, Department van Kolonien, *Kolonial Verslag* (annual series); Department van Oorlog, Geneeskundig Dienst der Landmacht, *Statistisch overzicht der bij het Nederlandsche leger in het year . . . behandelde zieken* (annual series).

[20] Spain, Ministerio de la Guerra, *Resumen de la estadistica sanitaria del ejercito española* (Madrid, 1884+); Portugal, Ministerio de Guerra, *Estatistica geral do servicio de exercito* (Lisboa, 1870–1+).

half of the century,[21] but the Ministère de la Guerre began its own regular annual series of *Statistiques médicale de l'armée metropolitaine et de l'armée coloniale* beginning in 1862. Volumes for 1869–71 were not published because of the Franco-Prussian War, but otherwise the series continues down to 1913. A French navy series later joined it, but, until the late 1890s, the navy published no regular returns for the *troupes de la marine* (later *troupes coloniales*) who actually did most of the fighting in the nineteenth-century tropics.

The Geography of Relocation Costs

In spite of gaps, the record shows certain major trends for the better part of a century. Table 1.1 provides a point of departure, because it shows the earliest data available for most of the listed territories. The significant data are in three categories: the death rates of soldiers at home, those of soldiers overseas, and the difference between them. This difference (the *relocation cost* in deaths of removing a person to a new setting, different from his childhood disease environment) can be measured absolutely – as so many deaths per thousand – or relatively, as the percentage increase or decrease over the rates prevalent at home. Relocation costs, however, need not be measured in deaths only. They can also be recorded separately for any one of the other health indicators found in the army reports – discharge on grounds of health, repatriation from a foreign station, morbidity measured by hospital entries, or morbidity measured by the mean percentage of the force in hospital at any moment. The most telling of these indicators is death.

Table 1.1 is arranged by region. The variance within some regions is large, although the regional pattern is clear. The temperate countries (Map 1.1) are reasonably homogeneous – showing death rates from 15 per thousand in the northern United States to 20 per thousand in France. Once beyond Europe and North America, the result of movement was generally negative – relocation exacted a *cost*. The one exception is a part of the southern and tropical Pacific, where relocation was a *benefit* to European soldiers.

Relocation Benefits

Epidemiological theory suggests that people moving as adults to a new disease environment will suffer for lack of the immunities they would have acquired in childhood. Nineteenth-century European opinion

[21] Jean Boudin, "Statistique médicale de l'armée anglaise," RMMM, 12(3d ser.): 369–89; 12:1–22 (1864–5); "Statistiques coloniale. Mortalité des troupes," RC, 10(2d ser.):473–81 (1853).

Table 1.1. *Mortality of European Troops Overseas, 1817–38*

Region	Nationality of Troops	Date of Sample	Deaths per Thousand	Relocation Costs or Benefits (percent)
Pacific Islands				
Tahiti	French	1845–9	9.50	50.01
New Caledonia	French	c. 1848	11.40	21.14
New Zealand	British	1846–55	8.55	44.12
Europe and North America				
France	French	1820–2, 1824–6	20.17	
Great Britain	British	1830–6	15.30	
Northern United S.ates	American	1829–38	15.00	
Canada	British	1817–36	16.10	
Mediterranean climate				
Algeria	French	1831–8	78.20	−287.70
Gibraltar	British	1818–36	21.40	−39.87
Malta	British	1817–36	16.30	−6.54
Ionian Islands	British	1817–36	25.20	−64.71
Cape Colony	British	1818–36	15.50	−1.31
Southern United States and malaria-free islands				
Bermuda	British	1817–36	28.80	−88.24
Southern United States	American	1829–38	34.00	−126.67
Mauritius	British	1818–36	30.50	−99.35
Réunion	French	1819–36	32.12	−59.25

Table 1.1. (cont.)

Region	Nationality of Troops	Date of Sample	Deaths per Thousand	Relocation Costs of Benefits (percent)
Southern Asia				
Bombay	British	1830–8	36.99	–141.76
Bengal	British	1830–8	71.41	–366.73
Madras	British	1829–38	48.63	–217.84
Ceylon	British	1817–36	69.80	–356.21
Coastal Burma	British	1829–38	34.60	–126.14
Straits Settlements	British	1829–38	17.70	–15.69
Dutch East Indies	Dutch	1819–28	170.00	–1,011.11
West Indies				
Jamaica	British	1817–36	130.00	–749.67
Windwards and Leewards	British	1817–36	85.00	–455.56
Guadeloupe	French	1819–36	106.87	–429.85
Martinique	French	1819–36	112.18	–456.17
French Guiana	French	1819–36	32.18	–59.54
Tropical Africa				
Sénégal	French	1819–38	164.66	–716.36
Sierra Leone	British	1819–36	483.00	–3,056.86

Source: British: PP 1837–8. xl (138); 1839, xvi [C.166]; 1840, xxx [C.228]; 1842, xxvii [C.356]. Madras, Coastal Burma, and Straits Settlements: Committee Report on Madras, JSSL, 3:113–43, 4:137–55 (1840–1). All three belonged to the Madras Army, but are here disaggregated. New Zealand: AMSR, 1:114 (1859), relocation calculated on British data for 1830–6. American: Thomas Lawson, *Statistical Report on the Sickness and Mortality in the Army of the United States*, 3 vols. (Washington; D.C. 1840–60). French Interior, Benoitson de Chateauneuf, "Essai sur la mortalité dans l'infantrie française," AHPML, 10:239–316 (1833). The year 1823 is omitted because of French intervention in Spain. Colonies, *Revue coloniale*, 10(2d ser.):473–81 (1853). New Caledonia, Bertillon, "Acclimatment," DESM, 1:43. Tahiti: F. Burot and M. A. Legrand, *Les troupes coloniaux*, 1:66–7. Dutch: *Deutches Kolonialblatt*, 5:116 (1894). Relocation calculated from British home data.

Table 1.2. *Mortality of European Troops Overseas, 1909–13*

	Nationality of Troops	Dates	Deaths per Thousand	Change from Table 1.1 (percent)	Relocation Costs of Benefits (percent)
Pacific Islands					
Hawaii	American	1909–13	1.30		50.00
Tahiti[a]	French	1903–6	2.30	−24.20	20.14
New Caledonia	French	1909–13	2.33	−79.56	19.10
Europe and North America					
France	French	1909–13	2.88	−85.72	0.00
Great Britain	British	1909–13	2.55	−83.33	0.00
Continental United States	American	1904–13	2.60	−82.67	0.00
Mediterranean					
Algeria and Tunisia	French	1909–13	5.25	−93.29	−82.29
Morocco	French	1909–13	21.99		−663.61
Gibraltar	British	1909–13	2.21	−89.67	13.33
Malta	British	1909–13	2.53	−84.48	0.78
Cyprus	British	1909–13	1.66		34.90
Egypt	British	1909–13	3.97		−55.69
Formerly Malaria-free islands					
Bermuda	British	1909–13	2.21	−92.33	13.33
Mauritius	British	1909–13	4.53	−85.15	−77.65
Southern Asia					
India	British	1909–13	14.08		−452.31
Ceylon	British	1909–13	5.49	−92.13	−115.29
Straits Settlements	British	1909–13	4.75		−86.27
North China	British	1909–13	5.09		−99.61
Philippines	American	1909–13	3.27		−25.77

Table 1.2. (cont.)

	Nationality of Troops	Dates	Deaths per Thousand	Change from Table 1.1 (percent)	Relocation Costs of Benefits (percent)
South China	British	1909–13	3.81		−49.41
Cochinchina	French	1909–13	8.90		−209.03
Annam/Tonkin	French	1909–13	3.57		−23.96
Dutch East Indies	Dutch	1909–13	6.39	−96.24	−150.44
West Indies					
Jamaica	British	1909–13	7.76		−204.31
French Antilles	French	1909–13	4.93	−71.91	−71.11
Cuba and Puerto Rico	American	1904–9	3.59		−38.08
Tropical Africa					
French West Africa	French	1909–13	6.65		−131.04
French Equatorial Africa	French	1909–13	5.66	−95.96	−96.56
Madagascar	French	1909–13	5.67		−96.74
British West Africa	British	1909–13	5.56	−98.85	−118.04
South Africa	British	1909–13	3.84	−75.23	−50.59
Kamerun	German	1901–6	41.12		−1512.63

a No troops in Tahiti in 1909–13, but annual average mortality in 1903–6 was 2.3 per thousand.
Source: Netherlands: Central Bureau voor de Satistiek, *Statistisch Overziergt den Behandelde Zieken van het Nederlanisch Lager over het jaar 1913* (The Hague, 1915), p. 28. Kamerun: Germany, Kolonialamt. *Medizinal-Bericht über die Deutschen Schutzggebiete*, 1905–6, pp. 122, 385–9, 393–4, 410–11, 422, 430. Philippines, Cuba/Puerto Rico, Hawaii, and United States: United States; *Report of Surgeon General of the Army*, Annual series. 1904–13. French Colonies 1909–13: *Statistiques médicale des troupes coloniales*, annual series. Morocco and Algeria: Ministère de Guerre, *Statistiques médicales*, report for 1913. French Colonies 1909–13: *Statistiques médicale des troupes coloniales*, annual series. Netherlands and Germany: British mortality data used as proxy.

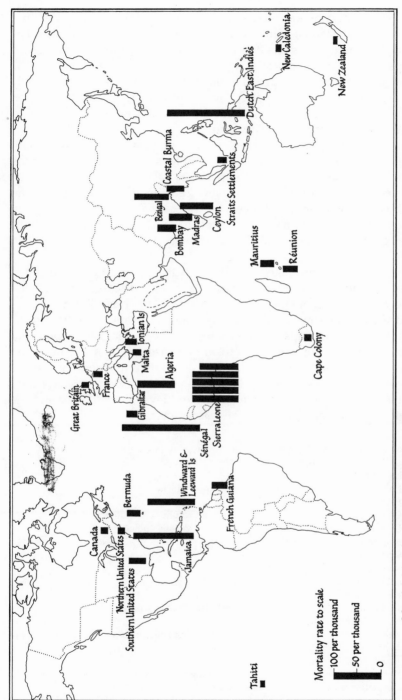

Map 1.1 Mortality of European Troops at Home and Abroad, 1817–38 (from numerical data in Table 1.1)

understood this phenomenon as the danger of a "tropical climate." But certain Pacific islands, some of them tropical, show the opposite. The most prominent and sustained example is Tahiti, which gave French troops a 100 percent mortality improvement over France itself in the 1840s and continued to produce mortality benefits on into the early twentieth century. Hawaii also joined the benefits group in the pre-war quinquennium. Our best evidence on a disease-by-disease basis, however, comes from New Zealand.

The Europeans rarely needed a large military force in the South Pacific, and therefore the size of the sample is restricted, except for the 1860s, when the New Zealand Land Wars called for a larger force. At mid century, the British force in New Zealand was barely more than a thousand men, and it showed the relocation benefit of 44 percent (Table 1.11). By 1859–63, it had risen to an annual average of 9,500 men, giving a far better statistical viability for the data reported in Table 1.3.

The new British nosology introduced in 1859, however, is a source of possible confusion. The largest class, "zymotic" diseases, implied that some form of fermentation was the cause. This class was then sub-divided into "miasmatic" diseases like malaria, blamed on "miasmas" from the soil, swamps, or other source; "enthetic," a graphic but appropriate term for sexually transmitted diseases; and the more obvious "dietic" and "parasitic" diseases. In spite of new terminology for disease classes, most individual diseases and disease groups kept their old names, although some categories like "fevers" or "diseases of the lungs" were subdivided for greater accuracy.[22]

---

[22] The British disease classification of 1859–68 was as follows:

Class I, Zymotic Diseases	*Modern Equivalents*
Miasmatic diseases	
Eruptive fevers	Smallpox, chicken pox
Paroxysmal fevers	Malaria, yellow fever
Continued fevers	Typhoid, typhus, and others
Dysentery/diarrhea	Included Asiatic cholera
Sore throat and influenza	
Ophthalmia	
Rheumatism	
Enthetic diseases	Syphillis, gonorrhea, etc.
Dietic diseases	Included scurvy and drunkenness
Parasitic diseases	Included Guinea worm
Class II, Constitutional	
Diathetic	Included lumbago, anemia, tumors, anasarca
Tubercular	
Class III, Local Diseases	
Nervous system	Including apoplexy and delirium tremens
Circulatory system	Mainly heart disease
Respiratory system	Pneumonia, but not tuberculosis of the lungs
Digestive system	Appendicitis, hernia, colic, enteritis,

The most unusual feature of military death in New Zealand over these five years was the fact that deaths from accident and battle exceeded deaths from disease – a situation that may be unique in European warfare of the nineteenth century.[23] The high number of deaths in battle is evidence of heavy campaigning, which usually brought a sharp increase in deaths from disease as well as battle. If, under this circumstance, deaths from disease were even lower than those in Britain, peacetime relocation benefits must have been still greater than Table 1.3 indicates.

Although New Zealand is not within the tropics, some tropical diseases might have been present, but they were not – no yellow fever, no malaria, no cholera.[24] This in itself removed some of the greatest dangers to European troops overseas. The telling evidence, however, is the killing incidence of diseases common in Europe as well. Table 1.3 shows relocation costs and benefits by disease in two ways. One is the difference in death rates per thousand between the colony and the mother country (column 3). The other is the relative contribution of each disease to the total relocation cost or benefit (column 4). The greatest sources of benefit were tuberculosis, pneumonia (the principal "disease of the respiratory system"), and smallpox (by far the most deadly of "eruptive fevers"). Together, these accounted for 60 percent of military deaths in Britain, but only 37 percent in New Zealand. Together, they accounted twice over for the total relocation benefit, because they were balanced by other diseases that showed relocation costs. These were the waterborne diseases that usually flourished on campaign – dysentery plus diseases of the digestive system, which together reduced benefits by 48 percent. "Continued fevers" (of the still undifferentiated typhus/typhoid group) took off another 20 percent. But either of these death rates was moderate compared with the usual campaign experience.

Urinary system	Including kidney disease
Reproductive system	Not including venereal diseases
Locomotive system	Including arthritis
Integumentary system	All kinds of skin diseases

Class V, Accidents or Violent Deaths
Accidents
In action
Punishment.

[23] See Louis C. Duncan, "The Comparative Mortality of Disease and Battle Casualties in the Historical Wars of the World," *Journal of the Military Services Institution of the United States*, 54:141–77 (1914).

[24] New Zealand and much of the Pacific basin were malaria-free because they had no Anopheline mosquitos to serve as vectors. The present division between malaria and malaria-free islands runs between the New Hebrides and New Caledonia and is thought not to have changed in recent times. This left all of Polynesia – including New Zealand, Hawaii, and Tahiti in the malaria-free zone (Boyd, *Malariology*, 1:725–6, 2:820–1).

Table 1.3. *Mortality of European Troops in New Zealand and the United Kingdom, 1859–63*

Disease	Deaths per Thousand			Contribution to Relocation Benefits (percent)	Percent of All Deaths from Disease	
	Britain	New Zealand	Difference in Rates		Britain	New Zealand
Miasmatic diseases						
Eruptive fevers	0.29	0.00	−0.29	32.22	3.48	0.00
Paroxysmal fevers	0.00	0.00	0.00	0.00	0.00	0.00
Continued fevers	0.40	0.58	0.18	−20.00	4.80	7.81
Dysentery/diarrhea	0.22	0.47	0.25	−27.78	2.64	6.33
Sore throat/influenza	0.04	0.00	−0.04	4.44	0.48	0.00
Rheumatism	0.08	0.00	−0.08	8.89	0.96	0.00
Enthetic diseases	0.11	0.00	−0.11	12.22	1.32	0.00
Dietic diseases	0.06	0.42	0.36	−40.00	0.72	5.65
Parasitic diseases	0.01	0.00	−0.01	1.11	0.12	0.00
Diathetic disease	0.14	0.16	0.02	−2.22	1.68	2.15
Tubercular disease	3.37	1.95	−1.42	157.78	40.46	26.24
Local diseases						
Nervous system	0.69	0.79	0.10	−11.11	8.28	10.63
Circulatory system	0.76	1.00	0.24	−26.67	9.12	13.46
Respiratory system	1.40	0.79	−0.61	67.78	16.81	10.63
Digestive system	0.50	0.68	0.18	−20.00	6.00	9.15
Urinary system	0.12	0.26	0.14	−15.56	1.44	3.50
Reproductive system	0.00	0.00	0.00	0.00	0.00	0.00
Locomotive system	0.02	0.00	−0.02	2.22	0.24	0.00
Integumentary system	0.09	0.16	0.07	−7.78	1.08	2.15

Other or not specified	0.03	0.17	0.14	−15.56	0.36	2.29
All diseases	8.33	7.43	−0.90	100.00	100.00	100.0
Accidents	0.62	1.84				
Battle	0.00	6.69				
Homicide/suicide	0.28	0.05				
Execution	0.01	0.05				
Punishment	0.00	0.00				
Grand total	9.24	16.06				

Note: The category "myasmatic diseases" is disaggregated in proportion to the annual data for household troops stationed in London and Windsor.
Source: AMSR for 1864, pp. 6; for 1860, p. 11; for 1861, p. 10; for 1862, p. 11; for 1863, p. 10.

Ironically, the European soldiers were spared from exactly the same European diseases they transmitted to the native population of the Pacific islands. The Pacific islanders' ancestors had come from Asia, but the island populations had been isolated for a thousand years or more. If they had ever had the full range of diseases prevalent on the Asian mainland, many of these diseases had long since died out, perhaps for lack of sufficient population density to keep them in circulation. Polynesian populations therefore lacked acquired immunities that might have protected them from the exotic diseases that swept the islands from the earliest European contact in the late eighteenth century. The demographic result is clear in New Zealand: The native population declined from about 100,000 to 200,000 in the late eighteenth century to 42,000 in 1896.[25] A similar decline took place throughout the Polynesian world, mainly from virgin-field epidemics of tuberculosis, pneumonia, venereal, and gastrointestinal infections.

Most Pacific islands were too small to call for a regular European garrison, apart from New Caledonia, which served France as a penal colony; but the force was so small – usually about 350 to 650 soldiers – that the evidence is only suggestive. Its relocation benefit was 21 percent around 1848, and 19 percent just before the First World War, although it had swung to a 72 percent relocation cost in 1903–9.[26] New Caledonian data are anomalous in another respect. The suicide rate there was extremely high – 2.88 per thousand in 1903–6 and 1.41 per thousand in 1909–13. Suicide was, indeed, the leading cause of death, and the death from homicide came to 1.23 per thousand in 1909–13. It is tempting to set New Caledonia aside as a special case, perhaps because of its role as a penal colony, but the data from Hawaii, Tahiti, and New Zealand suggest that a regional trend was also present.

Some aspects of this pattern extended to the western rim of the Pacific. The historical epidemiology of the Japanese civilian population suggests that, before the "opening" of Japan to the broader intercommunicating zone in midcentury, Japan also belonged among the relatively isolated societies in which both diseases and immunities were limited. Plague and typhus were absent. Dysentery was present, but it appeared seasonally and seems to have been fatal less often than it was in Western Europe. Measles was present from time to time in epidemic form, but not as an endemic childhood disease. In 1817–22, the first of the nineteenth-century cholera pandemics reached Japan, but the disease did not return until the late 1850s. Then, during the second half of that century, Japan, too, passed through the kind of disease crisis that had reached Europe long before. In the 1870s, the British sent a small

[25] Alfred W. Crosby, *Ecological Imperialism: The Biological Expansion of Europe, 900–1900* (Cambridge, 1986), esp. pp. 252–61.
[26] *Statistiques médicales coloniales*, 1903–6.

force to Japan, but its death rate by that date showed a relocation cost, not a benefit.[27]

Elsewhere on the Pacific rim, the Straits Settlements in the 1830s enjoyed a brief reputation for superior healthfulness – for European troops, curiously enough, but not for those recruited in British India. The death rate of European troops in Penang during 1829–38 was only 17.7 per thousand, although the mean strength of this force was too low to be significant.[28] Garrisons continued to be small, but the good reputation also survived with occasional mention through the rest of the century.[29]

The Regions of Relocation Costs

Most of the world falls into the category of relocation costs, although they were not always large. Climatically, the south shore of the Mediterranean was much like the north shore in Italy or southern France. On grounds of general climate, one might expect even smaller mortality differences than those reported on Table 1.1. The British posts at Gibraltar, Malta, and the Ionian islands, however, show a range of relocation costs from 7 percent to 65 percent, which seems to indicate that the disease environment was not much different from that of northern Europe. The high Algerian figure of 288 percent in the 1830s was certainly the result of campaigning in the conquest period. Within a decade or so, the Algerian death rate was closer to the rates of the Mediterranean islands. Indeed, by 1909–13, Gibraltar, Malta, and Cyprus had all begun to show small relocation benefits for British troops (Table 1.2).

The southern United States and certain subtropical or tropical islands – Bermuda, Mauritius, and Réunion – made up the second group. All of these fell within the range of 29 to 34 deaths per thousand. Of these, Bermuda and the southern United States were subtropical, and Bermuda was free of malaria as well. The two Mascarene islands – Mauritius and Réunion – had a fully tropical climate. They were the approximate antipodes of Jamaica, but they were malaria-free in the early nineteenth century.

The third group, in monsoon Asia, was also tropical, but the disease environment had its own peculiarities. It included endemic Asiatic cholera, missing from the New World before the nineteenth century,

[27] Ann Bowman Jannetta, *Epidemics and Mortality in Early Modern Japan* (Princeton, 1987), pp. 155–60, 188–207.
[28] "Second Report of a Committee . . . ," JSSL, 4:145 (1841).
[29] Asst. Surgeon A. Fergusson, "Sanitary Report for 1863," AMSR, 7:383–84 (1863). The force was usually small. In 1863, for example, it consisted of only eighty-one men. Among these, the only death was from heart attack, yielding the meaningless statistic of 12.35 deaths per thousand from this (and all other) causes. See Andrew Davison, *Hygiene and Diseases*, p. 131.

but it had no yellow fever. The very high mortality figure for the Dutch East Indies was unrepresentative for the same reason the Algerian figure was. These years included those of the Java War, with tough campaigns, high casualties from combat, and high disease rates. Otherwise, the range in India and Ceylon, from 37 per thousand for Bombay to 70 per thousand for Ceylon, is somewhat higher than the subtropical group and somewhat lower than the West Indies.

But southern Asia was a diverse region. Contemporaneous medical authorities were struck by the difference in death rates between the two sides of the Bay of Bengal. In the early 1840s, a committee of the Statistical Society of London studied the vital statistics of troops in the Madras Presidency – both European and "native." The Madras Army at that time served on both sides of the Bay – at Penang, Melaka, and Singapore in Malaya, and at Moulmein on what was then the Tenasserim Coast (now coastal Burma) – as well as in peninsular India. Death rates for European troops were much lower on the eastern than on the western side of the bay, although the reverse was true for Asian soldiers. Madras was worse than Burma for hepatitis, dysentery, and cholera, although slightly better statistically in deaths from "fevers." The authorities in Madras were so impressed that they proposed setting up a sanatorium in Burma to receive invalids from India, who might otherwise have been sent to England; and a few were actually transferred from Madras to Moulmein in lieu of medical discharge.[30]

In this period, as in the past, West Indian death rates for European soldiers were usually higher than they were in monsoon Asia, but erratically so. The main culprit was epidemic yellow fever, which was especially serious among new arrivals in the region but variable in its occurrence. It had a very high case-fatality rate but provided the survivors with permanent immunity.[31] In the sample years, the Jamaican death rate was exceptionally high (130 per thousand), whereas French Guiana was low (32 per thousand). In later decades, the order was reversed, with Jamaica low and French Guiana high (see Table 1.5).

Finally, tropical West Africa falls into a category all its own, with the highest morbidity and mortality rates for outsiders found anywhere in the world (see Map 1.2). The Sierra Leone rate of more than 400 per thousand was somewhat higher than usual, but peacetime rates of 100 to 200 per thousand had been common enough in the past and were to persist for several decades to come.[32]

---

[30] "Second Report of a Committee ...," JSSL, 4:144, 151(1841).

[31] For the epidemiology of yellow fever, see Macfarlane Burnet and David O. White, *Natural History of Infectious Disease*, 4th ed. (Cambridge, 1972), pp. 242–9; Thomas P. Monath, "Yellow Fever," in G. Thomas Strickland, *Hunter's Tropical Medicine*, 6th ed. (Philadelphia, 1984), pp. 176–80.

[32] K. G. Davies, "The Living and the Dead: White Mortality in West Africa, 1684–1732," in *Race and Slavery in the Western Hemisphere: Quantitative Studies*, ed. Stanley L.

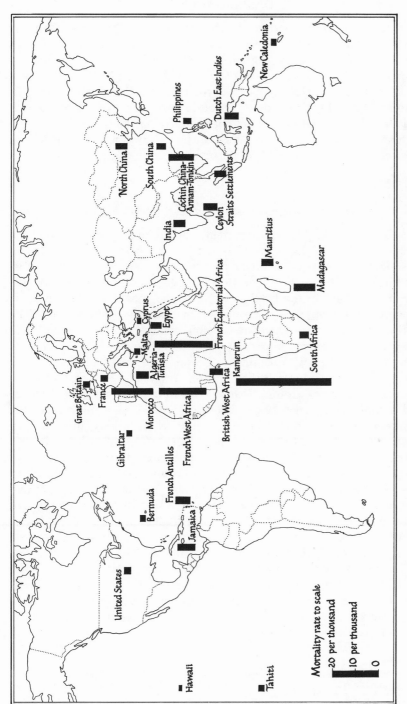

Map 1.2 Mortality of European Troops at Home and Abroad, 1909–13 (from numerical data in Table 1.2)

Table 1.2 provides another and similar baseline, this time at the end of the period – the last five years before the First World War, or as close to that as possible with the data available. The main lines of change are clear. Death rates had dropped everywhere – sometimes more rapidly for soldiers overseas than among those who stayed in Europe. As a result, although absolute relocation costs were down, relative relocation costs had not changed dramatically. They remained at more than 100 percent for the major European forces in Asia and in tropical Africa, and topped 50 percent in the West Indies and North Africa.

Change through Time by Cause of Death: Madras

The changes wrought by the mortality revolution are dramatic enough in themselves – as deaths per thousand – but their explanation lies in the changing cause of death in particular regions. Perhaps the most significant data are those for British India, which held the largest European armies in the tropical world. India, however, was an enormous territory embracing a number of discrete environments. The Madras Presidency itself was reasonably small and homogeneous, but most of the Madras army was stationed elsewhere. The political geography of British India under the *raj* was most complex. British India, the area of direct British control, originally consisted of three nuclear regions: one around Bombay, one in the hinterland of Calcutta, and a third based on Madras. These regions became the core of the presidencies, but with the expansion of British authority, literally hundreds of native states eventually came under British authority, although they were ruled by recognized Indian authorities on a day-to-day basis. Some were no larger than a group of villages. Others, like Mysore and Hyderabad in peninsular India, had the area and population of a medium-sized European state. All had their own police, and some had their own armies, although limited in size. The Madras Army, like the other two armies, therefore had the job of maintaining the security of British power outside the province of Madras itself. Just before 1860 its largest single force was, indeed, stationed in Hyderabad. As a result, the disease environment of the Madras Army was hardly homogeneous, but it was more homogeneous than the whole of India, and it was not much involved in intensive campaigning in the mid and late nineteenth century.

Engerman and Eugene D. Genovese, (Princeton, 1975), pp. 83–98; P. D. Curtin, "Epidemiology and the Slave Trade," 191–216 (1968); "The White Man's Grave: Image and Reality, 1780–1850," JBS, 1:94–110 (1961); *The Image of Africa: British Ideas and Action, 1780–1850* (Madison, 1964), pp. 177–97, 483–7.

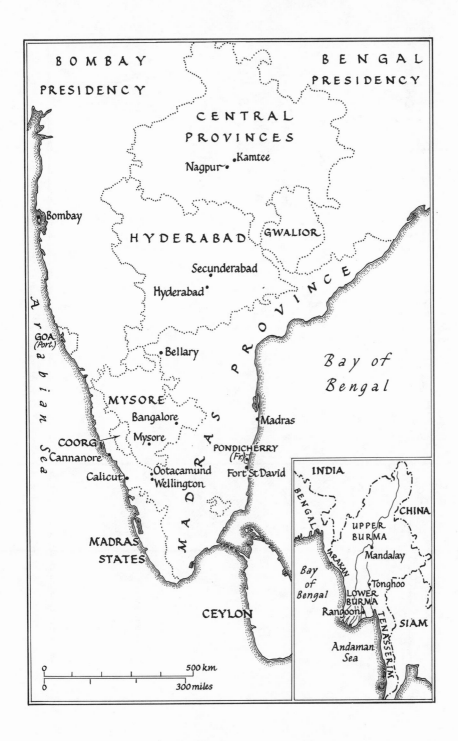

Map 1.3 South India and Burma – Early Nineteenth Century

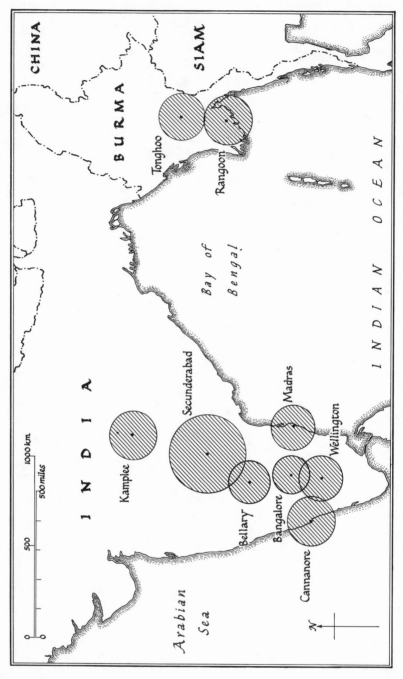

Map 1.4 Location of European Troops Attached to the Madras Army, about 1860

Table 1.4. *Military Mortality of the Madras Army, 1793–1838*

Years		Deaths per Thousand per Year
Wartime Service		
1793–98	Carnatic, India	59
1799–1800	Mysore, India	111
1801–5	Carnatic and the Deccan, India	88
1810–11	Java and Mascarene Islands, overseas	69
1817–19	Pindari War in the Deccan, India	73
1824–6	Burma, overseas	119
Peacetime Service		
1806–9		70
1812–16		57
1820–3		56
1827–38		48

Note: Rate of decline from 1812–16 to 1827–38 was 0.85 percent annually.
Source: "Report of a Committee of the Statistical Society of London...," JSSL, 3:124–5 (1840).

Data for Madras Presidency go back into the eighteenth century[33] (see Table 1.4). Over long periods, they reflect the mortality of field service in contrast to the lower rates of barracks life. Increased exertion, irregular food, and unsanitary water supplies all contributed to the mortality rates of the troops of Madras Presidency, which campaigned in the Mascarene Islands, Indonesia, and Burma as well as in southern and central peninsular India.

The peacetime segments of the record reflect a gradually declining mortality rate. The death rate for peacetime service in 1806–9 was unusually high at 70 per thousand. If that is set aside as atypical, the annual mortality rate dropped by 0.85 percent per year between 1812–16 and 1826–38. The committee of the Statistical Society, which compiled these data, recognized the mortality decline and attributed it (not quite accurately) to improving knowledge of tropical disease – and (far more likely) to general improvements in clothing, diet, quarters, and hospital care.[34]

Death rates in the other presidencies more nearly reflected the views

---

[33] These came mainly from the work of Dr. James Annesley, who had been president of the Madras Medical Board in the mid-1820s. The same committee of the Statistical Society that examined the returns from Burma and the Straits Settlements used Annesley's figures and assistance from Alexander Tulloch to bring them into line with the later official surveys ("Report of a Committee of the Statistical Society ...," JSSL, 3:113–43 [1840].)

[34] "Report of a Committee ...," JSSL, 3:122 (1840).

Mortality per Thousand of British Troops Serving in
Britain and Three Indian Presidencies, 1830–55

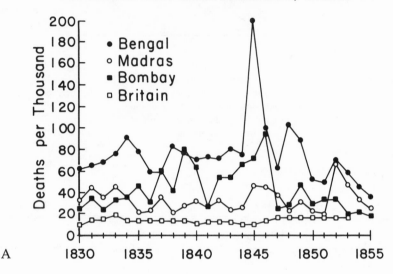

A

Trends in Percentage Relocation Costs for British
Troops Serving in Each Indian Presidency, 1830–53

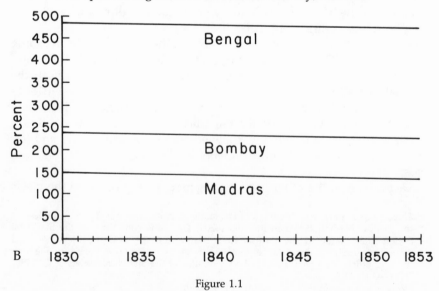

B

Figure 1.1

of the Royal Commission of 1863 – that past mortality rates fluctuated around 69 per thousand, a kind of plateau figure stretching indefinitely into the past.[35] The campaigns of the conquest, however, may well obscure a slow decline comparable to the Madras peacetime figures (see Figure 1.1, which is based on data in the appendix tables). Most authorities believe that British civilian mortality rates had also been declining slowly for about a century.

Figure 1.1 shows mortality from disease alone, and it reflects the high mortality of the wartime years. During the 1830s and 1840s, Britain established its "paramountcy" in India. Campaigning was frequent, especially in the two northern presidencies. The comparative peace for Madras accounts for its lower mortality rates. After 1852, death rates fell sharply in all three presidencies, again the probable result of relative peace in these years. Otherwise, death rates maintained a kind of stability from 1830 to 1855, and relocation rates produced a virtually horizontal trend line in all three presidencies, at nearly 500 percent for Bengal, just under 250 percent for Bombay, and 150 percent for Madras.

Change through Time: The Caribbean

In the West Indies (Map 1.5), circumstances were different; peace set in even before the fall of Napoleon in 1815 and continued for more than a century. Early in the century, British troops in the Caribbean were divided between the Windward and Leeward Command and the Jamaica Command. Of these, the Windward and Leeward Command is the preferred sample because it was numerically larger, and because the troops belonging to it were stationed in a greater variety of environmental settings. The central station was Barbados, but at times troops from the command served as far to the northwest as St. Kitts and as far to the southeast as British Guiana. But all West Indian mortality rates fluctuated annually, and no island was systematically much more healthy or less healthy than any other in the first half of the nineteenth century. The Lesser Antilles, French and British alike, were similar, with death rates a little lower than those of Jamaica yet substantially higher than those of French Guiana – which in earlier decades had the worst reputation in the Caribbean (Table 1.5).

As expected from campaign conditions, the death rates of all the islands had been high in wartime, but these levels continued into the

[35] The Royal Commission of 1863 arrived at the following annual average mortality figures by significant time periods: 1770–99, 55 per thousand; 1800–29, 85 per thousand; 1830–56, 58 per thousand. Mortality was again high in the years of the mutiny 1857–8, so that the overall figure from 1770 to 1863 was taken to be 69 per thousand (PP, 1863, xix [C.3184]. *Report of Commissioners Appointed to Inquire into the Sanitary Condition of the Army in India*, p. xi).

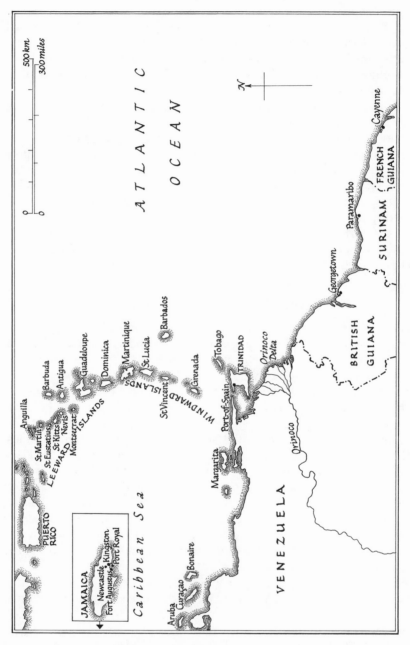

Map 1.5 The Eastern Caribbean

Table 1.5. *Mortality of European Troops in the Caribbean*

| | Deaths per Thousand per Year | | | | | Unweighted Average, All Colonies |
Years	Windward/ Leeward Command	Jamaica	Martinique	Guadeloupe	French Guiana	
1817–26	93	143	152	150	29	113.16
1827–36	65	102	73	67	32	67.74
1837–46	70	66	90	89	25	68.14
1847–56	70	33	51	26	53	46.52
1859–68	13	21				

Note: Rate of decline, all colonies, from 1827–36 to 1859–68 was 0.98 percent per year.
Source: British Caribbean, appendix tables. French Caribbean: *Revue Coloniale,* June 1852, pp. 474–5. French time per periods do not quite match. They are 1819–27, 1828–37, 1838–47, 1848–51.

immediate peacetime (Figure 1.2). The then-current military policy of keeping troops in the islands for a dozen years or more may be at fault to the extent that these men were veterans of the heavy fighting and the disease that went with it. By the 1830s and 1840s, however, death rates were more stable at a lower level. From 1827–36 to 1847–56, the overall mortality declined by 0.98 percent per year,[36] which is consonant with the similar rate of decline between peacetime periods in Madras Presidency.

The overall mortality, however, was higher than it was in India; the relocation costs for the Windward and Leeward Command indicated a stable trend line at more than 350 percent – higher than that of any Indian Presidency in spite of the fighting there. In Jamaica, however, the trend line shows a decline from nearly 600 per thousand to less than 200, but that downward trend actually reflects a sharp discontinuity in 1841. Before that, the trend of mortality had been rising slowly, from about 400 per thousand in 1830 to nearly 600 in 1831. After 1842, a new trend set in, moving from a little more than 150 per thousand in 1842 to less than 100 in 1852.[37] Military doctors at the time believed, probably quite correctly, that the change was mainly caused by the movement of most European troops in Jamaica to new barracks, only 15 miles from Kingston, but 3,800 feet above sea level – thought to be high enough to protect them from "fevers." A similar movement to Camp Jacob at 1,600 feet elevation in the highlands of Guadeloupe had a similar result. As we shall see, however, the panacea of seeking higher altitudes was not always quite so effective, and the pattern of "fevers" was less simple than it appeared to be early in the century.

Change through Time: Algeria

French troops first entered Algeria in 1830. They were then involved in military operations almost continuously to the end of the 1840s, and sporadically into the early 1870s. Their losses were therefore high even though the climate was similar to that of southern France. Mortality rates thus resembled those of the West Indies in peacetime, or those of southern India in wartime (Table 1.4).

The conquest of Algeria was a major military operation, compared with other nineteenth-century imperial wars. In the beginning, the French military promised to defeat the Dey of Algiers with 10,000 troops. By 1847, they needed more than 100,000 – more Europeans than the British used to conquer India.[38] The cost of empire in death from disease became a public issue from the 1840s, and it remained so until the twentieth century.

---

[36] Based on the unweighted average of the five commands shown in Table 1.5.
[37] Calculated from the data in Table A.9.   [38] Boudin, AHPML, 37:358–9.

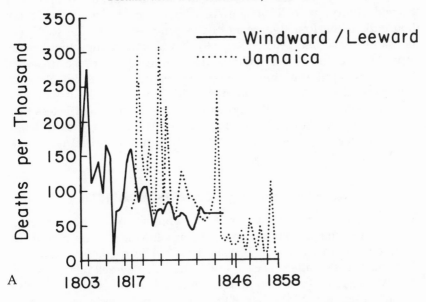

Mortality Rates for British Troops in
Britain and the Caribbean, 1803–58

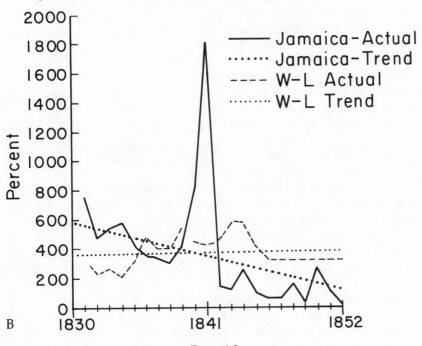

Relocation Cost for Movement from Britain to
Jamaica and the Windward/Leeward Command, 1830–52

Figure 1.2

The mortality rate for the French in Algeria dropped steeply over the midcentury, as it did in the West Indies and India – from 78 per thousand in the first five years of the conquest (1831–35) to 15 per thousand in the late 1860s (1863–69). It was this change that greatly impressed the British and made them look to Algeria for measures they themselves might apply in India (see Tables A.35 and A.36). And the change in relocation costs is indeed striking. Before 1848, it had been declining slowly, from a little more than 250 per cent to a little less than 200 (Figure 1.3). After 1862, it reappeared at an altogether different level – far lower, rising during the 1860s from around 50 percent to about 80 percent (Figure 1.4).

Changing Patterns of Disease: 1820s and 1830s

For the West Indies, the data for 1817–36 provide a point of departure for assessing changes still to come. Even allowing a wide margin for error, the contrast between British and Caribbean conditions was so stark that a basic pattern is clear (Table 1.6). The overall relocation cost was 593 percent, based on the unweighted mean of the two West Indian commands. More than 80 percent of that relocation cost came from tropical fevers, with another 15 percent classified under intestinal diseases – which included various forms of dysentery, along with typhoid fever, some hepatitis, and possible lead poisoning. The two West Indian commands, however, showed a marked difference. Yellow fever and malaria were far more serious in Jamaica than in the Lesser Antilles, where the soldiers died nearly as often from gastro-intestinal infections.

In contrast, more than half of all deaths in Britain were caused by diseases of the lungs – mainly pulmonary tuberculosis, with pneumonia in second place. Undifferentiated fevers would have been mostly typhoid. Epidemic cholera was unusual in Britain, but the period 1830–7 witnessed the passage across Europe of the second cholera pandemic in 1830–2. In more normal times, the death rate in Britain could have been 5 percent lower.

British troops on the Indian subcontinent before the mutiny in 1857 were in the service of the East India Company – and were administratively distinct from royal troops in either Britain or the West Indies. A committee of the Statistical Society of London assembled the Madras medical records for 1827–38 and readjusted the categories to conform to those used by Major Tulloch in his surveys of the Royal Army elsewhere (Table A.17). A direct comparison of Madras and British disease profiles is therefore possible (see Table 1.7). In contrast to the West Indies, the relocation cost in this decade was only 243 percent – less than half the West Indian figure, and "fevers" in the West Indies (in this case yellow fever and malaria) – accounted for the difference.

French Military Mortality in
Algeria and France, 1831–53

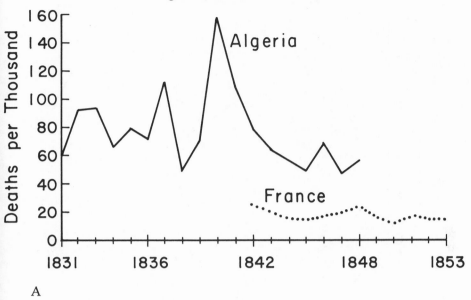

A

Relocation Costs in Deaths,
France to Algeria, 1842–48

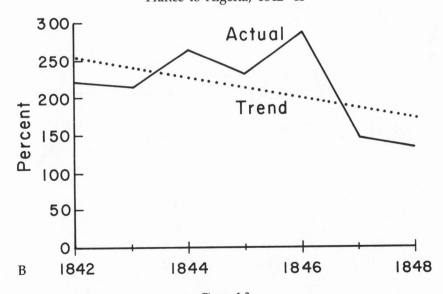

B

Figure 1.3

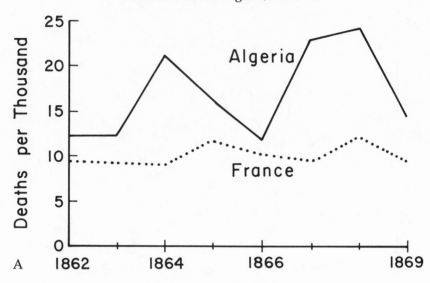

Mortality Rates of French Troops
in France and in Algeria, 1862–69

A

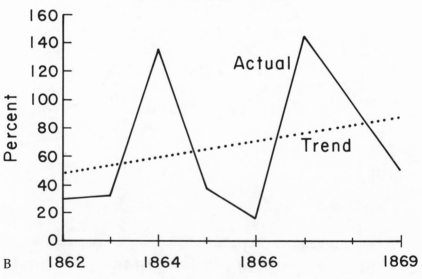

Relocation Cost for Movement
from France to Algeria, 1862–69

B

Figure 1.4

Table 1.6. Mortality of British Troops, United Kingdom and Windward and Leeward Command, 1817–36

Disease	Deaths per Thousand			Difference in Rates[a]	Contribution (percent)[b]	Percentage of Total Deaths from Diseases	
	Britain	Windward/ Leeward	Jamaica			United Kingdom	British West Indies
Fevers	1.40	36.90	101.90	68.00	81.49	10.00	71.22
Eruptive fevers	0.10	0.00	0.00	-0.10	-0.12	0.71	0.00
Diseases of the lungs	7.70	10.40	7.50	1.25	1.50	55.00	9.18
Diseases of the liver	0.40	1.80	1.00	1.00	1.20	2.86	1.44
Stomach and bowels	0.80	20.70	5.10	12.10	14.50	5.71	13.24
Diseases of the brain	1.20	3.70	2.60	1.95	2.34	8.57	3.23
Epidemic cholera	0.70	0.00	0.00	-0.70	-0.84	5.00	0.00
Dropsies	0.30	2.10	1.20	1.35	1.62	2.14	1.69
Other	1.40	0.00	0.00	-1.40	-1.68	10.00	0.00
All diseases	14.00	75.60	119.30	83.45	100.00	100.00	100.00
Wounds and injuries							
Other diseases/accidents	3.80	2.90	2.00				
Grand total	15.30	78.50	121.30				

[a] Difference between the mortality rate in Britain and the unweighted mean of the two West Indian commands.
[b] Contribution of each disease to total relocation cost in deaths.

Source: PP, 1837–8 (136), xi, pp. 4, 45; PP, 1839, xvi [C.166], p. 7. United Kingdom sample is Dragoons and Dragoon Guards, 1830–6. Windward and Leeward sample is all European troops in the command, 1817–36. Jamaica sample is all European troops in the command, 1817–36.

Table 1.7. Mortality of British Troops in the United Kingdom and in Madras Presidency, 1827–38, with Contribution to Relocation Cost

Disease	Deaths per Thousand		Difference in Rates	Contribution (percent)	Percentage of Total Deaths from Disease	
	Britain	Madras			United Kingdom	Madras
Fevers	1.40	5.57	4.17	12.24	10.00	11.59
Eruptive fevers	0.10	0.00	-0.10	-0.29	0.71	0.00
Diseases of the lungs	7.70	2.35	-5.35	-15.71	55.00	4.89
Diseases of the liver	0.40	5.62	5.22	15.33	2.86	11.69
Stomach and bowels	0.80	17.59	16.79	49.30	5.71	36.60
Diseases of the brain	1.20	1.70	0.50	1.47	8.57	3.54
Epidemic cholera	0.70	7.60	6.90	20.26	5.00	15.81
Dropsies	0.30	1.08	0.78	2.29	2.14	2.25
Pneumatic	0.00	0.95	0.95	2.79	0.00	1.98
Venereal	0.00	0.57	0.57	1.67	0.00	1.19
Abscesses and ulcers	0.00	0.22	0.22	0.65	0.00	0.46
Disease of the eye	0.00	0.06	0.06	0.18	0.00	0.12
Other	1.40	4.75	3.35	9.84	10.00	9.88
All diseases	14.00	48.06	34.06	100.00	100.00	100.00
Wounds and injuries						
Other diseases/accidents	1.30	0.57	-0.73			
Grand total	15.30	48.63	33.33			

Source: PP, 1839, xvi [C.166], p. 7. "Report of a Committee ...," JSSL, 3:127 (1840).

Had West Indian deaths from fevers been at the Madras rate, the West Indies would have been markedly healthier than India was. But Madras had cholera to set against the yellow fever of the West Indies. Madras also had five times the West Indian death rates for intestinal infections and abscesses of the liver (mostly from amoebic dysentery.) Unlike the British soldiers in the West Indies, where all diseases were more fatal than they were in Britain, those in Madras had one trade-off in the form of lower death rates from tuberculosis and pneumonia.

The most striking feature of this three-way comparison of Britain, Madras, and the West Indies is not the differing mortality rates but the differing disease profiles – the percentage of deaths attributed to each disease. In Britain more than half the deaths were from lung diseases; overseas, they were not more than 10 percent. In the West Indies, 71 percent of all deaths were from fevers; in neither Madras nor Britain did it reach 12 percent. In Madras, 64 percent of all deaths came from a trio of waterborne diseases – cholera plus diseases of the liver and intestines; the equivalent in Britain was only 19 percent, and 15 percent in the West Indies. These patterns were to change over time, but some remnant of the early nineteenth-century baseline survived for decades to come.

Changing Disease: 1840s to 1860s

The 1850s brought a decisive mortality change in Britain, and even greater improvement among European troops in the colonies. That makes it all the more unfortunate that both France and Britain interrupted their published statistics over the 1850s – largely because of the Crimean War. Only Jamaica later published annual mortality figures for the gap between 1847 and 1859.

Table 1.8 summarizes changes between the 1840s and the 1860s for principal causes of death in each of the four territories. In overall mortality, Britain and Madras were similar, with decreases close to 2.5 percent per year. Algeria and Jamaica were next with about 3.18 percent, while the Windward and Leeward Command did better still with 3.82 percent.

The cause of the Windward/Leeward advantage is clear. Death rates from each of the three principal causes of death – accounting for 80 percent of all deaths – dropped by 90 percent or more between the 1840s and the early 1860s. Only the decline of the diarrhea group in Algeria was as spectacular; it had accounted for 41 percent of all deaths, and mortality from that cause dropped by 87 percent. A third outstanding change was in Britain itself, where mortality from tuberculosis (which had accounted for 63 percent of military deaths) dropped by 75 percent.

Table 1.8 also suggests more general explanations. In all three over-

Table 1.8. *Mortality by Cause of Death, 1840s to 1860s: West Indies, Madras, Algeria, and Britain*

Disease	Percentage of All Deaths, 1837–46	Deaths per Thousand, 1837–46	Deaths per Thousand, 1859–67	Percentage Change	Change per Year
British troops in the Windward and Leeward Command					
Malaria/Yellow fever	50.01	34.66	3.28	−90.54	−4.21
Diseases of the digestive system[a]	22.07	15.30	1.17	−92.35	−4.30
Continued fever	7.56	5.24	0.54	−89.69	−4.17
Tuberculosis	7.53	5.22	1.60	−69.35	−3.23
All diseases	100.00	69.31	12.43	−82.07	−3.82
Jamaica Command, all diseases		66.44	21.15	−68.17	−3.17
British troops in the United Kingdom 1860–7					
Tuberculosis	63.38	12.58	3.16	−74.88	−3.48
Diseases of the respiratory system	8.16	1.65	1.32	−20.00	−0.93
Diseases of the digestive system[a]	3.22	3.08	0.77	−75.00	−3.49
All diseases	100.00	19.85	8.40	−57.68	−2.68
British troops in Madras					
Diseases of the digestive system[b]	41.44	17.20	7.03	−59.13	−2.75
Epidemic cholera	20.00	8.30	2.76	−66.75	−3.10
Fevers	9.16	3.80	1.51	−60.26	−2.80
Diseases of the lungs	6.99	2.90	2.86	−1.38	−0.06
Eruptive fevers	0.48	0.20	0.80	300.00	13.95
All diseases	100.00	41.50	19.86	−52.14	−2.43
French troops in Algeria		1847–8	1862–6		
Diseases of the digestive system	40.90	21.30	2.68	−87.42	−5.30
Remittent fevers	13.20	6.87	2.69	−60.84	−3.69
Typhoid fever	8.20	4.27	2.60	−39.11	−2.37
Pneumonia pleurisy	6.20	3.23	0.80	−75.23	−4.56
All diseases	100.00	52.07	14.04	−73.04	−4.43
French troops in Algeria		1836–46	1859–67		
All diseases		81.54	21.93	−73.11	−3.18

[a] Includes dysentery, diarrhea, and "diseases of the digestive system."
[b] Includes dysentery, diarrhea "diseases of the digestive system," and diseases of the liver.
Source: See Appendix tables.

seas territories, the outstanding improvement came in waterborne diseases. That larger category would include not only cholera and the gastrointestinal group, but also continued fevers, which would have been mainly typhoid where typhoid was not listed separately. In the 1840s, in all three territories, these diseases had accounted for at least 30 to 60 percent of all deaths. This group had been the most important cause of death, and its decline was the greatest source of improved mortality over the midcentury. The only exceptional gains from other causes were the quinine gains against malaria in the West Indies and the inexplicable drop in tuberculosis deaths in Britain itself.

The same data give a somewhat different picture if we ask how much each disease or disease group contributed to relocation costs in the 1840s and again in the 1860s (Table 1.9). In the West Indies, the decline of waterborne diseases meant that malaria and yellow fever, taken together, increased their share from 70 percent of relocation costs to a figure so high (120 percent) that the two tropical fevers alone accounted for the entire relocation cost and more – their weight being balanced by the fact that tuberculosis, pneumonia, and other diseases of the lungs now became less deadly in the colonies than they were in Europe. By the 1860s, the Windward and Leeward islands were a virtual health resort, with improved mortality in every category except malaria and "nervous and mental" diseases. Even the waterborne group were less deadly in the islands that they were in Britain itself.[39] The West Indies, in short, would have been in the "relocation benefits" column along with Tahiti and New Zealand, if it were not for the tropical fevers.

In Madras, malaria was less serious and yellow fever was absent, but malaria's share of relocation costs increased slightly. The combination of cholera and intestinal disease also held its dominant place, in spite of the overall drop in death rates from this cause.

Algeria provides no comparable data for the 1830s and earlier, but the pattern for the 1860s is both clear and markedly different from that of the other two colonies. Malaria accounted for half the relocation cost, far more than it did in Madras, but less than the West Indies. Intestinal infections accounted for another third, as they did in Madras. Typhoid fever (at 15 percent of relocation costs) was more important than it was anywhere else. Tuberculosis showed an improvement over Europe, as it did in Madras and the Caribbean; but the West Indies was

[39] The West Indian data for this period and later have to be taken with a larger allowance for error than would be the case for either Britain or Madras. The number of troops in the Windward and Leeward Command was only about 800. This means that, even with five-year averages, the numbers dying of a particular disease may be too small for the best statistical reliability, but nevertheless are worth considering. The usual strength of British troops in Madras during this period was about 10,000.

Table 1.9. Diseases Contributing to Relocation Cost in Deaths, Madras, West Indies, Algeria, 1837–46 and 1860s (percent)

Disease	Madras 1837–46	Windward/ Leeward 1837–46	Madras 1859–67	Windward/ Leeward 1859–67	Algeria 1862–6
Paroxysmal fevers	5.51[a]	70.12	6.11	81.39	55.12
Eruptive Fevers	-0.85	-0.59	4.29	-7.66	-0.01
Yellow Fever	0.00[b]	0.00	0.00	38.46	0.00
Continued Fevers	0.00[c]	5.66	7.07	2.98	20.93[d]
Diseases of the Lungs	-30.95	3.46	-6.02	-25.31	3.68
Tuberculosis	0.00[e]	-14.89	-8.12	-38.71	-11.7
Diseases of the Stomach and Bowels[f]	67.79	2.04	29.84	8.93	34.32
Epidemic Cholera	35.17	0.00	24.08	0.00	-0.46
Dysentery/Diarrhea	0.00[g]	27.42	24.75	0.9	0.00[g]
Diseases of the Brain	7.63	6.66	7.16	27.05	-2.86
Other	15.70	0.12	10.84	11.97	0.98
Total	100	100	100	100	100

[a] Simply fevers for Madras, 1837–42.
[b] Counted with paroxysmal fevers in Windward/Leeward, 1837–46.
[c] Counted as part of fevers.
[d] Typhoid fever, 14.62 percent; other continued fevers, 6.11 percent.
[e] Counted as part of diseases of the lungs.
[f] Includes diseases of the liver.
[g] Counted as part of diseases of the stomach and bowels.

unique in showing a similar improvement in smallpox and pneumonia as well.

While the dangers of fever in tropical stations was common knowledge, the improved colonial death rates from tuberculosis and pneumonia were not well known. Yet, for soldiers moving from Britain to Madras – either before or after the 1850s – the lower mortality from these lung conditions outweighed the increased mortality from malaria at least three times over. These mortality benefits nearly balanced the cost of cholera – although not the combined cost of cholera and other intestinal disease. Although deaths attributed to the gastrointestinal group dropped more rapidly than any other cause of death between the 1840s and the 1860s, they still accounted for half of the remaining relocation costs. In short, while the greatest advance was against waterborne diseases, the greatest challenge remaining in Madras was precisely those disease groups.

These mortality changes over the 1850s were among the most important of the nineteenth-century mortality revolution. Although detailed data are shown for only three overseas territories, they epitomize broader patterns. Some are easy enough to explain; others remain mysterious. Although scientific medicine in any full sense was still some time off, the achievements of the military doctors were spectacular. It is therefore all the more important to follow their search for a more general understanding of disease and their response to specific problems in specific places.

CHAPTER 2

SANITATION AND TROPICAL
HYGIENE AT MIDCENTURY

Most historians now believe that a mortality revolution took place
between the middle of the eighteenth century and the early twentieth,
but they disagree about its probable causes. One early view was that
often unspecified "advances of medical science" deserved most credit,
such as inoculation against smallpox introduced in the first half of the
eighteenth century and vastly improved Jennerian vaccination in the
nineteenth. That view may still be correct, but the "advances of
medical science" have yet to be specified.

One idea that has gained favor in recent decades is that clinical
medicine, which saved the lives of those already attacked by disease,
played only a small part in the mortality revolution before the 1890s, at
the earliest. Yet the drop in mortality was unquestionable. An alternative theory that appeared in the 1950s was Thomas McKeown's suggestion that medical advances, including smallpox inoculation, could not
in themselves account for such steeply falling death rates.[1] After elim-
inating other potential causes, McKeown concluded that only nutrition
had the probable power to produce such an important result.

The problem with this argument is that it is based on a series of
negatives followed by a guess. Thus, if A, B, C, D, and so on did not
bring about the observed effect, the cause must have been X – X being
nutrition. No one doubts the important relationship between nutrition
and health, but whether it was the fundamental cause of the mortality
revolution is impossible to demonstrate empirically. There is little evidence about actual levels of nutrition in the past, and the consequences
of nutrition are almost impossible to disaggregate in retrospect from
the whole context of health – either for the individual or for whole

---

[1] Thomas McKeown, *The Modern Rise of Population* (London, 1976), for a summary of the
case and reference to earlier works. Robert I. Rotberg and Theodore Rabb (eds.),
*Hunger in History: The Impact of Changing Food Production and Consumption Patterns on
Society* (Cambridge, 1983), contains articles by McKeown and others dealing with more
recent stages of the controversy.

populations. McKeown's case is therefore unprovable, although it could nevertheless be partly correct.

Its critics have followed several lines of attack.[2] Some concede that medical advances may not have been all-important, but neither is improved nutrition, which can combat some diseases, but not others. Good childhood nutrition is also effective sometimes – and sometimes not.[3] Some diseases – tuberculosis in early nineteenth-century Britain, for example – rose steeply as a cause of death during the same decades when improved nutrition was supposed to be reducing mortality; and tuberculosis is a disease in which malnutrition causes increased morbidity and mortality. In a few rare instances, indeed, the host's resistance to viral infection may be enhanced by malnutrition.[4]

Other critics have argued that McKeown overlooked the contribution of preventive medicine[5] or improved insect control.[6] Much disease in northwest Europe, for example, is transmitted by houseflies. Beginning in the eighteenth century, the environmentalist movement demanded better drainage, better ventilation, and the abolition of obvious filth from the cities. These measures were mainly aesthetic in intent, and they brought aesthetic benefits; but the by-product was fewer insects – and incidentally less infectious disease.

Some of the data on military mortality explored in Chapter 1 also have some bearing on European mortality in the nineteenth century. For one thing, soldiers serving at home are a statistically significant sample of the whole population in the sense that they were recruited mainly from young, working-class males who had had about the same childhood diet. They also served in similar conditions, with similar medical care, and with far better medical reporting on morbidity or on the cause of death than was the case for civilians. Once in the service, they also received the same food rations. That diet changed very little in the middle decades of the nineteenth century (Chapter 6). For this group, at least, nutrition can be taken as a constant for certain periods

---

[2] For a recent review of other possible influences on the mortality revolution, see James C. Riley, *The Eighteenth-Century Campaign to Avoid Disease* (London, 1987). For a bibliography of this literature, see Robert Fogel, *Nutrition and the Decline of Mortality since 1700: Some Preliminary Findings* (Cambridge, National Bureau of Economic Research, Working paper 1402, 1984), pp. 103–18.

[3] Rotberg and Rabb (eds.), *Hunger in History*, pp. 305–8, examines the relationship between particular diseases and nutrition.

[4] R. K. Chandra and P. M. Newberne, *Nutrition, Immunity, and Infection: Mechanisms of Interactions* (New York, 1977), pp. 7–8.

[5] See George Rosen, *A History of Public Health* (New York, 1958).

[6] James C. Riley, "Insects and European Mortality Decline," AHR, 91:833–58 (1986); Riley, *Eighteenth-Century Campaign*; Robert Woods and P. R. Andrew Hinde, "Mortality in Victorian England: Models and Patterns," JIH, 18:27–54 (1987), pp. 52–4 (1987); Robert Woods and John Woodward, *Urban Disease and Mortality in Nineteenth-Century England* (London, 1984), pp. 27–33.

in the four decades or so that bridged the middle of the nineteenth century.

At the same time, the military also had some disadvantages as a sample. Because armies rejected men who were not physically fit, the sample represents the initially healthy – not the entire population. It is also limited to a particular age range, roughly twenty to forty years. These people had lower death rates than the very old or the very young. Medical improvements, either prevention or cure, would affect this group most drastically. Thus, although the military sample was atypical of the whole population, it should have been especially sensitive in its response to changing incidence of infectious disease.

The data in Chapter 1 thus can shed some light on the importance of nutrition in the mortality revolution. First, nutrition cannot possibly account for the enormous differences between death rates at home and those overseas. As noted earlier, the death rate for British troops in Britain fell by 58 percent between 1837–46 and 1860–7, with no observable differences in nutrition to account for it (Table 1.8). The death rate from tuberculosis fell by 75 percent over that same period. Although good nutrition is known to provide some protection against tuberculosis, there is no observable difference in the levels of nutrition either during army service or in childhood to account for the change in those decades. In fact, we have no precise explanation of that remarkable change. However, the improved ventilation in barracks, which is documented, is a more likely partial explanation than improved nutrition, for which we have no evidence. The other striking improvement, a 75 percent drop in diseases of the digestive system, could also be attributed to nutritional improvement, if it were not for the fact that no known nutritional improvement took place. One place to begin looking for this and other mortality improvements is to see what army and other medical authorities at midcentury thought and did about them.

Tropical Health, Statistical Surveys, and Medical Reforms

Europeans had long distinguished between what conduct was permissible in Europe and what was permissible in the tropics. The rules they established in this regard constituted a form of preventive medicine, but with heavy moral overtones – rules to live by in the tropics. The prescriptions varied greatly from one authority to another, but all drew from the prevalent humoral theory, still fundamental to medical thought, although it had several different versions. Most medical authorities associated human health with human passions and habits of life. Heat was associated with fever; tropical heat was associated with moisture as well. Heat and exercise brought on perspiration, and perspiration affected the humoral balance of the body. The rules of hygiene therefore governed the intake and expulsion of liquids. They also recommended or forbade particular kinds of exercise. They recommended various kinds of temperature control – how to remain cool in the tropical heat, but also how to insulate the body against sudden changes of temperature. Some recommendations called for light and looser fitting clothes, but others called for insulating materials like flannel.[7] These prescriptions were often contradictory and they were often based on theory alone.

The empirical study of medical topography began in the late eighteenth century and continued strongly through the nineteenth. Each investigator examined a particular place, noting the climate, meteorological conditions, prevalence of diseases among the local population and visiting Europeans – sometimes with warnings or hygienic hints for travelers.[8] By the mid nineteenth century, worldwide surveys on medical topography had begun to appear.[9] When the *Dictionaire encyclopédique des sciences médicales* was first published in Paris in the 1860s, it contained an article on the medical topography of each country in the world on which information was available.

Balfour and Tulloch began their surveys against the background of this medical topography, which they tested against statistical fact. In the first volume, Alexander Tulloch compared the "common knowledge" of popular medical topography with his data from the West Indies. Medical topography often associated heat with high mortality, but, as he pointed out, heat was fairly constant from year to year, whereas disease fluctuated greatly. The same was true of soil and marshes. Moisture was also often blamed for tropical death, but Tulloch found that rainfall correlated poorly with death rates from disease. Miasmas generated on the South American mainland were sometimes blamed for ill health on the Caribbean islands, but British Guiana on the mainland was no more dangerous than the other colonies.

Altitude correlated somewhat better with safety from disease and death, but the correlation was far from perfect. Places 600 to 700 feet above sea level were often less healthy than the seaside. Stoney Hill in Jamaica at 1,360 feet was no better than the plains, although Maroon Town at 2,000 to 2,500 feet was much safer. And, forts on sand spits like Fort Augusta at the entrance of Kingston harbor, or the post at

[7] Philip D. Curtin, *The Image of Africa* (Madison, Wisc., 1964), pp. 74–87.
[8] See Riley, *Eighteenth-Century Campaign*, pp. 31–53. The following can serve as samples of the genre: Davidson, "Medico-Topographical and Statistical Report of the Convalescent Depot at Wellington, India, for the Year 1870," AMSR, 12:474–85 (1870); James Africanus Beale Horton, *The Medical Topography of the West Coast of Africa, with Sketches of Its Botany* (London, 1859); Jean Christian Marc François Joseph Boudin, *Essai de géographie médicale ou étude sur les lois qui préside à la distribution géographique des maladies, ansi qu'à leurs rapports topographiques entre elles. Lois de coincidence et d'antagonisme* (Paris, 1843).
[9] Auguste Frédéric Dutroulau, *Traité des maladies des Européens dans les pays chauds*, 2d ed. (Paris, 1868).

Lucea on the north coast, were comparatively safe. These observations led to the establishment of a new Jamaican barracks for European soldiers at Newcastle, high in the mountains behind Kingston.[10]

The early statistical surveys corrected other misconceptions. It was commonly believed that old soldiers were healthier than young soldiers, whereas in fact mortality increased with each additional year of service. This discovery eventually helped to change British enlistment policies. Until 1847, British soldiers enlisted for life, or until they "invalided" or retired for reasons of health. Normally they would be invalided after twenty-one years of service, even if their health continued to be good. The Limited Enlistment Act of 1847 allowed voluntary discharge at the end of ten years' service in the infantry or twelve years in the cavalry or artillery. Reenlistment for a second term would earn a pension after twenty-one or twenty-four years, depending on the branch of service.[11] The new act helped to reduce the average age of soldiers. By reducing numbers with high age-specific death rates, the act probably reduced crude death rates, even for service in Britain.

Tulloch had made another suggestion even before the statistical results came in. He argued that the usual ration of salt meat should be supplemented with fresh meat, since the better-fed officers had better mortality than enlisted men in the Windward and Leeward Command. Here is a case in which nutritional change may have made some difference overseas but would not have influenced the pattern of army rations at home.[12]

"Seasoning" was another tenacious bit of medical lore. It was "common knowledge" that newcomers to the tropics had to pass through a "seasoning sickness." It exacted its price in immediate mortality, but those who survived were then partly "acclimatized" to the new setting. This was similar to the common experience in Europe, where "childhood diseases" were rare among adults precisely because they left their victims immune to a future attack. The implication for military policy was clear – troops should be kept in tropical posts for long periods, as much as ten years, so that they could become acclimatized – and this had been British policy for troops in India and the West Indies.

Tulloch and Balfour disagreed, and so did Arthur S. Thomson using data based on the experience of troops in India. Their data seemed to

[10] PP, 1837–8, xl (138), pp. 101–3; T. G. Balfour, "Summary of the Reports on the Health of the Army Published Previous to 1859," AMSR, 2:131–41 (1860), p. 131.
[11] Report of the Committee on the Preparation of Military Statistics, PP, 1861, xxxvi (366), pp. 12–13.
[12] M. J. Cullen, *The Statistical Movement in Early Victorian Britain* (New York, 1975), p. 48. Salt meat has negligible quantities of vitamin C, which is one reason for the prevalence of scurvy on long sea voyages. Overcooked fresh meat is also low in vitamin C, but lightly cooked meat or fish is not (Kenneth J. Carpenter, *The History of Scurvy and Vitamin C* [New York 1986], pp. 221–18).

show that mortality rose with each additional year of service overseas, especially service beyond five or six years in the tropics. Tulloch and Balfour convinced the government that, instead of sending military units to the Caribbean for ten or eleven years, it should establish a regular rotation of three years' service in the tropics. For a time, the British army also sent troops to the relatively healthy stations of Bermuda or Gibraltar as "seasoning" preparation for further service in the humid tropics, although it later abandoned this measure as ineffective.[13] In retrospect, Tulloch and Balfour believed that this shift to short-term rotation was their most important contribution to improved mortality in the tropical world of the 1840s and 1850s.

Although they were no doubt correct that shortening service in the tropics saved lives, the need for "seasoning" or acclimatization remained questionable. It was difficult to separate the role of increasing age from that of increasing length of service in a particular place. The army's health surveys for 1830–7 and again for 1837–47 showed that deaths increased with age in Britain as well as overseas.[14] In France at midcentury, on the other hand, death rates dropped with each successive year of military service. In 1864, the French Ministry of War suggested that improved military mortality over the previous ten years had been largely due to the greater number of long-service men in the ranks.[15]

The data on length of service for troops overseas were somewhat different. For Jamaica in 1830–7, the death rate was 118 per thousand in the first year, dropping to 110 in the fifth year, before it began to rise again. But this was a time of yellow fever epidemic, and yellow fever was a seasoning sickness par excellence. Although the case-fatality rate was high, those who recovered had a lifetime immunity. In the Windward/Leeward Command, where yellow fever was less prevalent, the pattern was different. Mortality per thousand was much lower; it rose in the second and third years of service, but later fluctuations were irregular and inconclusive, as might be expected for a place with a high annual variance of death rates.[16]

In India, the pattern was much the same. Arthur Saunders Thomson brought together data on death rates and length of service for civil servants, army officers, and enlisted men who had served in India

[13] Sir R. Martin, *Lancet*, 1868 (1), p. 6.

[14] Graham Balfour, "Summary of the Reports on the Health of the Army Published Previous to 1859," AMSR, 2:131–41 (1860), p. 138–9.

[15] J. C. M. F. J. Boudin, *Traité de géographie et de statistique médicale et des maladies endémiques*, 2 vols. (Paris, 1857), 2:161–7; Boudin, "Statistique médicale de l'armée anglaise," RMMM, 12(3d ser.):369–89; 13:1–22 (1864–65) 12:380.

[16] According to PP, 1837–8, xI (138), pp. 92–3, the mortality rate per thousand in the Windward and Leeward Command, was as follows for each year of service: first, 77; second, 87; third, 89; fourth, 63; fifth, 61; sixth, 79; seventh, 83; eighth, 73; ninth, 120; tenth, 109.

during approximately the first third of the nineteenth century. In each case, the death rate tended to rise with increasing length of residence, but with occasional suggestions of a seasoning process as well. The death rate for Bengal civil servants, for example, was lowest among those who had served for eleven to fifteen years. The rate for those with twenty-one to twenty-five years of service was three time as high, but these men were already in their forties or early fifties.[17] The 1863 Royal Commission on the health of the army in India found a similar pattern of high mortality in the first year, which declined by about a third to a fifth before beginning to rise again.[18] These figures seem to confirm the existence of a seasoning period in the first years of overseas duty, but they also support the short-service recommendation for tropical duty.

In France, the seasoning question was part of another controversy. French colonization of Algeria had brought high mortality rates among the settlers as well as the soldiers. As a result, many argued that the whole Algerian operation should be abandoned. Others countered that, despite the initial losses, acclimatization would occur with the passage of time. Troop mortality was high during the first months of service in Algeria, but then it tapered off, although it remained higher than it would have been in France.[19] Some of the participants in this argument also used statistics, although the samples were small – they consisted of deaths in a particular hospital or deaths from dysentery in a particular hospital. Meanwhile, others observed that death rates fell with each successive year and therefore concluded that keeping troops in Algeria for ten years at a time saved lives.[20]

Both sides used Tulloch's and Balfour's statistics for the British experience. The leading antiacclimatizationist was Jean Christian Boudin, who argued that lasting adjustment to an alien climate was impossible. Like Balfour and Tulloch, he claimed that short service was the prime cause of decreased mortality in the tropics.[21] Many argued that the new rotation system was needed, but they still used the

---

[17] Arthur S. Thomson, "On the Doctrine of Acclimatization," *Madras Quarterly Medical Review*, 2:69–72 (1840).

[18] PP, 1863, xix [C.3184], p. xii.

[19] A. E. Foley and Martin, *De l'acclimatement et de la colonisation en Algérie* (Paris, 1847) are the chief protagonists. See also Louis Laveran, "Algérie," DESM, pp. 763–6; Adolphe Armand, *L'algérie médicale: topographie, climatologie, pathogénie, pathologie, prophylaxie, hygiène, acclimatement et colonisation* (Paris, 1854), pp. 505–20. For broader aspects of the acclimatization controversy, see David N. Livingstone, "Human Acclimatization: Perspectives on a Contested Field of Inquiry in Science, Medicine, and Geography," *History of Science*, 25:359–94 (1987).

[20] Félix Jacquot, and Topin, *De la colonisation et de l'acclimatement en Algérie* (Paris, 1849), pp. 49–54.

[21] J. C. M. F. J. Boudin, "Étude sur la mortalité et l'acclimatment de la population françaises en Algérie," AHPML, 37(2):358–91 (1847), pp. 373–4; "Statistique médicale de l'armée anglaise"; *Traité de géographie et de statistique médicale et des maladies endémiques*, 2 vols. (Paris, 1857), 2:150–61.

Tulloch and Balfour data to support seasoning. The seasoning issue was to remain unsettled during the rest of the century, although armies continued to collect data without a definitive conclusion (see Chapter 6).

Altitude and Hill Stations

The Europeans' oldest measure of protection in the tropics was altitude. The Spanish in Middle and South America had known since the sixteenth century that malaria and yellow fever were less common, even unknown, at high altitudes. Lind's classical early work on tropical medicine stressed the importance of moderate heights. He recommended only enough altitude to bring the daytime temperature down to 70°F, with the nights no less than 54°.[22] The British in India and the Dutch on Java also recognized the value of hill stations and used them systematically for protection from disease during the hot season. By the early nineteenth century, the literature on tropical medicine was filled with detailed and localized advice, and Tulloch decided that altitude was a factor to be tested statistically. He concluded that at least 2,500 feet of altitude was necessary for real safety – the same figure Von Humboldt had set as the upper limit of yellow fever in his survey of Spanish America.[23]

In 1845, Edward Balfour, whose personal experience had been in India, summarized the combined results of medical topography and the early statistical surveys. He recognized that altitude tended to make for better health, but not in all cases. In Ceylon, he found that the mortality of Galle on the southwest coast was less than a third that of Badulla in the highlands.[24] In fact, the relative salubrity of the southwest coast had to do with the local vector for malaria, *Anopheles culicifacies*, which thrives in puddles in relatively wet regions, but whose larvae are washed away by the heavy rains of the southwest before they have time to develop.[25]

Balfour was also impressed by the findings of medical topography (incorrect, as it turned out) that biological race was a more important source of immunity than childhood environment or acquired immunity. Thus, he concluded that whites were reasonably healthy in Gibraltar, which was fatal for West Indians. Europeans were healthy in

---

[22] James Lind, *Essay on the Diseases Incidental to Europeans in Hot Countries*, 6th ed. (London, 1808), pp. 117–28. Originally published 1768.

[23] PP, 1837–8, xl (138), pp. 101–3. See also Robert Lawson, "Observations on the Outbreak of Yellow Fever among the Troops at Newcastle in 1856," *British and Foreign Medico-Chirurgical Review*, 59:445–80 (1859).

[24] Edward Balfour, *Observations on the Means of Preserving the Health of Troops by Selecting Healthy Localities for their Cantonments* (London, 1845).

[25] Gordon Harrison, *Mosquitoes, Malaria, and Men* (New York, 1978), pp. 205–7; Leonard Jan Bruce-Chawtt, *Essential Malariology* (London, 1980), pp. 135–40, 162.

certain highland stations of Ceylon, which were fatal to Indians and even to Sinhalese.

The India Mutiny roused further fears about the health of European troops in India. Sir J. Ranald Martin, an authority on tropical medicine and later a member of the Royal Commission on the health of the army in India, had an elaborate plan for keeping all European troops in the heights, while "natives" policed the plains. The European troops would become, in effect, guards over the guardians of peace – moving down into the plains for only a few months of exercises during the cool season.[26] The Royal Commission went part way and recommended that a third of the European force should be kept in hill stations on rotation, although strategic points in the plains had to be occupied, "whether healthy or unhealthy." The commission also observed correctly that hill stations could preserve the health of troops stationed there, but did little to cure those who had already contracted disease in the plains.[27]

Even so, the Madras Presidency followed only some of these suggestions. Its principal hill station for military personnel was at Wellington, about 70 miles due east of Calicut and 6,000 feet above sea level – only a few miles from Ootacamund, the presidency's warm-weather capital for a few months each summer. Any health advantages the location might have had were obscured in the statistics by the fact that it received convalescent soldiers from all over the presidency, even from as far away as Burma. By the late 1860s, the greatest source of hospital admissions at Wellington was malaria contracted in the plains below; the death rate from malaria was often as high as or higher than that of other stations at lower altitudes.[28]

Nor did the Madras authorities find it possible to keep even a third of the force in the hills. Medical authorities of the early 1860s divided their territory into epidemiological zones. The single hill station held 9 percent of the total force. The seacoast, principally at Madras on the east coast and Cannanore on the west, had 22 percent. Twenty percent served in Burma, while fully half was distributed to various stations in the peninsular tablelands, mainly at an elevation of 1,000 to 3,000 feet. From south to north these were Bangalore in Mysore, Bellary in the presidency between Mysore and Hyderabad, Secunderabad in Hyderabad itself, and Kamptee in what was to become the Central Provinces. The authorities expected better health in the hills and plateau country, where the temperatures were lower. By the 1860s, indeed, Bangalore

[26] Martin, Lancet, 1868 (1), pp. 340–2.
[27] Great Britain, Royal Commission on the Sanitary State of the Army in India, Report of the Commissioners Appointed to Inquire into the Sanitary State of the Army in India ..., 2 vols. (London, 1863), 1:lxxi, lxxxi.
[28] Davidson, "Medico-Topographical and Statistical Report of the Convalescent Depot at Wellington, India, for the Year 1870," AMSR, 12:474–85 (1870).

was already a preferred residence for civilian retirees, and for more than a thousand military veterans who stayed in India[29] – a reputation it maintained for more than a century.

In fact, death rates in the tablelands were much higher than those on either coast, or in coastal Burma. This can be explained in part by the distribution of vectors capable of transmitting malaria. The coastal regions of the presidency were generally more free of malaria than the highlands, and dominant vectors also varied greatly. *Anopheles culicifacies* was an important carrier in northern India, and in Punjab. On the west coast of peninsular India, however, it could not breed because the heavy rain washed the larvae away before they could hatch – just as it did in southwestern Ceylon. As in Ceylon, too, *A. culicifacies* was active in the drier interior.

The situation in Burma was also contrary to European expectations. Fevers caused frightful mortality among British troops operating in Arakan in the 1820s, but the coastal strip from Rangoon southward was nearly malaria-free. In Bengal and on the northeast coast of India, fevers were a serious problem because *Anopheles sundaicus* breeds in brackish water that is plentiful there. South of Orissa and near the city of Madras, malaria was and is rare.[30] From the 1860s, these tendencies are fully reflected in the sanitary reports of the military in Madras. Rangoon or the southern coasts of Burma showed a high incidence of malaria only among units recently returned from service in central India. Contrary to the published evidence, however, many British medical officers still associated malaria with low altitudes, heavy rainfall, and swamps.[31]

Not all of the West Indian islands had possible sites for a hill station, but Jamaica did. Even before the 1840s, some troops had been kept at Maroon Town, but the new station at Newcastle made an immediate reputation.[32] The death rate for European troops on Jamaica dropped from 128 per thousand in 1817–36 to 60.8 per thousand in 1837–46, a change credited to the move – no doubt correctly.[33] The local vector was *Anopheles albimanus*, which lives in the low country, where it breeds in cane fields and irrigated areas.[34] It was not a very effective carrier, in any case, but it was numerous. It rarely reached into the Blue Mountains, although the troops in the mountains did suffer from

[29] *Report of the Commissioners*, 1: xxvi.
[30] Mark F. Boyd, (ed.), *Malariology: A Comprehensive Survey of All Aspects of This Group of Diseases from a Global Standpoint*, 2 vols. (Philadelphia and London, 1949) 2:812; 2:214–15.
[31] AMSR, 1860, p. 127; AMSR, 1863, p. 138; AMSR, 1869, p. 163.
[32] For Jamaica, unlike other stations in the tropics, the British authorities published annual mortality statistics for the period 1848–58 as part of a special investigation of yellow fever conducted in the mid-1860s (see Table A.2).
[33] Balfour, "Summary of the Reports," p. 131.
[34] Boyd, *Malariology*, 2:769–70.

the cholera epidemic of the mid-1850s and from periodic yellow fever.

The Windward and Leeward Command had no land at any such altitude. In 1859, a yellow fever epidemic broke out at the central barracks near Port-of-Spain on Trinidad. The authorities appointed a commission to look into the possibility of a hill station. It found the most eligible site at 2,200 feet – 300 feet short of the preferred range of 2,500 to 4,000 feet. The commission also wanted a high plateau rather than the peak or ridge site Trinidad had to offer. On those grounds, it recommended against any hill station at all.[35]

French experience in the Caribbean was comparable to that of the British, owing to the success of Camp Jacob on Guadeloupe. In Algeria, on the other hand, altitude brought no such advantage. In the 1840s, several military posts at 2,000 to 3,000 feet above sea level suffered serious malaria epidemics.[36] In fact, malaria occurs in the Atlas Mountains at altitudes up to 8,000 feet, with *Anopheles hispaniola* as the most likely vector, but Algeria had a wealth of vectors. *Anopheles sargenti* flourished so efficiently in the desert oases that both the towns-people and the desert nomads were heavily parasitized. The most serious endemic malaria, however, came in the humid coastal belt, where *Anopheles labranchiae* flourished over the whole range from Morocco in the west to Tunisia in the east.[37] Military medical authorities soon recognized that altitude and aridity might well bring safety elsewhere, but not in Algeria.

Waterborne Disease

By the early nineteenth century, water and health had already had a long association in European thought. Greek cosmology had a universe made up of the four basic elements – earth, air, fire, and water. The humoral theory of medicine grew, in turn, from this concept, featuring the four equivalent body fluids – blood, phlegm, black bile, and yellow bile – hence such manipulations of the bodily fluids as bleeding and purging. Bathing in or drinking waters of special repute had been common in western Europe since the time of the Roman Empire. From the late seventeenth century, English spas like Bath or Harrogate emerged as health resorts, although with some dispute about the precise qualities that made these waters valuable.[38]

In the eighteenth century, both chemists and minerologists were

---

35 AMSR, 1:169–70 (1859).
36 Armand, *Algérie médicale*, pp. 123–30.
37 Boyd, *Malariology*, 2:794.
38 Noel G. Coley, "Physicians and the Chemical Analysis of Mineral Waters in Eighteenth-Century England, MH, 26:123–44 (1982); Anne Hardy, "Water and the Search for Public Health in London in the Eighteenth and Nineteenth Centuries," MH, 28:250–82 (1984).

intensely interested in the chemical content of water, still seen as one of the four fundamental elements. The popularity of spas and health cures based on particular *kinds* of water, gave the analysis of water a commercial value that was otherwise rare.[39] Short of chemical analysis, the criteria of water quality were taste and appearance, and authorities could go to some length describing these qualities and associating them with particular sources of desirable dissolved gases and minerals.

As early as 1752, however, John Pringle had associated dysentery with sanitation – and decaying organic matter from putrefying animals as a source of disease.[40] In 1789, Antoine Lavoisier's *Traité élémentaire de chimie* opened the investigation still further with the discovery that water was not an element after all, but was made up of what we now call hydrogen and oxygen.[41] Others developed increasingly intricate means to identify material in solution, mainly inorganic materials. Some were also concerned with "impure water" – meaning chemically impure, since bacteria were not yet known – and one of the first impurities to be discussed was organic matter, since organic wastes could be associated with the same kind of decay that produced the miasma of malaria. In 1858, a respected French authority on military medicine explained how, "decomposed and fermented organic principles act in the same manner as paludic effluvia, and the same consequences may be caused equally by one or the other means of transmitting the infecting substances."[42] Diseases, in short, do not have causes specific to each. Rather, generalized causes of ill health operate equally to further all forms of disease.

The mode of drinking water was also important. The authoritative A. Grellois believed that water, like wine, should be drunk in moderation, especially in hot weather.[43] Warm water was also said to be dangerous because it thinned the blood without quenching the thirst, thus encouraging the individual to drink more than was good for him. Warm water was said to cause diarrhea, dysentery, an enlarged liver, jaundice, gastroenteritis, cholera morbus, and putrid fever.[44] Grellois's list of waterborne diseases was not entirely inaccurate, but he saw the fault as *warm* water, not impure water. He thought that iced water was equally dangerous; in New York alone, he claimed, more than 100 people died each summer from drinking iced water.[45]

By the early nineteenth century distilled water became available on

[39] Rachel Laudan, *From Mineralogy to Geology: The Foundations of a Science* (Chicago, 1987).

[40] John Pringle, *Observations on the Diseases of the Army* (London, 1752).

[41] Frederick Lawrence Holmes, *Lavoisier and the Chemistry of Life: An Exploration of Scientific Creativity* (Madison, 1985), esp. pp. 199–223.

[42] M. Grellois, "Étude hygiènique sur les eaux potables," RMMM, 2(3d ser.):120–212 (1859), p. 1854.

[43] Grellois, "Étude hygiènique," pp. 184–5.

[44] Grellois, "Étude hygiènique," pp. 145–6.

[45] Grellois, "Étude hygiènique," p. 148.

public sale, along with home distillation devices and systems for filtering turbid water. The basic principle of home filtration was first to allow the water to settle and precipitate any solids it might contain, then to pass it through a filtering medium – usually sand or gravel of varying coarseness.

Other forms of purification also had their advocates. Vinegar or lemon juice could be added for taste. Alum would speed the precipitation of solids in suspension. Better still, various tonic substances would provoke the body to necessary reactions that could counter any bad qualities of water. Wine, brandy, rum, and vinegar were all mentioned as useful tonics, although the French army found that vinegar could also cause indigestion. The minister of war, on the recommendation of the Sanitary Council of the Armies, prescribed brandy in place of vinegar – added to the troops' drinking water in the proportion of 3.125 milliliters per liter.[46]

The public and the medical profession were greatly concerned about clean water, but the association of water with disease was slow to come, though a few, like Pringle, had spoken early. In 1797, William Lambe in Britain had written about the danger of poisoning from lead pipes. He moved on to insist that distilled water was the only safe drink. In 1828, a royal commission investigated the public water supply in London, but no action followed. In the same year, however, a private water company serving the district of Chelsea installed the first slow sand filter.[47]

The distinction between kinds of filtration is significant. A rapid sand filter is a physical filter, like a piece of filter paper. It can remove silt and other suspended matter, but not impurities in solution – nor bacteria. The slow sand filter, on the other hand, is a biological filter in which living matter purifies the water. Recent versions begin with a settling basin, where solids can precipitate, reducing bacteria. Algae can also begin to grow, increasing the dissolved oxygen. Water is then allowed to seep slowly through a series of sand and gravel filter beds. Most important, at the point of entering the first sand layer, it encounters a layer of microorganisms adhering to the sand particles. This layer, called the filter skin, consists of bacteria, algae, and other forms of life that trap, digest, and break down the bacteria and organic matter in the raw water, leaving simple organic salts. As the water passes through the deeper sand beds, suspended impurities are strained out and further bacterial action takes place. Finally, aeration restores the oxygen used in the purification process and dissipates the carbon dioxide that was a by-product. The purification in this case is per-

[46] Grellois, "Étude hygiènique," pp. 140, 211–12.
[47] Hardy, "Water in London," 260–4; L. Huisman and W. E. Wood, *Slow Sand Filtration* (Geneva, 1974), pp. 9–26.

formed by biological agents, bacteria acting on bacteria, as in a septic tank.[48]

The people who installed the first sand filter in 1828 could not have known how or why it worked. That knowledge had to wait until bacteria were studied seriously more than a half-century later. Nor can we know in retrospect just how effective these early slow sand filters were. Today, however, with other forms of water purification available, many authorities still believe that a properly designed and operated slow sand filter is the best means of purifying water.

Sand, however, was early recognized as a "natural" filter. By 1858, sand-filtered water from the Garonne was available in Bordeaux. The Fonvielle filter – a cylindrical filter that passed water through two layers of sponges followed by seven levels of alternate fine sand and gravel – served many districts of Paris. It probably worked to some degree as a biological purifier. Other filters produced a tasteless and odorless product, but they were surely less effective in removing bacteria. The French Souchon filter was popular because it worked fast with little water pressure – hence was a rapid, not a slow filter. The filtering elements were heavy cloth and alternate layers of charcoal. The chief pharmacist of the French military hospitals recommended a similar filter for French troops in the field, but there is no reason to think that it would have had any effect on bacteria.[49]

A few researchers had nevertheless begun to associate disease with water – specifically with cholera. Cholera was endemic in India, especially in Bengal, and became more widespread in the nineteenth century as epidemics reached Europe and passed on to North America and the West Indies.[50] In the early 1850s, cholera reached British and French troops fighting against Russia in the Crimea, with important repercussions for military medicine. The high death rates brought wide publicity, which was heightened by the efforts of Florence Nightingale and then by the Herbert Commission and other parliamentary inquiries.[51]

In 1854, during the English cholera epidemic, Dr. John Snow was able to show the connection between a particular pump in London and several hundred cholera deaths. Snow's investigations also showed a

---

[48] Huisman and Wood, *Slow Sand Filtration*, pp. 27–46; John Pickford, "Water Treatment in Developing Countries," in *Water, Wastes, and Health in Hot Climates*, ed. Richard Feachem, Michael McGarry, and Duncan Mara (London, 1977), pp. 182–4.

[49] Grellois, "Étude hygiènique," pp. 136–9.

[50] No notice of cholera appears in these West Indian mortality data before 1846 or after 1859 (with the exception of Jamaica). The worst of the epidemic happened to strike during the period of missing data.

[51] PP, 1857–8, xviii [C.2318], "Report of the Commissioners Appointed to Enquire into the Sanitary Condition of the Army"; and PP, 1857–8, xxxviii, "Medical and Surgical History of the British Army Which Served in Turkey and the Crimea during the War against Russia in the Years 1854–55–56."

strong correlation between sources of water in London and the incidence of cholera. Even without knowing the causative agent, a strong empirical case could be made that cholera was caused by some waterborne substance.[52] But this kind of knowledge was fragile. Army doctors still believed water quality influenced overall health, but did not consider it a cause of particular diseases, and this attitude remained dominant until Robert Koch's bacteriological discoveries of the 1880s.[53] Advance from knowledge to action was equally slow in civilian circles. In 1861, a medical researcher returned to Dr. Snow's famous Broad Street pump and found that it its water still contained 1.92 grams per liter of organic matter derived from sewage.

Scientific research moved primarily in another direction, toward the chemical analysis of water. "Hardness" or the presence of bicarbonates of calcium or magnesium was sometimes regarded as dangerous; in fact is was merely inconvenient for washing. Military doctors developed techniques for field analysis. The French army published tests for chlorine, sulfuric acid, sodium, magnesium, and nitric acid. Good drinking water should contain no more than 0.250 grams per liter nor less than 0.150 grams per liter of minerals. With less, water becomes insipid and unnutritious, like distilled water; with more, it becomes hard, and lacks the good taste it should have.[54]

Some of this chemical research produced valuable results. Researchers correctly identified lead as a poison, although they disagreed on the threshold of danger – which some placed as low as 0.00721 grams per liter and others as high as 0.0564 grams per liter.[55] They also recognized that organic matter in general was a possible danger, and, in 1862, Dr. Woods, a British Army staff-assistant surgeon developed a test for the organic content of water using potassium permanganate – a test still in use.[56] In retrospect, of course, not all organic matter was truly dangerous (tea and soup are heavy in vegetable organic matter), but it was the best guide chemical analysis could offer at the time.

By the late 1860s, British military doctors recognized that cholera and

[52] John Snow, *On the Mode of Communication of Cholera*, 2d ed. (London, 1855). For a survey of cholera, see Roderick E. McGrew, *Encyclopedia of Medical History* (New York, 1985), pp. 59–64, esp. p. 63. See also Hardy, "Water and Public Health," pp. 268–70; Margaret Pelling, *Cholera, Fever and English Medicine* (London, 1978), pp. 203–28.

[53] Alfred Keogh, "The Results of Sanitation on the Efficiency of Armies in Peace and War," JRAMC, 12:357–785 (1909), pp. 362–3.

[54] Morin, "L'essai des eaux en campagne," RMMM, 9(3d ser.):310–16 (1863).

[55] E. A. Parkes, "Review of the Progress of Hygiene during the Year 1861," AMSR for 1860, 2:349–51. The pollution was reported as 6.08 grains per gallon, but this and other such measures are here translated into the more common metric grams per liter. Recent WHO standards for lead content are considerably lower at 0.10 mg/l (WHO, *International Standards*, p. 33).

[56] E. A. Parkes, "Review of the Progress of Hygiene during the Year 1862," AMSR for 1861, 3:308–34, pp. 313–15; John Pickford, "Water Treatment in Developing Countries," p. 168.

perhaps typhoid may have been carried in water by some agent that could not be detected by chemical or microscopic analysis. The Broad Street pump, which delivered tasteless water, had helped to destroy the old belief that taste was a reliable test of safety. Military doctors also knew that foul-tasting water could be safe.[57]

Action followed these discoveries somewhat unevenly. In the colonial world, soldiers were often at the mercy of public water supplies. In the West Indies, the general loss of life in the cholera epidemics of the 1850s was especially alarming. In the wake of slave emancipation, governments believed the plantation economy was threatened by a labor shortage, and many colonial governments subsidized labor migration from India or China. A safe water supply for the whole population was not a mere convenience; it was a necessity and worthy of support from the dominant planting class, for, if cholera returned, the loss of life would cost far more.

Public action followed in many of the British Caribbean colonies.[58] By 1860, the army barracks in Demerara, British Guiana, were supplied by artesian wells. On Barbados, the Bridgetown Water Company began to tap artesian wells inside limestone caves, which supplied the barracks as well as the town. Water became so plentiful that the military could use it to flush the drains to the sea. Trinidad also had piped water, which came from the Maraval reservoir high in the mountains above Port-of-Spain, with flushed drains and a swimming pool for the troops.[59]

Only Jamaica lacked an assured supply of reasonably safe water. The troops high in the mountains at Newcastle had piped water from mountain streams. Although the water looked clear and was filtered through "dripstones" as well, Newcastle's record for waterborne disease suggests pollution near the source. Troops in Kingston and Port Royal depended on piped water from a reservoir near the head of the Hope River, a source that was even more doubtful.[60]

The results of these changes are borne out by the declining death rates. In the Windward and Leeward Command, the death rate of European soldiers from diseases of the digestive system dropped from 15 per thousand in 1837–46 to 1 per thousand in 1859–67. Improvements in the water supply brought lower mortality from gastrointestinal disease everywhere, but the decrease of Windward/Leeward military mortality by more than 92 percent was greater than that of the

[57] E. A. Parkes, "Report on Hygiene for 1867," AMSR, 9:296–317 (1866), pp. 153–4.
[58] Kenneth F. Kiple, "Cholera and Race in the Caribbean," *Journal of Latin American Studies*, 17:157–77 (1984), p. 176.
[59] AMSR, *Reports*, 2:262 (1860); 5:322 (1863).
[60] Johnson, R. J. O'Flaherty, and Lt.-Col. Gain, "Report of the Commission Appointed to Investigate the Origin, Progress, and Results of the Epidemic of Yellow Fever in the Island of Jamaica in 1866 and 1867," AMSR, 9:224–48 (1867), p. 228.

Madras Presidency (59 percent), Jamaica (54 percent), or of Britain itself (75 percent).[61]

In Algeria, the high death rates of settlers brought a sense of crisis and a demand for public action and public spending similar to that of the West Indies and greater than in France itself. By the 1840s, the French settlers in Algeria had begun to exploit mineral springs as health resorts.[62] By the mid-1860s, the Algerian government worked systematically to tap new artesian wells and to improve the water supply for Algerian towns. Its goal was to have piped water with filtration at the point of use, following the pattern of French cities at the time,[63] although French and British cities did not fully achieve piped water until the 1880s and even later.

In Madras, the water supply was organized in traditional Indian ways, and the army normally followed these, rather than trying to copy the latest European recommendations. At Wellington, the Madras hill station, for example, drinking water came from wells in the hillsides above the barracks, was piped to the vicinity of the barracks, and then carried by men and bullocks in hide bags called *mussacks* to the barracks itself. Once there, it was filtered through three ceramic pots filled with fine sand and charcoal and mounted on tripods. The system was open to contamination at several points, and diarrhea and dysentery were more of a problem in Wellington than in other Indian hill stations.[64]

Sewage Disposal

The intense urbanization of the nineteenth century meant crowding, just as military life meant crowding, and this multiplied the problems of sewage removal. The normal solution in the past, and into the early decades of the nineteenth century, was the cesspit. People threw human excreta and other household wastes into unlined holes in the ground. These cesspits were emptied periodically at night and the contents disposed of in streams, on nearby agricultural land, or sold for processing into fertilizer. In spite of the bad odor, cesspits had an advantage that was not recognized at the time. They began a natural

---

[61] See Chapter 1, Table 1.6. For Jamaica see AMSR, 2:135 (1860) and 10:85 (1868).

[62] Alfred Étienne Victor Martin, *Manual d'hygiène à l'usage des Européens qui viennent d'établir en Algérie* (Alger, 1847), pp. 56–9.

[63] Joshua Paynter, "Report upon the Sanitary Condition of French Troops Serving in Algeria," AMSR, 7:437–51 (1865),p. 441; J. Sutherland, J. Paynter, C. B. Ewart, and R. S. Ellis, "Report on the Causes of Reduced Mortality in the French Army Serving in Algeria," PP, 1867, xv [Cd.1947], pp. 31–45; Edmond Kolb, *Étude sur l'hygiène de l'Algérie* (Montpellier, 1859, pp. 101–3. For water supply in metropolitan France see Jean-Pierre Goubert, *La conquête de l'eau; l'avènement de la santé à lâge industriel* (Paris, 1986).

[64] Davidson, "Wellington," AMSR, 12:477 (1870)

process of biological purification, not unlike that of a modern cesspool. The less fortunate fact was that material from the cesspits leaked into the water table before the bacterial action was complete, and thus found its way into nearby wells.

The earliest sewers were not for human waste; they were urban drains used to carry rainwater into nearby rivers or streams. It was only natural, however, to use these drains for other wastes as well. In the early nineteenth century, cities grew, water closets became increasingly popular, and nearby bodies of water became polluted far beyond their natural capacity to purify wastes by bacterial action. Rivers became the equivalent of gigantic cesspits.

Urban sewage became a critical problem in Western Europe from the 1830s onward. People might not be conscious of the need for pure water, or of what made water safe or unsafe, but they had no problem discovering what made sewage unpleasant to have around, even though they might not know precisely why it was dangerous. Different countries, even different urban districts, approached the problem in their own ways. In England of the 1840s, the movement for improved sanitation is associated with the name of Sir Edwin Chadwick.[65] Chadwick's solution was to find ways to spread human waste over the land as fertilizer.[66]

In 1862, a House of Commons committee argued against adding human waste to sewage water. It simply moved the pollution to the rivers and streams. An enormous amount of water was required to carry the load of sewage from a moderate-sized town, which meant an additional expense in the water supply. Some objected that water carriage dilutes the human waste to the point of destroying its potential value for agriculture.[67] One possible course was to separate solid waste from liquid, deodorize it with carbolic acid or other suitable chemical agent, and sell it for fertilizer. A prolonged debate ensued, between those who favored the "water system" and those who favored the "dry earth system."[68]

The dry earth system was not very different from the ancient Chinese system of "night soil" collection and removal, which was also practiced in some parts of Europe. Urine was disposed of separately, and feces fell into a receptacle, where dry, sifted earth with a high clay

[65] E. Chadwick, *Report from the Poor Law Commissioners on an Inquiry into Sanitary Conditions of the Labouring Population of Great Britain* (London, 1842).

[66] G. M. Fair, J. C. Geyer, and D. A. Okun, *Water and Wastewater Engineering*, 2 vols. (1966), 1:1-1 to 1-16.

[67] For problems of landspreading sewage, see Joel A. Tarr, "From City to Farm: Urban Wastes and the American Farmer," *Agricultural History*, 598–612; Wylie D. Burge and Paul B. Marsh, "Infectious Disease Hazards of Landspreading Sewage Wastes," *Journal of Environmental Quality*, 7:1–9 (1978).

[68] Parkes, "Hygiene in 1862," 19–22.; E. A. Parkes, "Report on Hygiene for 1863," AMSR, 4:335–54 (1862), pp. 339–41.

content was immediately added as a deodorizing agent. Toilets on this principle were already in use, with a container of dry earth rigged to supply an appropriate quantity on demand. By 1862, about thirty towns in England had schemes to separate solid matter from liquid sewage before it was dumped into streams. Several treated the dry sewage with chemical deodorizers before selling it for agricultural uses.[69] Some skeptics claimed that dry earth was not a perfect deodorizer. Others objected that the labor cost of removing the waste-and-earth mixture was too high for the modest agricultural value of the product. The two systems remained in competition up to the end of the century.

British military sanitary engineering was an extension of civilian work, with two additional problems – troops had to be able to take the field away from fixed facilities, and they had to confront tropical diseases – but military recommendations followed the main trends in civilian thinking. In practice, this meant that they wavered between the competing recommendations, although the "water system" was preferred in theory. In 1860, water-flushed latrines and sewers to carry the waste were the approved recommendation. Whenever possible, the sewage water was to be used on the fields for irrigation and fertilization, but only at a safe distance from the barracks.[70]

But practice differed from place to place. In the Windward and Leeward Command, piped water and the convenient proximity to the sea made the "water system" with its flush toilets a natural choice.[71] In India, however, a nonsewer system of latrines was an ancient tradition. In 1858, the standard latrine plan of the Bengal government called for a row of seats with holes over a movable pan 8 inches deep under each hole. Behind the seats was an enclosed space where "sweepers," or Indian servants, were in constant attendance. After the latrine was used, a sweeper immediately removed the pan, emptied it into a larger container, rinsed it with water, which he emptied into the same container, then added two inches of clean water and replaced the pan under the seat. Urine was collected in a separate container. The airtight receptacles for urine and other excrement were removed daily to pits at least a half mile from the nearest barracks, where the waste was mixed with quicklime and buried. This system was clearly labor-intensive. Each eight-seat privy served 100 soldiers, and required at least one sweeper.

With such a system already in use, it was only natural for Indian medical authorities to modify it on the basis of the dry earth recommendations, rather than to change it wholesale. By the mid-1860s, Madras authorities reported favorably on the "dry earth conservancy

[69] Parkes, "Hygiene in 1862," pp. 319–22.
[70] Parkes, "Hygiene in 1860," p. 343.
[71] AMSR, 11:86, 88 (1869).

system," as it was then called, but not without some criticism. The Army Sanitary Committee on the Cleansing of Indian Stations looked into the Madras proposals and found them wanting. As the committee pointed out, wastewater from rain and washing had to be removed from any military station whatever system was used for the latrines. The dry earth system required a separate additional system that, in effect, duplicated sewage lines that had to be there in any case. For each thousand men, this meant the separate removal by cart of 3,500 pounds of dry earth plus waste each day, not to mention the labor of sweepers required to manage the latrines.

There were other objections as well. In 1866, both the standard text on military hygiene and the Army Sanitary Commissions recommended flush toilets for all permanent military establishments.[72] The reasoning had nothing to do with bacteria, since the danger of bacteria had not yet been discovered. The problem was the dangerous gases thrown off by decomposing sewage. Fresh feces were not harmful: "It is only during the process of decomposition, that fæces become pernicious; hence, any circumstance which retards decomposition, prevents the occurrence of evil effects." The decomposition gases were reported to be so injurious that men could be struck down merely by looking into a sewer.[73] The dry earth system nevertheless won out in Madras. In 1880, it was used in every station, and it continued in general use in India and in Jamaica.[74]

The more serious problem with the dry earth system was that if the fecal material was exposed to air in the absence of screening, as it was in India and Jamaica, it was also open to contact with flies, which in turn had contact with food in the unscreened cook houses and mess halls. It was an easy route for the transmission of disease, especially typhoid fever.[75] As early as 1860, medical authorities recognized the difference between typhus and typhoid. Dr. William Budd had already shown that typhoid was contagious, and that the contagion passed from the victim's intestinal tract into sewage. As Dr. E. A. Parkes of the British Army Medical Service wrote in 1860, "The grand fact is clear that the occurrence of typhoid fever points unequivocally to defective removal of excreta, and that it is a disease altogether and easily preventable. Typhoid fever ought soon to disappear from every return of disease."[76]

If "soon" mean a half-century, he was right. Meanwhile, the prob-

---

[72] Charles Alexander Gordon, *Army Hygiene* (London, 1866), pp. 484–5.
[73] Gordon, *Army Hygiene*, pp. 445, 479.
[74] "Dry Earth Conservancy, Madras," AMSR, Report for 1867, pp. 216–23; AMSR, 22:247 (1880).
[75] James C. Riley, "Insects and European Mortality Decline," AHR, 91:833–58 (1986), p. 845; Hardy, "Water and Public Health;" Alfred Keogh, "The Results of Sanitation on the Efficiency of Armies in Peace and War," JRAMC, 12:357–785 (1909), pp. 363–5.
[76] Parkes, "Hygiene in 1860," p. 361.

lem was alternatives. Until understanding of sanitary engineering and the cause of disease advanced beyond the level prevalent in the 1860s, little more could be done to prevent certain diseases – especially typhoid fever, where the dry earth system was clearly implicated in the continued high mortality.

Ventilation

Air, in humoral theory, was as important as water. Miasma arising from the ground or from swamps contained both air and water. "Contagion" in mid nineteenth-century usage was similar. It could be an emanation from bodies of those who were ill, but also from those who were not ill.[77] This generalized contagion might reach dangerous levels if the air were not changed frequently enough.

In their first reports, Tulloch and Balfour were concerned about the ventilation of barracks. Public concern heightened during the Crimean War and continued through a long series of commissions and investigations in both France and Britain, rising to a peak in the 1860s. These investigations also took in other public accommodation and places of notoriously polluted air, like coal mines. Some of the research concentrated on chemical impurities and suspended matter in the air – parallel to the investigation of chemical impurities in water – and some took into account the process of fermentation. Pasteur had only recently shown that heating air to 125°C would destroy whatever property was responsible for the fermentation of liquids. At the time, many diseases were considered to be "xymotic" or yeast-associated, as they were in the British disease classification introduced in 1859.[78]

Commissions on public accommodation recommended specific standards of space and air movement for particular conditions. A French commission of 1861, for example, recommended ventilation at the rate of 1,060 cubic feet per person per hour in public buildings during daytime, 2,120 cubic feet per person at night, and 2,624 cubic feet per hour for hospitals – but 4,237 cubic feet in spaces where wounds were being dressed, and 5,649 cubic feet during epidemics.

The military conducted similar investigations. Tulloch had shown just how crowded barracks could be. One example on Tobago in 1827 had rooms 12 feet high, but each man was allowed the length of his body plus a width of 22 to 23 inches. This was far too narrow for beds, even camp cots, so the men slept in hammocks packed as close as was

---

[77] See Charles E. Rosenberg, "The Therapeutic Revolution: Medicine, Meaning, and Social Change in Nineteenth-Century America," *Perspectives in Biology and Medicine*, 20:485–506 (1977); "Florence Nightingale on Contagion: The Hospital as a Moral Universe," in *Healing and History: Essays for George Rosen*, ed. C. E. Rosenberg (London and New York, 1979), pp. 116–36.

[78] Parkes, "Hygiene in 1860," pp. 343ff.

physically possible – for a total space allowance per man of only 231 cubic feet.[79]

A royal commission established after the Crimean War recommended 600 cubic feet per man for barracks in Britain, 1,200 cubic feet for hospitals in Britain, and 1,500 cubic feet for hospitals in the tropics. By 1863, Indian regulations already called for a barracks standard of 1,000 cubic feet, to which authorities added a minimum floor space of 80 square feet per man. In low or poorly-ventilated barracks, however, 1,500 cubic feet plus 100 square feet of floor space were required.[80] In Jamaica, the yellow fever commission recommended raising the space per man at Newcastle Barracks to 800 cubic feet and 75 square feet of floor space – approximately the area of three standard double beds.[81]

By the late 1860s, British army research had expanded still further, especially under F. De Chaumont, professor of hygiene at the Army Medical School at Netley. He began with the assumption that all indoor air was chemically different from "pure" outdoor air and was to some degree poisonous, causing fevers and other illness. He was especially concerned with carbon dioxide, which increased with human breathing in a confined space. His solution was to increase natural ventilation, rather than space alone, to 3,000 cubic feet per man per hour.[82] If fact, carbon dioxide at the level Chaumont feared was not poisonous, and the cost of heating air to the level needed to meet Chaumont's recommendation in a cold climate would have been prohibitive. In general, midcentury standards ranged from 600 to 1,000 cubic feet per man, and these remained in effect until after the First World War. They no doubt helped reduce the transmission of some disease, especially of respiratory infections and tuberculosis, and they would certainly have made barracks life more pleasant for the occupants.

These multipurpose public health measures – altitude, clean water, clean air, and sewage disposal – almost certainly accounted for the most important mortality changes in midcentury, the decrease in water borne infections. In addition, the move to hill stations certainly reduced the death rate from malaria in places where a suitable site could be found. But medical personnel also sought more specific solutions to tropical disease – or disease in general. Consequently, greater attention was focused on the most spectacular and (for Europeans) the most exotic causes of death, especially malaria, yellow fever, and cholera.

[79] PP, 1837–8, xl (138), p. 3

[80] PP, 1863, xix [C.3184], pp. liii–liv.

[81] Johnson, O'Flaherty, and Gain, "Report of the Commission," pp. 243–7.

[82] F. De Chaumont, "Amount of Fresh Air Required to Reduce the Normal Standard of Carbonic Acid in Air Vitiated by Respiration," Lancet, 1866 (2):230–1 (Sept. 1, 1866); "On Ventilation and Cubic Space," Edinburgh Medical Journal, 1867 (1):1024–34 (May 1867).

CHAPTER 3

KILLING DISEASES OF THE
TROPICAL WORLD

Many of the principal killers of Europeans overseas were killers in
Europe as well. But Europeans overseas also met a range of diseases
they thought were peculiar to the tropical world – even though these
might occasionally turn up in Europe in less serious form. The greatest
single cause of death in the nineteenth-century tropics was malaria – as
it is today. But the great epidemic diseases, yellow fever and cholera,
also posed special problems, as did the tropical variants of common
diseases, poisons, and deficiencies – like typhoid, lead poisoning, and
beriberi. Each had its place in European medical thought and therapy
during the first two-thirds of the nineteenth century. Only tuberculosis
provided Europeans with a clear relocation benefit.

Malaria

The most obvious medical victory of this period was against malaria.
Even in Madras, where malaria was less serious than it was in Algeria
or the West Indies, deaths from fevers dropped by 60 percent between
the 1840s and the 1860s, more rapidly than the general decline in
mortality (see Table 1.6). In Algeria, mortality from fevers dropped by
61 percent – a significant decline, although less than the 87 percent decline in intestinal disease. By 1859–67 in the Windward and Leeward
Command, "paroxysmal fevers" (which were a combination of yellow
fever and malaria) dropped by more than 90 percent over the same
period, and the Jamaican death rate from these fevers was even lower
by the 1860s.[1]

Quinine contributed to the decline of fever deaths everywhere. It
was the first "wonder drug" that could attack a specific disease, but its
acceptance was neither universal nor simple. Cinchona bark from the
Andes had been known to Europeans since the middle of the seventeenth century, but it had varied reception. Some cinchona had the
characteristic bitter taste, but might contain little or none of the ef-

[1] It was 3.1 per thousand for Jamaica, 3.28 for the Windward/Leeward Command
(AMSR, 10:76, 83 [1868]).

fective antimalarial alkaloids. Medical practitioners were then dis-
appointed, as they were when they found the bark was ineffective
against yellow fever or typhoid, neither of which was very clearly
distinguished from malaria in the eighteenth century. This disappoint-
ment helped to give bark a bad name and raised the uncertainty about
appropriate dose, timing, and possible effectiveness as a prophylactic
as well as a cure.[2]

The new chemistry of the early nineteenth century brought an important breakthrough for several medicines previously used in their
natural state. Chemists had isolated morphine from opium as early
as 1804, but the process was later lost and had to be rediscovered.
In 1817, Joseph Pelletier isolated emetine from ipecacuanha, a South
American root. Emetine was widely used as an emetic and, in modified
form, as an antidysenteric. In 1820, Pelletier and Joseph Caventou
isolated quinine and the other antimalarial alkaloids from cinchona
bark.

Medical men began to experiment with the new drug almost immediately, first in France, then in the United States. In 1823, the first
commercial production began in Philadelphia, where doctors at the
University of Pennsylvania had also begun using it. The widest distribution in the early years, however, came in the Mississippi Valley,
where Dr. John Sappington of Arrow Rock, Mississippi, distributed it
as "Dr. Sappington's Anti-Fever Pills." He also encouraged regular
prophylactic use of the new medicine, advising his customers to take a
pill at the same time each day, when church bells rang.[3]

The new uses of cinchona prompted a renewed search for cinchona
supplies, especially for species of trees with a high quinine content
in their bark. By the 1840s, bark searchers in the forests east of the
Andes had collected so much bark that the Bolivian government
banned further export for a time. In 1849, Richard Spruce, an English
naturalist, returned from South America with seeds of red cinchona or
Cinchona succirubra. In 1860, the seeds reached India, and planters
began growing the trees in Madras and Ceylon. *C. succirubra* was not
the species highest in quinine, but it yielded three other alkaloids with
antimalarial properties. When all four were extracted, the yield in
effective antimalarials could be as high as 11 percent of the bark. This
combination became available as totaquine in India during the 1860s for
as little as one rupee per ounce.[4] Meanwhile, the use of quinine spread
sporadically because of conservative opposition.

In the sphere of French military medicine, the dominant voice in the

[2] Dale C. Smith, "Quinine and Fever: The Development of the Effective Dosage," JHM,
30:343–67 (1974), pp. 343–56; Philip D. Curtin, *The Image of Africa* (Madison, 1964).

[3] Smith, "Quinine and Fever," pp. 355–8; Norman Taylor, *Quinine: The Story of Cinchona*
(New York, 1943), pp. 4–5.

[4] Marie L. Duran-Reynals, *The Fever-Bark Tree: The Pageant of Quinine* (Garden City, NY,
1946).

early nineteenth century was that of François Broussais, professor at Val-de-Grâce Hospital in Paris, where most of the French army doctors of the mid nineteenth century received their training. Broussais was a proponent of the debilitation theory for the treatment of fevers. He believed that all fevers were essentially the same, and that differences in symptoms were merely accidental. All were caused by inflammation of an organ, and inflammation arose from irritation. The appropriate treatment was therefore a restricted diet, heavy bloodletting, and heroic doses of mercurial and opium preparations. Broussais and his followers considered quinine still another irritant, to be withheld in early stages of a fever and then given only in minute doses.[5]

In the early 1830s, François Maillot, a French army doctor serving in Algeria at Bône (now Annaba), broke with the Broussais school and started treating fever victims with large doses of quinine from the beginning of the illness. Where Broussais would have administered 30 to 40 centigrams of quinine, Maillot recommended one gram per day and up to three or four grams in serious cases.[6] He found that quinine was effective even against some apparently continuous fevers, where the intermissions were too weak for clear diagnosis, and he made his bow to tradition by moderate blood letting as well. His reform was so important that several authorities later credited him with the success of the French conquest of Algeria, though he recommended sulphate of quinine only as a cure for malaria.[7]

British experiments with quinine came a little later than those of the Americans and French. A naval surgeon on the ill-fated British Niger Expedition of 1841–2 experimented with doses of about 17 centigrams a day, which he later increased to 60 centigrams. Finally, in 1842, he began giving himself 0.5 to 1 gram a day prophylactically, which prevented fever until he got back to England and stopped the drug. He then came down with fever.[8]

In 1847, Alexander Bryson, the chief medical officer of the British Navy in West African waters, ordered a shift from wine and cinchona bark to wine and quinine as a prophylactic against malaria. The dosage was 30 centigrams of quinine in 1 ounce of wine to be taken daily for fourteen days after exposure to fever on shore duty. And he suggested

[5] Hamet, "Malaria and Military Medicine during the Conquest of Algeria," MS, 25:24–33 (1932), pp. 26–8; Erwin H. Acherknecht, "Broussais: Or a Forgotten Medical Revolution, BHM, 27:320–43 (1953).
[6] Recent recommendations would be on the order of 2 grams the first day, followed by 1.3 grams per day for the rest of the first week, for a total of 10 grams (Smith, "Quinine and Fever," 352, 366).
[7] Hamet, "Malaria," p. 30; Smith, "Quinine and Fever," p. 320; Léon Colin, Traité des fièvres intermittentes (Paris, 1870), pp. 376–7; Dr. Bordier, National, 5 October 1881, quoted in Maillot, "Garnison de Bône," p. 176.
[8] T. R. H. Thomson, "On the Value of Quinine in African Remittant Fever," Lancet, 1846 (1), p. 244.

that merchant vessels on the West African coast be required to do the same, just as they were required to issue lime juice as an antiscorbutic. By 1848, the director general of Army Medical Services sent out a circular recommending "copious doses" early in the course of a fever. Prophylactic quinine thus became widely used in the British armed forces during the 1850s. At least some ships in the French Navy were also using prophylactic wine with quinine at 2 grams per liter of wine – a lighter mixture than Bryson's, but the daily dosage was unspecified. Early in the American Civil War, the federal Sanitary Commission recommended prophylactic quinine as well, citing the British practice on the coast of China in 1858 as a precedent.[9]

Recommendations, however, were not always followed. Quinine, even disguised in wine, has an unpleasant and bitter taste. Large doses could produce undesirable side effects. Interestingly, Campari and other bitter wines, now admired for their taste, began as medicines. Many medical men in Algeria followed Maillot's principal recommendations, and the settlers used quinine freely.[10] Dutroulau's authoritative text on tropical medicine not only recommended quinine at Maillot's dosage for actual cases of fever, but also advised a daily intake of quinine in wine as a prophylactic, although some others said that coffee was just as good. As late as 1861, however, the principal British authority on medical practice for India allowed quinine to be used only in small quantities and argued that "depletion" by bleeding was still the best possible remedy for fevers.[11]

In the 1860s, despite quinine's limited success, Europeans were still attributing tropical fevers to miasma arising from soil, especially from marshes. The French in Algeria launched a major drainage program, an empirical form of mosquito control that also saved lives. Records from the military hospital at Bône suggest the comparative effectiveness of draining as against quinine. Prophylactic quinine was not used. A drop in hospital entries for malaria therefore roughly measures the effectiveness of mosquito control. Hospital entries from malaria

[9] Alexander Bryson, "On the Prophylactic Influence of Quinine," MTG, 8(n.s.):6–7 (Jan. 7, 1854); Gold Coast Annual Report for 1849, PP, 1850, xxxvi [C.1232], pp. 95–6; Daullé, Cinq années d'observations médicales dans l'éstablissement français de Madagascar (Paris, thesis no. 179, 1857), pp. 54–5, 64–5; E. A. Parkes, "Review of the Progress of Hygiene during the Year 1861," AMSR for 1860, 2:367.

[10] A. Rozier-Joly, "Considerations générale sur les constitutions médicales des pays marécageux," GMA, 4:33–, 51–, 101– (1859); 5:4–, 42–, 62–, 157–, 178– (1860); 6:2– (1861); 7:45–, 80–, 147– (1862); 8:47–, 65–, 78–, 91– (1863) 5:64–5 (1960); J. B. L. Baudens, Rélation de l'expédition de Constantine (Paris, 1838), pp. 10–11; Colin, Fièvres intermittentes, pp. 417–19; Joshua Paynter, "Report upon the Sanitary Condition of French Troops Serving in Algeria," AMSR, 7:437–51 (1865) p. 438.

[11] Auguste Frédéric Dutroulau, Traité des maladies des Européens dans les pays chauds, 2d ed. (Paris, 1868), pp. 238–54; Alphonese Laveran, Traité des maladies et épidémies des armées (Paris, 1875), p. 106; James Ranald Martin, The Influence of Tropical Climates in Producing the Acute Endemic Diseases of Europeans, 2d ed. (London, 1861), p. 384.

were high in the 1830s, became high again in the epidemic years of 1852–3, but dropped to about a fifth of that level by the 1860s.[12] Drainage therefore gained an 80 percent drop in morbidity from malaria. Quinine was used to cure malaria, once acquired. A drop in the case-fatality rate roughly measures its impact. The case-fatality rate dropped from a range of 5 to 23 percent in the 1830s to a range of 2 to 3 percent by 1852–3. Mortality, in short, began to fall by the late 1840s (presumably from the use of quinine), although the drop in morbidity came only in the 1860s (as the drainage works began to control mosquitos). These figures apply only to the vicinity of Bône, but the military death rate from malaria for Algeria in general dropped by 61 percent between 1846–8 and 1862–6 (Table 1.8).

French medical authorities gave most of the credit to draining, clearing, and cultivation by French settlers. In 1866, the British mission to investigate French methods accepted that conclusion, although it noted in passing a number of minor contributions, such as field hospitals, better rations, better clothing for the troops, and well-drilling for the sake of improved water supply. Quinine was one of these minor improvements. Even Maillot, looking back from the 1880s on the medical advances in Algeria, argued that the role of drainage was equal to that of quinine. Alfonse Laveran, six years before he identified the plasmodial protozoa in human blood, gave drainage and cultivation priority over other preventive measures.[13] This emphasis on drainage helped to control malaria, but it may also have helped delay full use of prophylactic quinine until the early twentieth century.

Like the British in India, the French in Algeria recognized relocation costs. Their particular concern was to explain, and to prevent if possible, further deaths among colonists in Algeria. The acclimatization controversy led scientists to distinguish between diseases that were susceptible to seasoning and those that were not. Dr. Alfred E. V. Martin, editor of a medical manual for the colonial government, took the optimistic view that, although seasoning gave no protection against "marsh disease," that disease could be controlled by draining the land. Hepatitis and diseases of the intestinal track, on the other hand, were "acclimatization diseases," which declined after proper seasoning. In the long run, then, Frenchmen would be able to live as safely in Algeria as they did in Europe.[14]

[12] François Clement Maillot, "État sanitaire de la garnison de Bône, de 1832 à 1881," *Gazette des hôpitaux*, 1884 (2):266–7, 175.

[13] J. Sutherland, J. Paynter, C. B. Ewart, and R. S. Ellis, "Report on the Causes of Reduced Mortality in the French Army Serving in Algeria," PP, 1867, xv [Cd.1947], pp. 16–31; Maillot, "Garnison de Bône," *passim*; A. Laveran, "Maladies des armées," pp. 193–203.

[14] Alfred Etienne Victor Martin, *Manual d'hygiène à l'usage des Européens qui viennent d'ètablir en Algérie* (Alger, 1847), pp. 127–71.

The Algerian experience also led French medical thought into a cul de sac. Europeans generally associated malaria with marshes; but that association was not accurate for Algeria, where the variety of anopheline vectors allowed malaria to flourish in desert oases and high in the mountains. By the mid-1850s, doctors in Algeria were investigating other sources of miasma, hence of malaria. The most likely possibility was some condition of the soil itself, according to then-current ideas associating particular diseases with particular places. Léon Colin, a military doctor and professor at Val-de-Grâce conceded that malaria could come from marshes, but said it could also come from dry soil, especially from soil that has been dug up. This new danger was called *terrassements* in French, or "upturning" the soil in English. Once the soil had been planted and put into permanent cultivation, however, that very cultivation deprived it of its poison – just as it did in northern Europe where malaria had once flourished and had since disappeared. Colin thought the name of the disease should itself be changed from *intoxication palustre* (marsh poison) to *intoxication tellurique* (earth poison).[15]

Still another French idea about acclimatization was the doctrine of antagonism, which was first proposed centuries earlier by Thucydides. According to this doctrine, the epidemic appearance of one disease provided immunity against certain others. Jean Boudin applied it to the Algerian setting in his treatise on intermittent fevers and later gave it the status of a law. He believed that certain diseases oppose other diseases in the human body, so that wherever malaria is endemic, typhoid fever and tuberculosis of the lung are rare. Therefore, Boudin argued, Europeans could never become acclimatized to life in Algeria. Although they might well contract less malaria if they drained the swamps, they would have more typhoid.[16]

The doctrine of antagonism enjoyed a certain popularity in the 1840s and 1850s. The editors of the *Dictionaire Encyclopédique des Sciences Médicales* assigned it a separate article by Alphonse Laveran. He conceded that Boudin had made some important pathological observations, but they were not consistent enough to support the general proposition. Laveran went ahead on his own to identify more precisely the patterns of immunity revealed in the military mortality statistics. Many others at the time believed that race was a major immunizing factor, but he showed that childhood environment was more significant. During the British Niger Expedition of 1841–2, blacks recruited in Europe and America came down with fever. Blacks recruited on the African coast did not. In a series of yellow fever epidemics in Mobile, Alabama, blacks born in Africa showed greater immunity than

---

[15] L. Colin, *Fièvres intermittentes*, pp. v–xii, 461–90.
[16] Jean Chrisitan Marc François Joseph Boudin, *Traité de géographie et de statistique médicale et des maladies endémiques*, 2 vols. (Paris, 1857), esp. 1:76–97.

those born in America. In Jamaica, local whites showed an immunity to yellow fever, which attacked new arrivals from Europe. Acclimatization, Laveran concluded, was not necessarily impossible.[17]

The Epidemics: Yellow Fever

Nineteenth-century European medicine was sharply divided between contagionists and anticontagionists, who tended to see the cause of disease in generalized environmental conditions, or in miasmas. Europeans had known from antiquity, however, that certain diseases are transmitted from one person to another. This was clearly the case with syphilis and smallpox. Confronted with an apparently infectious disease, Europeans had for centuries responded in one of two ways – quarantine or flight. The word "quarantine" was first used to refer to the forty days' isolation that medieval Venice imposed on ships arriving from infected ports. Flight was not open to everyone, but it could save a fortunate few who succeeded in isolating themselves, like the characters in Boccaccio's *Decameron* who fled to escape the plague.

These old remedies could still be used against yellow fever and cholera, the main epidemic diseases of the tropical world. Yellow fever is mosquito-borne, like malaria, but the vector, *Aëdes aegypti* behaves differently from the malaria-carrying anophelines. It is essentially a domestic mosquito, at least in the Americas; it tends to stay around human habitations, breeding in any open container of water it can find. Its flight is short, less than 100 yards. During epidemics, the disease tends to spread only a few dozen yards at a time, often from house to house. *A. aegypti* can also live up to four months. Because it could survive long ocean voyages by sailing ship, epidemic yellow fever could reach North America or northern Europe and survive there at least briefly, until it died out with the first frost.[18]

The case-fatality rate is highly variable. With some, especially children, yellow fever may show no clinical symptoms at all, although it always leaves a lifelong immunity. For biostatistical purposes, therefore, the existence of a "case" is hard to establish, although tests can now indicate an acquired immunity, hence a prior infection. Nineteenth-century authorities recognized only cases marked by the peculiar symptoms of yellow skin color and "black vomit." These were a small part of the total. Aside from the subclinical cases, yellow fever was easily mistaken for a variety of other diseases, from malaria to influenza.

---

[17] A. Laveran, "Antagonisme," DESM, 5:229–45 (1867).
[18] William Coleman, *Yellow Fever in the North: The Methods of Early Epidemiology* (Madison, 1987), esp. pp. 3–14.

Yellow fever's pattern of immunity influenced its epidemiology. The immune ex-victim, whether diagnosed or not, was not only safe from further clinical symptoms; his blood would not support the virus. He could not, therefore, act as a "carrier" like some recovered victims of typhoid fever or tuberculosis. In order to survive at all, the parasites needed groups of nonimmunes concentrated within the flight range of *A. aegypti*. Otherwise the disease would die back into the forests, where nonhuman victims served to keep it alive until a better opportunity occurred. European soldiers newly arrived in the Caribbean were ideal; but the survivors in turn became immune, thus ending the epidemic.

In the nineteenth-century Caribbean, however, yellow fever struck somewhere nearly every year, and rarely returned to the same place until a few years had passed.[19] On Jamaica, for example, a serious attack occurred in 1841–2, when the highland barracks at Newcastle was built. It then returned in 1853–4, 1856–7, 1860, and 1867–8. The normal military response, once the disease reached a Jamaica port, was flight. The outbreak in 1856–7 was studied with great care.[20] When the disease appeared at Port Royal and Kingston, the soldiers stationed there were ordered to Newcastle, but they included men who were already infected. As a result, 83 per thousand of the man stationed at Newcastle died, presumably of yellow fever. The medical men who studied the disease believed, however, that the causes were local and not imported with the troops from the seacoast. In 1860, another infected ship arrived, and the troops stationed on the coast were immediately removed to Newcastle. This time, the only fatal cases among the military were patients in the naval hospital in Port Royal and one unfortunate soldier who happened to be in jail.[21]

Flight was an effective precaution only if none of the fleeing soldiers were already infected. In the Jamaican epidemic of 1867–8, the authorities waited more than six months after the first civilian cases appeared before moving the troops into the mountains. As a result, some carried the virus in their blood. *A. aegypti* lives perfectly well at high altitudes as long as the temperature stays well above freezing. The crowded barracks on the mountainside were nearly perfect for transmitting the disease at close quarters.

[19] A. Hirsch, *Handbook of Geographical and Historical Pathology*, 3 vols. (London, 1883–6). Translated by C. Creighton. 1:322–7 contains a list for the Caribbean from 1802 to 1877.

[20] Robert Lawson, "Observations on the Outbreak of Yellow Fever among the Troops at Newcastle in 1856," *British and Foreign Medico-Chirurgical Review*, 59:445–80 (1859).

[21] H. Johnson, R. J. O'Flaherty, and Lt.-Col. Gain, "Report of the Commission Appointed to Assemble to Investigate the Origin, Progress, and Results of the Epidemic of Yellow Fever in the Island of Jamaica in 1866 and 1867," AMSR, 9:228 (1867); AMSR, 2:74 (1860).

Some, at least, of the military doctors recognized that yellow fever was contagious in the same sense smallpox was. They scattered the soldiers by dividing them among as many huts as possible, setting up tented camps wherever a flat space could be found. But the retrospective Jamaica Yellow Fever Commission disagreed. It held that the yellow fever epidemic of 1867–8 was the result of a "general epidemic influence" of unknown origin, which caused "all febrile disorders to assume, under its influence, the character of yellow fever." This, the commission concluded, was aggravated by the crowded conditions. As supporting evidence, they noted that the most crowded huts at Newcastle had the worst morbidity and mortality rates. By the time the epidemic finally died out toward the end of 1868, more than half the force had been admitted to hospital with some kind of fever, and 55.53 per thousand had died of fever, which equaled 80 percent of all deaths.[22] Given the fact that Newcastle was normally malaria-free, almost all of these deaths must have been caused by yellow fever.

The tactic of flight was widely practiced on other islands, even when a hill station was not available. Between May and November 1861, yellow fever broke out in Georgetown, British Guiana, The medical officer immediately moved the troops to Belfield, 15 miles from town, where they were kept "under canvas" until the epidemic had passed. None died. If the epidemic had reached Belfield, the medical officer planned to move them on to Barbados.[23]

The next year, yellow fever appeared in Bridgetown, Barbados. The medical officer first moved the men from barracks to barracks and "under canvas" a short distance away, but he finally shifted them to Gun Hill, 7 miles from town, where they remained until the epidemic passed. Here again, the maneuver worked; the only soldiers who died were nine officers and five noncoms who stayed in town with the West Indian troops under their command. Ironically, the black troops' supposed immunity to yellow fever caused the death of their officers. Again in 1867, in a new epidemic, removal to Gun Hill saved the whole force.[24]

By the 1860s, timely flight had become an effective defense against yellow fever. In mid century that purely empirical strategy may well have saved as many lives as quinine did. But each remedy fell short of its potential, because the medical officers had no way of knowing why these empirical safeguards worked, when they did work; quinine was not always used prophylactically and systematically, and flight was sometimes delayed long enough to allow the parasites to move to the new camp along with the troops – as at Newcastle in 1867–8.

---

[22] Johnson and others, "Commission on Yellow Fever," AMSR, 19:228–40 (1867).
[23] AMSR, 3:62, 267 (1861).   [24] AMSR, 4:73, 256–8, (1862); AMSR, 9:70, 74 (1867).

The Epidemics: Cholera

Cholera attracted even more medical attention in the mid nineteenth century. It was not as fatal as yellow fever in the West Indies – or as the other waterborne diseases of the diarrheal group in India – but its appearance was far more spectacular. Its first symptoms were mental depression and internal distress, followed by vomiting, stomach cramps, and acute diarrhea marked by thin, "rice-water" stools. The victim often died of dehydration within a few hours of the first seizure. Some recovered, but the case-fatality rate was typically about 40 percent outside of the region of endemic cholera at the mouths of the Ganges. In its home territory, it still appears each year, affecting many times the number of people who actually develop clinical symptoms. The microbe *Vibrio cholerae* (originally called *V. comma*) is passed out in the vomit and stools and reaches further victims either through drinking water or food, with an incubation time of about two days. Unlike yellow fever, the residual immunity is imperfect – not enough to guarantee against possible later infection, still less against a subclinical case that nevertheless allows the victim to transmit the disease to others.[25]

Outside the endemic area along the Bay of Bengal, cholera is epidemic, killing large numbers in its spectacular way and then moving on. Cholera's disappearance after an epidemic occurrence is not well understood. It may be that *V. cholerae* is not long-lived away from its human victims. In water, it tends to die out in competition with other, harmless bacteria, unless renewed from fresh victims. In any event, the epidemic visitation has been cholera's characteristic appearance outside the Bengal region, especially from the nineteenth century onward.

Europeans in India had suffered from the disease since the sixteenth century, but it became more widespread toward the end of the eighteenth. In 1817–26, it broke out in the first pandemic to reach far beyond India, moving east through Southeast Asia and north to China and Japan. It also moved west along the trade routes but only as far as Persia and Mesopotamia. It was this pandemic that attacked British troops in Madras.

The next pandemic was far more serious. It began in 1829, moving westward into Egypt and north into Russia. In 1830–2, it made its first appearance in Europe and then reached across the Atlantic to New York late in 1832. By 1834, it had reached the Pacific coast and moved south into Mexico and Central America. In the Caribbean, it reached

[25] D. R. Nalin, "Cholera," in *Hunter's Tropical Medicine*, 6th ed., ed. G. Thomas Strickland (Philadelphia, 1984), pp. 305–12; Roderick E. McGrew, *Encyclopedia of Medical History* (New York, 1985), pp. 59–64.

Cuba, but not Jamaica or the Lesser Antilles. It is therefore absent from the West Indian data for 1817–36, although it may have killed as many as 8 percent of the Cuban slave population. In the Maghrib, it reached Oran in 1834 and Algiers the next year, but did not go east of Tunisia. By 1835, it had disappeared.[26]

The third pandemic, which was even more serious for Europe, began in the early 1850s and reached its highest death rate in 1854. It was then that Dr. John Snow was able to confirm that cholera was associated with London's water supply. This time cholera reached into the Nilotic Sudan and down the East African coast as far as coastal Tanzania. On Zanzibar it killed an estimated 38 people per thousand. There, as in the West Indies, it was more serious for the unaccustomed African population than it was for Indians or Europeans.[27] In North Africa, it attacked all of Algeria and Tunisia in 1849–50. In the Americas, it reached the Caribbean in 1850–2, where it killed an estimated 71 per thousand on Jamaica. Unfortunately, these years were not reported in detail for the British troops on the island, but in the Caribbean in general the death rate among blacks was higher than among whites.[28] After one more visit in 1867, which affected only Cuba, epidemic cholera died out in the Caribbean.

The fourth pandemic of 1863–75 was less serious than the third had been in Europe, North America, or the West Indies. It was far more disastrous, however, in Africa, where it extended down the east coast to Madagascar, killing 148 per thousand of the local population at the French post of Nossi-Bé, but comparatively few Europeans and even fewer Indians.[29] On the west coast of Africa, it may have been even more severe, although it was not reported in detail. In the European posts of Senegambia, it again killed few Europeans – who were few in number anyway – but it killed 50 per thousand among the *tirailleurs sénégalais*.[30] By contrast, the annual death rate of European troops in Madras in 1827–38, the period of the second pandemic, was only 7.6

---

[26] Charles E. Rosenberg, *The Cholera Years: The United States in 1832, 1849, and 1866* (Chicago, 1962), pp. 13–38; Roderick E. McGrew, "The First Cholera Epidemic and Social History," BHM, 34:61–2 (1960); Kenneth F. Kiple, *The Caribbean Slave: A Biological History* (Cambridge, 1984) p. 146; M. A. Vincent and V. Collardot, *Le choléra d'après les neuf epidémies qui ont règné à Alger, depuis 1835 jusqu'en 1865* (Paris, 1867); Nancy Elizabeth Gallagher, *Medicine and Power in Tunisia, 1780–1900* (Cambridge, 1983), pp. 44ff.

[27] James Christie, *Cholera Epidemics in East Africa* (London, 1876), pp. 111ff.

[28] Kiple, *Caribbean Slave*, pp. 146–7; George W. Roberts, *Population of Jamaica: An Analysis of its Structure and Growth* (Cambridge, 1957), pp. 177–8.

[29] Jean-Baptiste Barnier, "Note sur l'épidémie de choléra qui a sévi dans l'ile de Nossi-Bé," AMN, 16:190–8 (1871), pp. 190–5; Christie, *Cholera Epidemics*, pp. 118–267, 441–4.

[30] P. F. A. T. Carbonnel, *De la mortalité actuelle au Sénégal et particulièrement à Saint-Louis* (Paris, thesis no. 10, 1873), p. 14. The rate is an annual average for 1868–70.

per thousand or 4.04 per thousand for the Indian troops, which was a common level for troops in India.[31]

For Algeria and Tunisia, the fourth pandemic was the most serious of all – but for the Africans, not the Europeans. The longstanding French concern about acclimatization of soldiers and colonists extended into the 1850s. Until 1855, the Europeans still sustained a net natural decrease, but in the early 1860s the excess of births over deaths produced a respectable population increase of 1.22 percent. Immigration pushed the total growth rate even higher.[32]

As the French settler population recovered, the native Algerians passed into a severe demographic crisis. It began in 1864–5, when the French suppressed a rebellion in southern Oran Province. Then, in 1866–70, came desert locusts, drought, epidemic cholera, and epidemic typhus, all in rapid succession. Authorities disagree about the actual size of the population loss, but estimates suggest that somewhere between one-third and one-fifth of the Algerian population died, with great variation from one region to another. A few isolated regions even managed to sustain a growing population during the crisis period, just as the colonists from Europe did.[33]

French military losses in Algeria from cholera were slight compared with those of the Algerians. In 1868, the year of combined typhus and cholera, French military death rates jumped by 38 percent over the levels of the recent past, but the next year they sank even below those of the early 1860s,[34] presumably because men of military age had already survived two cholera pandemics in France itself.

Particular units, however, shared the fate of the colonized. In July 1867, cholera arrived at the oasis town of Biskra. Within two weeks, it killed more than 20 percent of the native population and half of the French military detachment, forcing the French to evacuate altogether by the end of the month.[35] During the next two years typhus was harder on the French forces in Algeria than cholera had been, but there, too, the expected pattern failed to emerge.

The British in India had been accustomed to periodic cholera since the eighteenth century, and they monitored it carefully. Even though it

---

[31] "Report of a Committee of the Statistical Society of London, Appointed to Collect and Enquire into Vital Statistics, upon the Sickness and Mortality among the European and Native Troops Serving in Madras Presidency, from the year 1793 to 1838," JSSL, 3:127 (1840).

[32] Annie Rey-Goldzeiguer, *Le royaume arabe: La politique algérienne de Napoléon III, 1861–70* (Alger, 1977), p. 374.

[33] Rey-Goldzeiguer, *Royaume arabe*, pp. 450–74; André Nouschi, *Enquête sur le niveau de vie des populations rurales constantinoises* (Paris, 1961), pp. 338–77; Djilali Sari, *Le désastre démographique* (Alger, 1982), pp. 55–9; Gallagher, *Tunisia*, pp. 69ff.

[34] Laveran, *Maladies des armées*, 1:149.

[35] Nouschi, *Enquête*, p. 345.

was not the most important single killer, it was the most spectacular.[36] By midcentury, medical authorities in Madras had identified a regular route that epidemics had followed from the locus of the infection at the mouths of the Ganges since the first pandemic of 1818. As the disease spread, it moved first toward the regions of dense populations and intense commercial traffic. From coastal Bengal it passed first to the west across the Central Provinces, then southward through parts of Bombay Presidency and on down the west coast, although only the most virulent epidemics crossed over to Ceylon. Those that reached the core area of Madras Presidency, did so from the southwest. Mountains held up the spread of cholera. The Himalayas were a serious barrier, but lower mountain chains like the Western Ghats behind the west coast of peninsular India also seemed to slow its spread. Only after it had crossed these hills could it move freely through the rest of Madras Presidency.[37]

Some of the epidemiology of Indian cholera is explicable in the light of recent knowledge. *V. cholerae* was endemic in lower Bengal because of the water storage systems there. Water, even warm water, is to some degree self-purifying. Microorganisms die out in competition with each other, as in a septic tank. *V. cholerae* is tolerant to high alkalinity in water, however, which would be fatal to most other microorganisms. It can thrive in water with a pH up to 10.5. This characteristic gave it an ecological niche in the large ponds or tanks in the Ganges delta. The water in these tanks is alkaline and static during the dry season, the season for the local cholera outbreaks. In the monsoon season, fresh inputs of water reduce the pH and hence the *V. cholerae*, but they also spread it abroad, where it can be sustained by rapid passage from one victim to the next. An extremely dry season, however, can also reduce the numbers of *V. cholerae* by reducing the growth of algae on which they live.[38]

Wherever cholera struck in the nineteenth century, people wanted to know how it had been transmitted and how it could be prevented. There were contagionist and anticontagionist schools of thought, as in the case of yellow fever. The contagionists, a minority, and sometimes a small minority, believed that cholera was transmitted from one per-

---

[36] The Royal Commission on the health of the army in India, for example, produced a table of deaths over the period 1825–44, singling out cholera in relation to other causes of death. Overall, it showed that cholera accounted for 13 percent of all deaths among the company's European troops and 19 percent of all deaths among the company's native troops. *Report of Commissioners Appointed to Inquire into the Sanitary State of the Army in India*, 2 vols. (London, 1863), p. xcvi. Also printed in part in PP, 1863, xix, [C.3184].

[37] W. R. Cornish, *A Record of the Progress of Cholera in 1870, and Resumé of the Records of Former Epidemic Invasions of the Madras Presidency* (Madras, 1871), pp. 3–5.

[38] Aiden Cockburn, *The Evolution and Eradication of Infectious Diseases* (Baltimore, 1963), pp. 176–85; Nalin, "Cholera," pp. 306–7.

son to another like smallpox and syphilis. Their opponents tended to think that an epidemic grew out of local conditions of the same miasmatic nature as those that caused other diseases. They recognized that the "natives" were especially susceptible on account of squalid living conditions, and, in the West, that the poor were also susceptible. After Snow's discoveries of the 1850s, drinking water was more clearly implicated, but not to the satisfaction of all, and not necessarily as a triumph for contagionists generally.[39]

The contagionist doctrine in the mid nineteenth century was associated in the professional mind with an older, less scientific kind of medicine. This school recommended quarantine measures but otherwise did not consider the spread of contagion to be preventable. The doctrine could therefore be used to justify sitting back and letting the poor and the "natives" die, since nothing could be done about it in any case.[40] By the 1860s in Algeria, however, contagionism had also become a cry for action. Some doctors argued that, although nothing could be done about contagion itself, the disease could be attacked through its predisposing causes. It was possible to isolate the victims, to take strict care in disposing of their excrement, to control the entry of strangers, and to create a piped water supply with underground drains for wastewater.[41]

The anticontagionists often came up with much the same remedies. Dr. Inglis, in his sanitary report for Madras 1863, suggested that cholera was caused by "peculiar physical and atmospherical states operating on the decomposing vegetable and organic products at the low fluvial level described, and the sudden cessation, to the removal of all fermenting elements requiring meteorological conditions for their development" (sic).[42] But he then described the workings of these emanations in ways that sounded empirically correct and quite contagionist:

It is well known that the emanations, both exhalent and secretive, and other collective pollutions evolved from the persons of large congregations of human beings in India, conduce to outbreaks of cholera, and, as in Madras as well as sister Presidencies, we have our fairs and sacred places resorted to by thousands of devotees, wherein, under the favouring conditions adverted to, the choleraic germ is in-cubated; so have we when the pilgrims return homewards, radiating in every direction from a contaminated centre, the lethal products conveyed along our lines of road and deposited in village and district,

---

[39] Rosenberg, Cholera Years, pp. 72–81; John W. Cell, "Anglo-Indian Medical Theory and the Origins of Segregation in West Africa," AHR, 91:307–35 (1986), pp. 322–6.

[40] Erwin H. Ackerknecht, "Anticontagionism between 1821 and 1867," BHM, 22:562–93 (1984).

[41] Vincent and Collardot, Le choléra, pp. 125 ff, 195.

[42] AMSR, 7:375 (1863).

bazaar and encampments far and wide, rendering such routes unsafe for indefinite periods.[43]

His prescription was to avoid marching troops through known cholera zones, changing routes if necessary, and moving troops by train whenever possible.

These measures added up to something very close to those in standard use against yellow fever. When, in either case, the disease appeared in barracks, the men were moved under canvas. An infected post would be evacuated altogether for a time. Non-Western authorities took similar measures. In 1849–50, for example, when the cholera pandemic first reached Tunisia, the Bey of Tunis moved his residence under canvas to the garden of one of his ministers in Carthage, taking his guards with him.[44]

The cholera danger passed its peak after the 1850s. It never returned to the British West Indies. After the 1870s, it was no longer a serious problem in Europe and Algeria, mainly because pandemics leave behind a partly immune population. During the 1860s, the cholera death rate for European soldiers in India fluctuated from an extreme high of nearly 17 per thousand in 1861 to a little more than 1 per thousand in the best years. The disease was not controlled as well as might have been possible, but its deadliness was reduced. Its symptoms still attracted attention, but it was a declining threat.

Tuberculosis

In the 1860s, tuberculosis killed more soldiers in France and Britain than any other disease, but it was the most important single source of relocation "benefits" in the British West Indies, Algeria, Madras, and New Zealand (see Tables 1.7 and 4.2). In 1837–46, tuberculosis had accounted for half the deaths among British troops in Britain. In the 1860s, it still accounted for 38 percent of all deaths of British troops in Britain, and 22 percent of the death of French troops in France. By contrast, it accounted for only 7 percent of deaths in Madras, Algeria, and the Windward and Leeward Command in the 1840s.

From the 1850s, the tuberculosis death rate began to drop steeply in all five samples – most of all in Britain itself and the West Indies. This was the beginning of a slow decline of the disease in Europe in general. The reason for the decline remains obscure, in spite of the medical advances that have recently brought tuberculosis under control.[45] Nineteenth-century medical authorities sometimes com-

[43] AMSR, 7:376 (1863).
[44] Gallagher, *Tunisia*, pp. 44 ff.
[45] McGrew, *Encyclopedia of Medical History*, pp. 336–46; R. J. S. Simpson, "Tuberculosis in the British Army and its Prevention," JRAMC, 12:18–27 (1909).

mented on the decline of tuberculosis at home or abroad, but that was all. Good fortune was a nonproblem by definition; research went into problems that were serious or growing.[46]

Poisons, Deficiencies, and Mysteries

Various mysteries intrude on the otherwise explicable data for European mortality overseas up to the 1860s. For example, the tables for Madras in 1837–46, show a death rate of 4.5 per thousand from diseases of the liver – down only slightly from the 5.62 per thousand reported in 1827–38. "Hepatitis and abscess of the liver" was to remain a serious problem for several decades to come. The obvious possibilities in modern terms are hepatitis A and B, and other similar viruses not yet identified. Hepatitis A produces the common appearance of jaundice, but it rarely kills. Hepatitis B sometimes does, and it may be transmitted by sexual contact, insects, or water. Infected individuals can act as carriers for long periods of time, and the present incidence of carriers in the population is markedly higher in parts of Asia than it is in South and Central America or Europe. It can also lead to chronic liver disease and to cancer of the liver.[47] The "abscesses of the liver" reported from Madras, however, were far more acute. It seems likely that the vast majority of these deaths were not caused by a hepatitis virus at all, but were untreated amoebic dysentery.

Beriberi, caused by vitamin B_1 deficiency, became increasingly common in the second half of the nineteenth century. Under its Japanese name, Kaké, it is described as early as the second century, and the Dutch physicians on Java encountered it there in the eighteenth century. It first appears in British military mortality discussions in 1845, in an article by Balfour, who classified it as a form of "dropsy," and estimated that it accounted for 0.20 deaths per thousand among British troops on tropical duty. Brown rice normally contains B_1, but machine milling of rice and other grains became common in the nineteenth century. By the mid nineteenth century the disease was scattered through the tropical world.[48] It was more common in Asia than anywhere else, but prominent in nineteenth-century Brazil and among civilians in the Caribbean.

The disease takes two different forms among adults. Dry beriberi is marked principally by signs of degeneration of the nervous system. Wet beriberi, on the other hand, features cardiovascular functions. In the early nineteenth century most doctors would probably have classi-

---

[46] L. Laveran, "Algeria," DESM, p. 778–9; Martin, Manuel d'hygiène, pp. 163–71.

[47] A. J. Zuckerman, "Viral Hepatitis," in Strickland, Tropical Medicine, pp. 133–43.

[48] T. Graham Balfour, "Comparison of the Sickness, Mortality, and Prevailing Diseases among Seamen and Soldiers, as Shown by the Naval and Military Statistical Reports," JSSL, 8:77–86 (1845), p. 84; Hirsch, Handbook, 1:569–603.

fied it under dropsies, as Balfour did, but one symptom is also an
enlarged, tender liver.[49] Many medical authorities who dealt with the
disease toward the end of the century called it "neuritis" or a "disease
of the nervous system," stressing the symptoms of the dry variety.[50] It
is therefore unclear from the published statistics how serious it actually
was, since it could turn up under several different headings, and it
could occur in combination with other vitamin deficiency diseases,
especially scurvy.

The category "diseases of the brain" (or "diseases of the nervous
system" after 1837) is a problem category in its own right, with beriberi
as one possible cause. A high death rate from nervous disorders,
moreover, was found in both India and the West Indies – the West
Indian rate being five to six times that of the United Kingdom.[51]
Medical men at the time listed epilepsy, "sunstroke," and a large range
of nervous disorders as the most prominent causes of death under this
heading, sometimes including delirium tremens. One British doctor in
the Caribbean attributed four out of five deaths from diseases of the
nervous system to delirium tremens and estimated the direct and
indirect death rate from drink at 42 per thousand.[52]

Such a high figure is clearly impossible, but the problem remains.
Few of these diseases of the nervous system are fatal today among men
of military age. Heat stroke is rare, although it has a high case-fatality
rate when it does occur. Another possible explanation is cerebrospinal
meningitis, notoriously an epidemic disease of the military in Europe,
but its usual death rates are much lower than those listed for nervous
disorders in either India or the British West Indies. Heat stroke may
also have accounted for some of these deaths in India, and beriberi still
seems to be an insufficient explanation.

Lead poisoning had long been recognized and associated with lead
pipes in distilleries and cider crushing. As long ago as 1767, Sir George
Baker had published a paper indentifying lead as the cause of the
disease known in the British apple country as "Devonshire cholic."[53]

---

[49] McGrew, Encyclopedia of Medical History, p. 32; G. Thomas Strickland (ed.), Hunter's
Tropical Medicine, 6th ed. (Philadelphia, 1984), p. 850.
[50] Tatsusaburo Yabé, "Disparition du Kakké (Béribéri) dans la marine japonaise," Archives
de médecine navale, 73:58–1 (1900), p. 48; David E. Anderson, The Epidemics of Mauritius
(London, 1918), p. 222.
[51] Diseases of the brain or nervous system were reported as follows in deaths per
thousand (see appendix tables):

	1816–37	1837–46	1859–63
United Kingdom	0.7	0.59	0.69
British West Indies	3.7	3.88	2.11
Madras	1.7	2.6	1.59

[52] AMSR, 1:72 (1859).
[53] William Augustus Guy, Public Health, A Popular Introduction to Sanitary Science: Being a
History of the Prevalent and Fatal Diseases of the English Population from the Earliest Times to
the End of the Eighteenth Century, 2 vols. (London, 1870–4), 1:9–12.

Evidence of lead poisoning is found in the skeletal material of slave cemeteries of the Caribbean, but not in North America.[54] The principal, but not the sole explanation of this difference is the fact that lead piping was used in the West Indies to distill cheap grades of rum. Soldiers in the West Indies no doubt drank the same rum the slaves could afford.

Lead poisoning appears in contemporaneous records as "dry belly-ache," in the African as well as the American tropics.[55] In the French colonies it was listed as "colique." In 1850, Dutroulau called it one of the five principal illnesses in the French tropical empire, although it was not an important cause of death.[56] In Madras of 1827–38 under the East India Company, colic, identified as such, accounted for 7 percent of hospital entries by European troops, but only 0.16 percent of deaths.[57]

Although the danger of lead pipes was known in the eighteenth century, they were still common on ships with the shift to steam power after the 1830s. By midcentury, it had become a problem for the French Navy and on shore in Guyane and Sénégal, and French authorities warned against lead containers.[58] By the 1860s, British military medicine recognized that both cholic and paralysis could be produced by lead.[59] By the 1880s, most had come to believe that the dry colic of the tropics was in fact "lead-colic," its new name – although a few still claimed that it was another disease with the same symptoms and a different source.[60]

As medical authorities became aware of the nature and source of lead poisoning, lead dropped out of use in the West Indies, and "diseases of nervous system" dropped to British levels in the Lesser Antilles and Jamaica alike by the early 1880s – although remaining comparatively high in India. The best one can do with the evidence at hand is to attribute some part of the nervous and mental disorders in India to beriberi, and to assign part, perhaps a large part, of the same category in the West Indies to lead poisoning.

---

[54] Arthur C. Aufderheide, J. Lawrence Angel, Jennifer O. Kelley, Alain C. Outlaw, Merry O. Outlaw, George Rapp, Jr., and others, "Lead in Bone III. Prediction of Social Correlates from Skeletal Lead Content in Four Colonial American Populations ...," *American Journal of Physical Anthropology*, 66:353–61 (1985).

[55] Lind, *Hot Climates*, p. 59.

[56] Dutroulau, *Maladies des européens*, pp. 13, 16, 40–1, 58, 69, 77.

[57] "Report of a Committee ...," JSSL, 3:127 (1840).

[58] A. Chevalier, "Sur la nécessité de proscrire les vases de plomb ...," AHPML, 50:314–36 (1853); A. Laveran, *Maladies des armées*, pp. 96–9.

[59] Charles Alexander Gordon, *Army Hygiene* (London, 1866), p. 425.

[60] Hirsch, *Handbook*, 1:265–78.

CHAPTER 4

RELOCATION COSTS IN THE LATE NINETEENTH CENTURY

In the middle decades of the nineteenth century, military death rates in the tropical world dropped more rapidly in absolute terms than they would ever do again. Between 1837–46 and 1859–68, the annual average death rate in the Jamaica Command declined by 45 per thousand; in Algeria, by 61 per thousand; in India, by 31 per thousand.[1] These figures for India and Algeria may overstate the case somewhat, because they are based on a period of frequent warfare, on one hand, and a period of comparative peace, on the other; but even at half that figure, the proposition would still be true. Experience made these achievements possible. Medical authorities responded to empirical observation, even though the underlying general principle was barely suspected – if not completely misunderstood.

The half-century before the First World War was different. Empirical advances continued, but their consequences were statistically less impressive through the 1870s and 1880s. The annual decline in death rates over the midcentury had been in the range of 2.5 to 4.5 percent per year. The annual decline in death rates from the 1860s to the 1890s fell to 0.9 to 1.6 percent per year. Over the midcentury, the greatest gains in mortality occurred overseas, in the West Indies and Algeria. From the 1860s to the 1890s, the greatest gains were in Europe itself.

Then, in the 1880s, Western microbiologists discovered the germ theory of disease. As this knowledge spread, the scientific base of medical practice changed beyond recognition. By 1914, medicine rested on the same experimental base that persisted to the present.[2] Some of the early consequences are reflected in the mortality figures. Between the 1890s and 1909–13, the percentage decrease in mortality was higher than ever, in the range of 3.88 to 5.5 percent per year. And again, the greatest gains occurred overseas in India and Algeria. This chapter

[1] See Tables A.31–A.36. The Indian data for 1837–46 are the unweighted mean of annual average mortality for all three presidencies.
[2] For a convenient summary of the history of medicine through this period, see Robert P. Hudson, *Disease and Its Control: The Shaping of Modern Thought* (Westport, Conn., 1983), pp. 121–225.

deals with the quantitative weight of these changes – leaving most explanations to the two chapters still to come.

Changing Mortality Patterns

Statistical reporting on the health of the armies, resumed by Britain in 1859 and France in 1862, provides annual time-series of mortality by cause of death for France, Great Britain, Algeria, India, and the British West Indies over more than fifty years before 1914. The long series of mortality reports from the Dutch East Indies also continued, but without such extensive cause-of-death reporting.[3]

All of these records must be considered against a background of changing recruitment policies. In the period 1847–70, British enlistments were limited to ten or twelve years (depending on the branch of the service), but reenlistment was possible so that military service could last a total of twenty-four years. Then, after 1870, a new "short service" system replaced this "long service" regime. Enlistments still lasted about twelve years, but part of that time would be spent in the reserves – in effect a return to civilian life. Actual service with the colors tended to be about seven to nine years.

The French service drew on more men for shorter periods under a system of universal conscription. The state periodically called up all males by date of birth. Many were rejected for physical or other reasons, but the liability to serve remained. This meant that the French army tended to be slightly younger than the British. The actual age of British soldiers, however, was not as variable through time as the changing regulations might suggest. Between 1860 and 1905, the number per thousand under the age of thirty was never lower than 672 (in 1875), nor higher than 854 (in 1895). Most of the time, it lay in the range of about 725 to 825 per thousand.[4]

Health conditions overseas continued in the established pattern of extreme diversity (see Tables 1.1 and 1.2). Table 4.1 summarizes mean mortality levels for the five sample areas discussed in the earlier chapters – plus the Netherlands Indies – for the period from about 1860 to the First World War. Mortality rates fell steadily, but these averages and their standard deviations show some important regional differences. French soldiers in Algeria or British soldiers in the the West Indies died at about twice the rate of those who stayed at home. Those

---

[3] The annual series of reports of the Army Medical Service (later Department) cover, of course, a much greater range of British forces overseas, as reported in Tables 1.1 and 1.2. For present purposes, however, India and the West Indies are taken to be representative of their particular climatic zones.

[4] R. J. Simpson, "Tuberculosis in the British Army, and Its Prevention" JRAMC, 12:19–20 (1909).

Death by Migration

Table 4.1. *Mortality Levels of European Troops in Six Representative Regions,*
c.1860–1914

Country	Mean Mortality per Thousand	Standard Deviation
Great Britain, 1859–1914	6.01	2.52
France, 1862–1913	6.66	2.57
British West Indies, 1859–1914	12.32	9.52
Algeria, 1859–1913	21.61	7.51
British India, 1859–1914	17.20	8.67
Dutch East Indies, 1859–1914	39.15	30.94

Source: British Army Medical Service, *Reports*, Annual Series. Ministère de Guerre.
Statistique médicale de l'armée metropolitaine et de l'armée coloniale (annual series). For the
Dutch East Indies, *Kolonial Verslag* (annual series). For 1895–1900, *Geneeskundig Tidjschrift*
voor Nerlandische Indie (annual series). See appendix tables.

in India died at nearly three times the home rate, while those in the
Dutch East Indies died at six times the home rate.

The pattern of year-to-year variation reflected in the standard deviations was widely recognized by medical authorities. Variance of death
rates in the humid tropics – in Indonesia or the Caribbean – was
highest, followed by the rates in North Africa and India, and then
Europe itself. Epidemic cholera, yellow fever, and the incidence of
military campaigns account in part for this situation. Britain, France,
and the West Indies were generally at peace during this period.[5] The
heaviest campaigns in the conquest of India and Algeria had already
taken place in the first half of the century, although fighting continued
off and on. In southeast Asia, however, some of the most serious
fighting still remained, especially the Dutch campaigns for the conquest of Sumatra.

Figure 4.1 shows this annual movement of death rates on semilog
charts at two different scales. With the logarithmic scale of the vertical
axis, the angle of rise or fall in the series indicates percentage change
regardless of the absolute values. (For numerical equivalents see
appendix tables.) Each chart shows mortality changes in two of the
overseas territories compared with the mortality of European troops in
Britain. India and the Dutch East Indies show the expected spectacular
decline in death rates, but mortality in the Dutch East Indies began
higher than in British India before dropping to roughly the same level.
The Dutch East Indies rate was also more variable – high but fluctuating down to the mid 1870s, then dropping steeply over the quarter-
century 1875 to 1900. The death rate in British India was variable, with

[5] France was involved in the Franco-Prussian War, but wartime conditions prevented the
publication of medical statistics for those years and are not included in these samples.
Although the Anglo-Boer War was fought outside of Europe, it did influence the
British death rates, which included deaths of repatriated soldiers from South Africa.

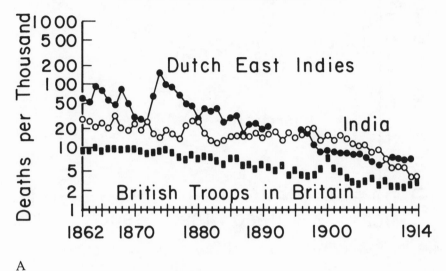

European Troop Mortality in India
and the Dutch East Indies, 1862–1914

A

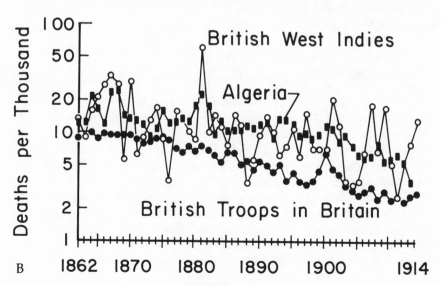

European Troop Mortality in Algeria
and the British West Indies, 1862–1914

B

Figure 4.1

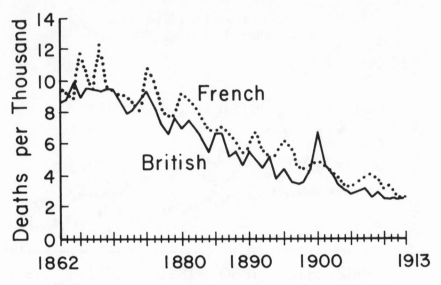

Figure 4.2. Mortality Rates of European Troops in Europe, 1862–1913

a slow decline to 1903, then falling more steeply down to 1910, and more steeply still in the immediate pre-war years.

In contrast, Algeria and the British West Indies were at nearly the same, more moderate, level, although the level in the West Indies varied more from year to year. Both had improved drastically over the midcentury decades. Further progress was only gradual until about 1900, when the Algerian death rate repeated the spectacular drop experienced in British India. After 1895–1904, the West Indian data lose their credibility. The only European force left in the British Caribbean was a reduced Jamaica Command – which was too small to be statistically viable. In 1905, an earthquake and fire in Kingston destroyed the building that housed the military records, and the reporting for the next few years was erratic and unreliable.

Figure 4.1 uses military mortality in Britain to represent Europe in general. Figure 4.2 shows that French and British death rates moved more or less together throughout this period, although the British rate was a little lower than the French. The striking exception is the British surge in death rates from 1899 to 1902, which coincided with the Anglo-Boer War – and was, in fact, a consequence of that war, as soldiers repatriated from the war zone died of disease contracted in the field. Neither the French nor the British showed more than a moderate decline in mortality down to about 1880, followed by a steeper fall over the next thirty-five years. On the French side, mortality rates dropped especially steeply between 1895 and 1904, and again between 1908 and 1913.

These trends and their association with particular diseases appear more clearly in Table 4.2, which shows changes in the annual average death rates by region and disease from the early 1860s to the decade centered on 1899. This was the period in which the sharpest mortality declines occurred in Britain and France, not overseas. The cause is clear, but its explanation is not. As of the 1860s, tuberculosis was the most important cause of death among men of military age in Europe, but then tuberculosis death rates dropped by about 2 percent per year in both countries. No one knows why. Otherwise, the mortality gains were distributed over several diseases, with a notable drop in gastro-intestinal deaths in France, but rather a slow improvement for pneumonia in both countries. The most significant victories over disease in these decades were won by Algeria and the West Indies against malaria, and by Algeria and France against the gastrointestinal group.

The deaths listed under the "mental and nervous" category remain unexplained, as in the earlier part of the century, when they had been overshadowed by more important causes of death. The great midcentury drop in other death rates gave them a new prominence everywhere, except in Algeria. From the 1860s, however, they led the general decline in death rates in Britain, India, and the West Indies.

Typhoid fever was a significant new factor. The British statistics of the 1860s still left it obscurely within the category "continued fevers," but in Algeria and France it rose from less than 10 percent of all causes of death in the 1840s (Table 1.8) to about 20 percent by the 1860s. By the 1890s, it had become the principal cause of death in India, France, and Algeria alike – and an important killer in Britain and the West Indies, although it was far less serious there than elsewhere. Nor was the new prominence a mere consequence of declining deaths from other causes; death rates per thousand also rose – more than threefold in India between the 1860s and the 1890s. This increase alone accounts for India's slow rate of mortality decline in this period.

Table 4.3 shows a pattern of remarkable change in the first fifteen years of the twentieth century.[6] Progress was now most marked over-

[6] The West Indian data are omitted from the table because of their unreliability and the small sample size, but they are as follows:

European Troops in the British West Indies

Disease	Percentage of all Deaths, 1895–1904	Deaths per Thousand 1895–1904	Deaths per Thousand, 1908–13	Percentage Change	Change per Year
Yellow fever	20.46	1.52	0.00	−100.00	−8.70
Malaria	19.94	1.48	1.52	2.70	0.24
Typhoid fever	11.79	0.88	1.03	17.05	1.48
Tuberculosis	9.62	0.71	0.52	−26.76	−2.33
Digestive system	8.68	0.64	0.52	−18.75	−1.63
Circulatory system	5.78	0.43	1.03	139.53	12.13
All disease	100.00	7.42	7.24	−2.43	−0.21

Table 4.2a. *Mortality by Cause of Death, 1860s to 1890s*

Disease	Percentage of all Deaths, 1859–67	Deaths per Thousand, 1860–7	Deaths per Thousand, 1895–1904	Percentage Change	Change per Year
British troops in the United Kingdom					
Tuberculosis	37.62	3.16	0.59	−81.33	−2.26
Respiratory	15.71	1.32	0.99	−25.00	−0.69
Circulatory	11.90	1.00	0.41	−59.00	−1.64
Nervous	8.57	0.72	0.26	−63.89	−1.77
Continued fevers[a]	5.00	0.42	0.21	−50.00	−1.39
All disease	100.00	8.40	3.52	−58.10	−1.61
British troops in Madras, India[b]					
Digestive	19.94	3.96	1.90	−52.02	−1.45
Dysentery	15.46	3.07	0.79	−74.27	−2.06
Cholera	13.90	2.76	0.55	−80.07	−2.22
Nervous system	7.75	1.54	0.33	−78.57	−2.18
Circulatory system	6.60	1.31	0.41	−68.70	−1.91
Continued fevers[a]	6.19	1.23	5.62	356.91	9.91
All disease	100.00	19.86	13.25	−33.28	−0.92
European troops in the British West Indies					
Yellow fever	21.63	3.43	1.52	−55.69	−1.53
Malaria	20.23	3.21	1.48	−53.89	−1.48
Nervous system[c]	10.99	1.74	0.14	−91.95	−2.52
Continued fever[a]	9.70	1.54	0.88	−42.86	−1.17
Circulatory system	7.89	1.25	0.43	−65.60	−1.80
Digestive system	6.26	0.99	0.50	−49.49	−1.36
All disease	100.00	15.87	7.42	−53.25	−1.46

seas – mortality improved more in Algeria than in France, and more in India than in Britain. The greatest single cause of improvement was the victory over typhoid fever – especially in the immediate pre-war years, so that the average for 1909–13 understates the achievement that took place between 1909 and 1913. The other notable improvement was the malaria death rate, which now fell more rapidly in India than it had done in the mid nineteenth century, when quinine was first introduced. In Algeria as well, malaria deaths declined almost as rapidly as they had done a half-century earlier – 3.22 percent per year in contrast to 3.69 over the mid nineteenth century (Table 1.8). (See Chapter 6 for some of the reasons why these changes took place.)

Trends in Relocation Costs

Figures 4.3 through 4.6 show the main lines of mortality change for three national armies – English, French, and Dutch – in four overseas regions – India, Netherlands Indies, the British West Indies, and Alger-

Table 4.2b. *Mortality by Cause of Death, 1860s to 1890s*

Disease	Percentage of all Deaths, 1862–6	Deaths per Thousand, 1862–6	Deaths per Thousand, 1892–6	Percentage Change	Change per Year
French troops in France					
Tuberculosis[d]	21.85	2.09	0.85	−59.33	−1.98
Typhoid fever	20.23	1.93	0.98	−49.22	−1.64
Digestive system	11.91	1.14	0.28	−75.44	−2.51
Pneumonia/pleurisy	12.18	1.02	0.80	−21.57	−0.72
Nervous system	4.19	0.40	0.21	−47.50	−1.58
All disease	100.00	9.56	4.31	−54.92	−1.83
French troops in Algeria					
Malaria	19.13	2.69	0.75	−72.12	−2.40
Digestive system	19.06	2.68	0.71	−73.51	−2.45
Typhoid fever	18.50	2.60	3.66	40.77	1.36
Tuberculosis[d]	10.81	1.51	0.86	−43.05	−1.43
Pneumonia/pleurisy	5.72	0.80	1.01	26.25	0.88
All disease	100.00	14.04	8.51	−39.39	−1.31

[a] Recorded as enteric fever in 1895–1904.
[b] From Madras Presidency only in 1859–67; from all of British India in 1895–1904.
[c] Includes totals listed under nervous and mental system and under cerebrospinal fever.
[d] For 1862–6, includes pthisis of the lung and bronchitis, then a common designation in France for chronic tuberculosis.
Source: Appendix tables.

ia. Each figure contain two charts. The first shows the annual mortality rates at home and abroad from 1860 to 1914. The second shows the annual relative relocation cost expressed as a percentage of home death rates, along with a trend line indicating the level and direction of change in relocation costs over the entire period. Part of the pattern is expected; death rates were higher abroad than they were at home, although both declined steeply during this half-century. Another part is less expected: although relocation costs fluctuated widely over time, the trend was mainly level or slightly rising.

In India, the relocation trend was virtually flat at nearly 200 percent over the period 1859–1914 (Figure 4.3). For the West Indies (Figure 4.5), it rose slightly, from a little less than 100 percent to a little more than 110 percent by 1898, the last year of the general West Indian Command. In Algeria it also rose (Figure 4.6) from a little more than 50 percent to a little more than 100 percent – although Algerian relocation costs started downward after about 1902. Only the Netherlands East Indies showed a long-term trend of declining relocation costs – and then only because the very high mortality rates of the 1860s and 1870s set such a high point of departure. A separate trend line for the period

Table 4.3a. *Mortality by Cause of Death, 1890s to 1909-13*

Disease	Percentage of all Deaths, 1895–1904	Deaths per Thousand, 1895–1904	Deaths per Thousand, 1908–13	Percentage Change	Change per Year
British troops in the United Kingdom					
Respiratory system[a]	28.13	0.99	0.06	−93.94	−8.17
Tuberculosis	16.76	0.59	0.25	−57.63	−5.01
Circulatory system	11.65	0.41	0.29	−29.27	−2.55
Digestive system[b]	9.09	0.32	0.28	−12.50	−1.09
Nervous system	7.39	0.26	0.17	−34.62	−3.01
Typhoid fever	5.97	0.21	0.06	−71.43	−6.21
All disease	100.00	3.52	1.95	−44.60	−3.88
British troops in India					
Typhoid fever	42.42	5.62	0.62	−88.97	−7.74
Digestive system[b]	20.30	2.69	1.01	−62.45	−5.43
Tuberculosis	5.81	0.77	0.24	−68.83	−5.99
Respiratory system	5.74	0.76	0.10	−86.84	−7.55
Malaria	4.68	0.62	0.18	−70.97	−6.17
Cholera	4.15	0.55	0.13	−76.36	−6.64
All disease	100.00	13.25	4.87	−63.25	−5.50

Table 4.3b. *Mortality by Cause of Death, 1890s to 1909-13*

Disease	Percentage of all Deaths, 1892–6	Deaths per Thousand, 1892–6	Deaths per Thousand, 1909–13	Percentage Change	Change per Year
French Troops in France					
Typhoid fever	22.80	0.98	0.27	−72.45	−4.26
Tuberculosis	19.78	0.85	0.76	−10.59	−0.62
Respiratory system	18.47	0.80	0.75	−6.25	−0.37
Influenza	7.05	0.30	0.04	−86.67	−5.10
Scarlet fever	6.59	0.28	0.14	−50.00	−2.94
Digestive system[b]	6.43	0.28	0.19	−32.14	−1.89
All disease	100.00	4.31	2.93	−32.02	−1.88
French troops in Algeria					
Typhoid fever	43.05	3.66	1.50	−59.02	−3.47
Respiratory system	11.84	1.01	0.77	−23.76	−1.40
Tuberculosis	10.14	0.86	0.73	−15.12	−0.89
Malaria	8.78	0.75	0.34	−54.67	−3.22
Digestive system[b]	8.29	0.71	0.50	−29.58	−1.74
All disease	100.00	8.51	4.81	−43.48	−2.56

[a] Includes listing for pneumonia and brocho-pneumonia when listed separately.
[b] Includes listing for dysentery plus diseases of the digestive system.
Source: Appendix tables.

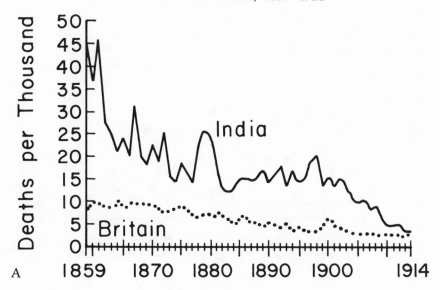

British Army Mortality per Thousand
in Britain and in India, 1859–1914

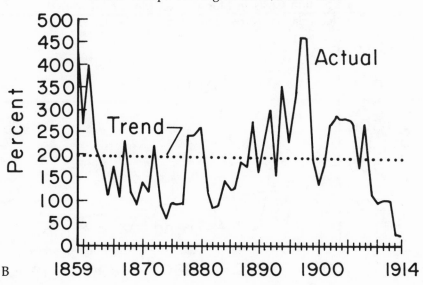

Relocation Costs in Mortality for
British Troops Serving in India, 1859–1914

Figure 4.3

Death by Migration

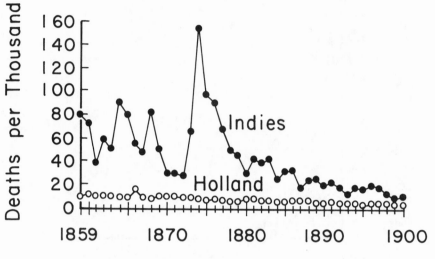

Dutch Military Mortality in the Netherlands
and the Netherlands East Indies, 1859–1900

A

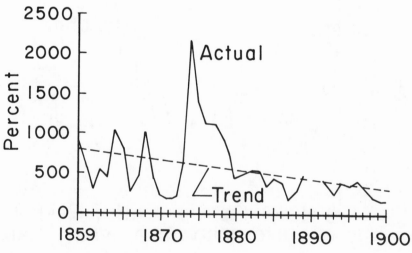

Relocation Costs in Mortality on Movement from
the Netherlands to the Netherlands Indies, 1859–1900

B

Figure 4.4

Mortality of British Troops Serving in
Britain and in the British West Indies, 1859–98

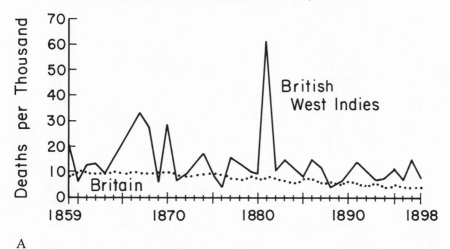

A

Relocation Cost in Mortality for British
Troops Serving in the West Indies, 1859–98

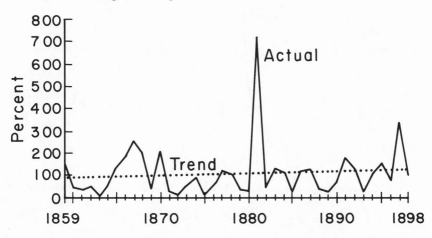

B   Figure 4.5

French Army Mortality in France
and in Algeria, 1863–1913

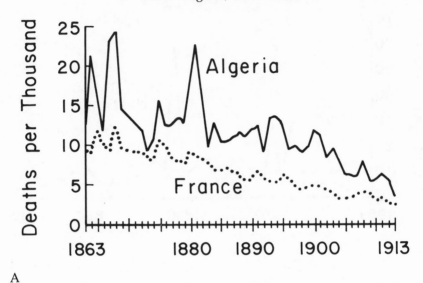

A

Relocation Costs in Deaths, French Army
in France and Algeria, 1863–1913

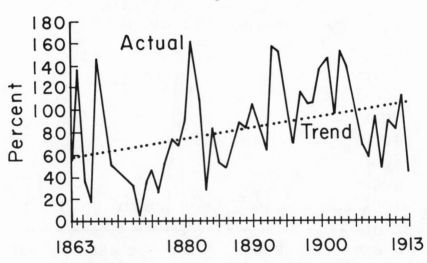

B   Figure 4.6

Table 4.4. *Representative Disease Profiles: France, Great Britain, India, Algeria, and the British West Indies*

Disease	Sample Periods from the 1860s				
	Great Britain, 1860–7	France, 1862–6	Algeria, 1862–6	Madras, 1860–3	British West Indies, 1859–63
Malaria	0.00	2.25	19.13	3.52	20.23
Yellow fever	0.00	0.00	0.00	0.00	21.63
Continued fevers	5.00	21.06	21.02	6.19	9.70
Cholera	0.00	5.49	3.59	13.00	0.00
Tuberculosis[a]	37.62	21.85	10.81	11.23	10.18
Nervous system	8.57	4.19	1.94	7.75	10.99
Circulatory system	11.90	2.36	1.62	6.60	7.89
Respiratory system	15.71	6.67	5.72	3.17	2.75
Digestive system	9.21	11.91	19.06	35.40	8.08
Other	11.99	24.22	17.11	13.14	8.55

	Sample Period 1909–13				
	Great Britain	France	Algeria	India	Jamaica
Cerebrospinal fever	0.51	2.38	0.97	0.00	7.18
Typhoid fever	3.08	9.08	31.12	16.40	14.23
Influenza	0.51	1.12	0.40	0.00	0.00
Malaria	0.00	0.00	7.16	4.67	20.99
Cholera	0.00	0.00	0.00	3.44	0.00
Pneumonia[c]	14.87	16.08	11.92	7.14	7.18
Tuberculosis[a]	12.82	23.82	12.63	6.35	7.18
Nervous system	8.21	4.08	3.14	5.03	0.00
Circulatory system	14.87	2.70	3.69	8.73	14.23
Respiratory system	6.15	6.19	4.22	2.65	0.00
Digestive system[b]	14.36	6.61	10.33	21.16	7.18
Other	24.62	27.94	14.42	24.43	21.83

[a] For France and Algeria, includes cases listed as bronchitis.
[b] Includes cases listed as dysentery.
[c] For France and Algeria, includes cases listed as brochopneumonia.
Source: Appendix tables of comparative mortality.

from 1880 onward (not illustrated) would approximate the flat trend of the other three examples.

Disease Profiles

Nineteenth-century Europeans wrote as though one set of diseases occurred in Europe, and another overseas, in the tropical world. That view was not entirely wrong; but disease profiles for men in the army could vary greatly even within Europe, while those overseas differed from place to place even more (Table 4.4; see also Tables 4.2 and 4.3).

In the 1860s, the French disease profile resembled the Algerian more than the British – although the Algerian death rates were, on the whole, markedly higher. The similarity of conditions on the two shores of the Mediterranean helps to explain that pattern, but the climatic similarity on the two shores of the English Channel had less effect. The French deaths from "continued fevers" (that is, mostly typhoid) were more than four times the British rate. The percentage of British deaths from tuberculosis were more than twice the French, and the pro-portional British deaths from "respiratory diseases" (mostly pneumonia) were nearly three times the French.

Differences among the three overseas territories are to be expected. Men died of malaria in Algeria and the Caribbean – but much less so in India. They died of yellow fever in the West Indies and nowhere else. They died far more often of cholera and gastrointestinal infections in Madras than anywhere else, and the death rates from tuberculosis everywhere overseas were less than half those in either European sample.

By the pre-war decade, many of these characteristics had changed radically. The five disease profiles now had more in common, partly because of improved medical knowledge, but also because diseases could travel along the routes of more intense intercommunication. The convergence of disease profiles was not an isolated phenomenon; it was part of a more general convergence within the European-controlled world – in matters as distant from epidemiology as chang-ing commodity prices or the mutual adaptation of cultures. But some disease patterns persisted. British soldiers in Britain, like French sol-diers in France and Algeria, still died of nearly the same combination of diseases. Malaria held approximately its earlier position in all three of the overseas territories. So, too, did diseases of the digestive system. The absolute drop in deaths caused by the worst killers, however, opened the way for cancer and heart disease ("diseases of the circula-tory system") to play a stronger role – for the first time among such a young age group.

Variation within Regions

The representative quality of the regions sampled is a problem in studies of this kind. As already mentioned, the data on the British West Indies for the twentieth century is highly questionable because of the small sample size and uncertain accuracy of the records them-selves. The same question must be raised about other regions. Broad generalizations such as "all troops stationed in France" or "European troops stationed in the Madras Presidency" merely suggest the sum of a range of subregions. If the disease patterns in these subregions are not sufficiently similar, we may find ourselves trying to add tamarinds

Table 4.5. *Distribution of Troops and Annual Average Death Rates Before 1860, Madras Presidency.*

	Size of Force	Percentage of Total Force	Annual Deaths per Thousand	Unweighted Regional Mean	Years of Observation
Seacoast					
Madras	919		28.93		16
St. Thomas Mount	248		12.09		1
Cannanore	1,128		31.65		17
Subtotal	2,295	21.65		24.22	
Tablelands					
Bangalore	424		24.39		17
Bellary	855		48.60		7
Secunderabad	3,059		56.78		8
Kamptee	915		47.72		7
Subtotal	5,253	49.56		44.37	
Hill					
Jackatalla	964	9.10	20.74	20.74	1
Burma					
Rangoon	1,174				
Tonghoo	913				
Subtotal	2,087	19.69	33.00	33.00	9
Total	10,599	100.00			

Note: Unweighted mean ≡ 33.77; standard deviation ≡ 14.58.
Source: AMSR, 2:125 (1860).

and mangoes. In that case, the individual subregions, not the larger aggregate, would be the proper focus for study.

This problem is not especially serious in the records of the United Kingdom or France, although regional differences existed in both. It becomes more serious in a place like India, which was about the same size as all of Western Europe and had far greater variety in its climate and physical environment. Madras Presidency was the sample chosen, rather than the entire subcontinent, for exactly that reason. Yet the Presidency was an extremely various place. It was smaller than all of India, but it was still large. From Cape Camorin to the northern tip of Burma is nearly 2,000 miles, and the range of latitude from about 8 North to 28 North is roughly equivalent to the difference between Algiers and Copenhagen, or Miami and Montreal.

Table 4.5 presents a geographical summary of the principal disease environments within the presidency during the two decades before 1860 – as the medical authorities at that time perceived them. Variance in death rates is considerable; the unweighted mean death rate was

Table 4.6. *Distribution of Troops and Death Rates, 1884–93, Madras Presidency*

	Size of Force	Percentage of Total Force	Deaths per Thousand	Unweighted Regional Mean
Seacoast				
Madras District	578		16.71	
St. Thomas Mount	326		11.82	
Cannanore	105		8.14	
Calicut	109		12.56	
Malapuram	145		13.25	
Subtotal	1,263	9.57		12.50
Tablelands				
Bangalore	2,114		7.35	
Bellary	661		8.61	
Belgaum	1,178		5.12	
Secunderabad	2,931		12.90	
Subtotal	6,884	52.17		7.03
Hill				
Wellington	1,110	8.41	10.06	10.06
Burma				
Rangoon District	2,029		14.87	
Mandalay District	1,910		20.81	
Subtotal	3,939	29.85		17.84
Total	13,196	100.00		

Note: Unweighted mean ≡ 11.85; standard deviation ≡ 4.36
Source: AMSR, 27:241 (1894). Stations of less than 100 men omitted.

33.77 per thousand, with a standard deviation of 14.58. On the other hand, the approximate distribution of troops within the presidency was remarkably constant from midcentury to the 1890s and beyond (see Table 4.6). Half of the Madras Army was kept in the tablelands of Mysore and Hyderabad, where the death rates were highest. Death rates were markedly lower at the hill station and on the coast (both along the Arabian Sea and the Bay of Bengal), and they were markedly lower in Burma. (This was to change later in the century when the British marched north into Upper Burma, but even then the Burma detachments were not usually a large part of the total force.) The aggregate, therefore, can be taken to stand for an approximately constant mixture of disease environments in south India and Burma during the second half of the nineteenth century – not perfect, but a useful basis for calculating relocation costs. It would not be a suitable basis for discussing epidemiological correlations between particular diseases and geographical or meteorological factors like heat, altitude, and rainfall.

By 1884–93 (Table 4.6), the size of the British force had increased by about 30 percent, and its distribution had shifted slightly. The table-lands and the hill station remained at the same levels. Numbers on the seacoast decreased by half, while those in Burma had doubled – following the conquest of Upper Burma. Mortality rates improved everywhere, but far more in the tablelands than anywhere else, and the differences in mortality among stations declined sharply. The Madras data can only be used up to 1895, when the presidency armies were abolished and aggregate data were reported only for the entire British army in India, although military subdivisions and certain posts can still be followed in detail.

Neither the British West Indies nor Algeria could compare with Madras, in sheer size and diversity, but some internal differences are noteworthy. The three provinces of Algeria – Constantine, Algiers, and Oran – were roughly the same size. Each contained a similar mixture of coastal plain, mountains, and transmontane desert. Health and mortality varied, however, from one to the other owing to the irregular incidence of military campaigns or epidemic disease.[7] The French army published more disaggregated records – region by region, even post by post – than the British did but if all of Algeria is used as a sample, the resulting set of time-series data is more consistent than those of any single province.

In the early nineteenth-century Caribbean, relative healthfulness had often alternated between the Windward and Leeward Command and the Jamaica Command. The British medical authorities were concerned about these differences. Between 1859 and 1863, for example, the annual average mortality of European troops in Jamaica was 19.64 per thousand, in contrast to 11.72 for the Windward and Leeward Command.[8] That difference was all the more disturbing because it followed the triumph of the 1840s, when the move to Newcastle barracks had reduced the death rate by half. After the 1870s, when the two West India commands were amalgamated, health conditions still differed between the two divisions of the united command, although neither was clearly better or worse off until the 1890s. Then, over the period 1891–95, Barbados was less healthy than Jamaica by some measures, but not by others. Jamaica had the higher mortality rate, but Barbados had more hospital admissions, more troops invalided, and more per thousand constantly sick. Barbados's total of dead plus in-

---

[7] At an early stage in this study, I tried having a single province, Algiers, stand for the range of conditions in all three. The experiment, however, yielded a number of erratic time series, which smoothed out when the three province were aggregated. The aggregation also produced a more satisfactory sample size, which consisted of as many as 35,000 as late as 1913.

[8] AMSR, 14:78–9 (1873)

valided on account of disease yielded a D + I index of 35.66 per thousand, compared to 24.08 per thousand for Jamaica.[9]

During 1895–1904, the last decade that Barbados had its separate military units, the balance shifted a little in the other direction. Jamaica now lost more men than Barbados (this time from typhoid and yellow fever), while Barbados, formerly reputed to be malaria-free, lost twice as many men from malaria as Jamaica did. The D + I index was 31.8 for Barbados and 36.65 for Jamaica (see Table A.15). In short, differences existed between the two commands, but they were not consistent over time; consequently, the aggregate of both is used whenever possible, if only to have a larger sample size.

Variation by Rank and Gender

Records for enlisted men form the principal data base for this study, for several reasons. Enlisted soldiers ("other ranks" in British terminology of the period) were more numerous; they served under uniform regulations; and statistical reporting about their health was more detailed than it was for their officers. It is important, however, to glance at health conditions of officers and women, if only to remove the possibility that enlisted men were somehow exceptional.

Only India provides an adequate sample of either officers or women. French military data did not take in women, although European women in Algeria were included in the ordinary civilian censuses. In the Caribbean, female dependents and officers alike were too few to produce reliable statistics, but a survey of 1865 suggested that differences between soldiers and their dependents were small.[10] The British force in India, however, was large enough to provide useful comparative information about both groups. Table 4.7, which summarizes Table A.50, gives annual admissions and deaths per thousand for female dependents, officers, and enlisted men in India from 1899 to 1913.

The differences were not very significant. Women turned themselves in at the hospital less frequently than men did, but they were free to remain home from work without being officially ill – which men were not. Officers were admitted less often than either women or enlisted men, perhaps for similar reasons. Women's death rates, however, were higher than men's, both in 1899–1908 and again in 1909–13. The most obvious explanation is that man had to pass a physical examination to enlist, whereas their dependents did not. Officers' death rates were also slightly higher than those of enlisted men, but the officer – enlisted man comparison becomes more complicated if invaliding is also taken into account.

[9] See the Appendix for an explanation of D + I indices. AMSR, annual series, reports for 1891 through 1895. See also Table A.15.

[10] "On the Sickness and Mortality among Soldiers' Wives," AMSR for 1865, pp. 155–65.

Table 4.7. *Admissions and Deaths of Female Dependents, Officers, and Other Ranks, 1899–1913, India*

Annual Average	Admissions per Hundred Thousand			Deaths per Thousand		
	Female Dependents	Officers	Other Ranks	Female Dependents	Officers	Other Ranks
1899–1908	7.22	7.51	9.70	12.97	11.97	11.63
1909–13	5.27	5.84	5.89	7.34	6.27	4.74

Source: AMSR, 49:103–4 (1908); 55:57 (1913).

Table 4.8 shows some of these relationships. Just after 1900, officers' hospital admissions were 25 percent less than those of enlisted men, although this difference virtually disappeared on the eve of the First World War. At the same time, officers' death rates, roughly equal to those of enlisted men at the beginning of the century, rose to be a third higher on the eve of the war. Medical authorities were greatly concerned, especially about typhoid fever, which was far more serious among officers than among other ranks. They found no good explanation, aside from the obvious fact that enlisted men were under far stricter control outside working hours. In any case, typhoid inoculation soon eliminated the problem (see Chapter 6). Not only were officers' death rates higher, their invaliding rates were higher still – roughly double those of other ranks – with the result that the D + I index for officers was 60 to 100 percent higher than it was for the enlisted ranks. This difference may reflect the officers' right to ask for repatriation in case of illness; or it may reflect the fact that just before the war medical authorities were trying to reduce the number of enlisted men being repatriated by sending them to convalescent centers in the Indian hills instead.

Relocation Costs and Disease

The total relocation cost in mortality was a balance between costs and benefits. Table 4.9 (pp. 102–3) summarizes costs and benefits for each major disease or disease group, measured by its contribution (either negative or positive) to the total relocation cost for each decade after the 1860s, and for each overseas sample area.

Certain general patterns stand out. In the 1860s through the 1880s, the cost in mortality from tropical diseases like malaria and yellow fever was high. These diseases were then so rare in Europe, if they existed at all, that soldiers had little or no acquired immunity. Their

Table 4.8. Death Rates and Invaliding of Officers and Other Ranks, 1900–13, India

Annual Average	Admissions, Rates per Hundred Thousand		Deaths, Rates per Thousand		Invalided, Rates per Thousand		D + I, Rates per Thousand	
	Officers	Other Ranks	Officers	Other Ranks	Officers	Other Ranks	Officers	Other Ranks
1900–4	8.08	10.52	12.78	13.05	65.91	35.04	78.69	48.09
Percent differential for officers	−23.16		−2.10		88.13		63.64	
1905–8	6.75	8.24	10.55	9.44	53.29	22.68	63.84	32.12
Percent differential for officers	−18.17		11.76		135.00		98.78	
1909–13	5.87	5.89	6.27	4.74	16.53	7.61	22.80	12.35
Percent differential for officers	−0.31		32.39		117.24		83.69	

Source: AMSR, 51:89 (1909); 55:56 (1913).

incidence diminished through time, however, with the more systematic use of quinine against malaria and mosquito control against yellow fever in the American tropics. In the pre-war years, these diseases not only killed fewer men per thousand, they also accounted for a smaller part of the total relocation cost.

A second group of diseases was endemic to Europe and the tropics alike. The most serious were the waterborne diseases – cholera, typhoid fever, and the dysenteries taken together. They were the most important single source of relocation costs for India, and for Algeria in most decades. They had been equally serious in the West Indies during the first half of the century, but were no longer so in the 1860s or later.

The third group of diseases were the benefits category – they were known both in Europe and overseas but were more often fatal in Europe. Tuberculosis and respiratory diseases, especially pneumonia, were outstanding in this respect in all three territories, but especially in the West Indies. With the passage of time, however, the benefits of relocation declined. In the West Indies of the 1870s, the sum of the benefits from individual diseases totaled 121 percent, which meant that the sum of the costs from individual diseases necessarily came to 221 percent. By 1909–13, the costs and benefits had both declined sharply, and benefits were negligible – as, indeed, they had been in the West Indies in the first half of the nineteenth century. In Madras, the benefit category was never that large, but it reached 42 percent in the 1880s; and it, too, became insignificant by 1909–13.

These three categories of disease appeared in different combinations in the three overseas territories. In Algeria, typhoid rose to account for 65 percent of relocation cost by 1909–13. Malaria, on the other hand, declined from 55 percent of relocation cost to only 18 percent. The role of the gastrointestinal group also fell by half over this period. For Algeria, unlike the other two cases, the role of "benefit" diseases was never significant.

In India, the pattern of diseases contributing to relocation costs was relatively constant from one decade to the next. Diseases of the digestive track were the leading cost in the first half of the period, and they remained important even afer they were overtaken by typhoid fever from the 1890s onward. The cost of malaria was less here than in the Caribbean or Algeria, and it was relatively constant over time. Cholera played a fluctuating role, as yellow fever did in the West Indies.

This broad pattern of shifting relocation costs began as a fact of nature. It was only slightly influenced by human interventions, either positive or negative. By the early twentieth century, however, human intervention had become the main determinant. That intervention was made possible by a revolution over these decades in European understanding of hygiene and tropical medicine.

Table 4.9. *Contribution to Relocation Costs in Death, by Disease, 1860s to 1910s*

	1860s	1870s	1880s	1890s	1900s	1909–13	Average All Columns
France/Algeria							
Malaria	55	63	60	18	19	18	39
Tuberculosis	–12	9	–8	0	0	–2	–2
Typhoid	15	3	0	64	71	65	36
Digestive diseases	34	20	31	10	5	16	19
Respiratory diseases	3	–2	–13	5	3	8	1
Other	5	7	30	3	3	–6	7
Total	100	100	100	100	100	100	100
	1859–67	1869–77	1879–84	1886–94	1895–1904	1909–13	
Britain–West Indies							
Malaria	43	42	25	26	37	29	34
Yellow fever	46	95	68	19	39	0	44
Tuberculosis	–21	–34	–10	–20	3	5	–13
Typhoid	15	61	10	70	17	18	32
Venereal disease	–1	–9	0	4	n.a.	10	1
Nervous system	14	17	1	1	–3	–3	5
Digestive system	6	6	9	–2	5	7	5
Respiratory system	–12	–45	–1	–18	–18	2	–15
Circulatory system	–3	–18	1	2	0	14	–1
Other	14	–15	–2	17	19	19	8
Total	100	100	100	100	100	100	100

Britain – Madras (through 1880s); India (1890s onward)

	1860–67	1869–77	1879–84	1886–94	1895–1904	1909–13
Malaria	6	4	5	8	6	10
Tuberculosis	-8	-9	-24	-1	2	-1
Cholera	24	16	22	11	6	7
Typhoid	7	13	27	54	56	31
Kala Azar						7
Venereal Disease	2	0	1	1	n.a.	2
Nervous system	7	14	17	0	1	1
Circulatory system	3	5	0	0	3	2
Digestive system	55	62	55	24	24	40
Respiratory system	-6	-8	-18	-4	-2	-2
Other	10	4	14	8	5	3
Total	100	100	100	100	100	100

Note: n.a. = not available. Typhoid listing for the 1860s and 1870s includes other "continued fevers". Pneumonia, where listed separately, is combined with "respiratory diseases." Dysentery and diarrhea are combined with "diseases of the digestive system."

CHAPTER 5

THE REVOLUTION IN HYGIENE AND TROPICAL MEDICINE

The climate of a country has a most important influence on the health and character of its inhabitants. It therefore requires careful study by those who, having previously lived in temperate zones, are suddenly transferred to a tropical country: and whose very change of environment necessitates a perfect knowledge of many rules and precautions, if they desire to maintain a standard of health at all commensurate with what they naturally expect to enjoy at home: as well as to ward off those diseases, the result of deteriorations of the functions of the body, which are the effect produced by long residence in tropical countries.

J. Lane Notter, "Hygiene in the Tropics"[1]

From the 1870s to the 1890s, military medicine, tropical medicine, and tropical hygiene experienced a revolutionary change. At core of the revolution was the germ theory of Robert Koch, Louis Pasteur, and other microbiologists, but the theory itself grew out of a new attitude toward experimentation – toward the systematic collection and dissemination of knowledge.

The growing body of knowledge led to a stream of manuals giving practical advice, each appearing in new editions every few years. For India, the base was James Johnson's, *Influences of Tropical Climates on European Constitutions* (1813). James Ranald Martin joined as coauthor in 1841, then as sole author of the revised edition in 1859, and still another in 1861.[2] William James Moore's *Manual of the Diseases of India* began a new series in 1861. New authors and new editions appeared in 1886, 1889, 1893, 1903, some with a subvention from the government of India. Successive editions in this case shifted emphasis from public to private hygiene – telling civilian expatriates how to protect their own lives.

For professionals, tropical hygiene took a different direction. In 1875,

---

[1] In Andrew Davidson (ed.), *Hygiene & Diseases of Warm Climates* (London, 1893), p. 25.
[2] James Ranald Martin, *The Influence of Tropical Climates in Producing the Acute Endemic Diseases of Europeans*, 2d ed. (London, 1861).

Henry King published *The Madras Manual of Hygiene*, covering the whole range of possible public action to protect the health of Europeans in the Madras Presidency. By 1894, William Ewing Grant had become the principal author and, with a bow to King's earlier contribution, turned it into *The Indian Manual of Hygiene*, a far larger, more detailed, and more authoritative work. It covered a range of information useful for tropical life – from domestic architecture, to ventilation, nutrition, and the design of a modern sewerage system. In all of these matters, its authors were fully aware of the best practices of sanitary engineering and public hygiene in Europe. The two editions – 1875 and 1894 – neatly span the crucial two decades in which the germ theory was first put forward and then accepted.

At the end of the century a new generation of influential publications began to appear, set still more firmly in the new theories of tropical medicine. Patrick Manson's manual of tropical disease first appeared in 1898 and reached five editions by 1914.[3] After the war still more editions appeared, with Philip Heinrich Manson-Bahr as the principal collaborator. Manson's work was essentially a manual for clinicians dealing with individual cases. Its counterpart for public health was W. J. R. Simpson's *Principles of Hygiene as Applied to Tropical and Sub-Tropical Climates*.[4] Simpson was Professor at King's College, London, and the work was based on his lectures at the London School of Tropical Medicine. Perhaps more significant was the fact that a school of tropical medicine now existed. There were, in fact, two in Britain, the other being at Liverpool.

Another succession of volumes was specifically concerned with military hygiene, which in Britain was nearly synonymous with tropical hygiene. Beginning in 1861, E. A. Parkes, a former medical officer in India became professor of hygiene at the Army Medical School and began a "Review of the Progress of Hygiene," as a feature of the army's annual statistical volume.[5] Each year's article noted important publications on military medicine in principal European languages and summarized new developments in hygiene. The series appeared almost every year down to 1907 and continued thereafter in the *Journal of the Royal Army Medical Corps*. Parkes also published a small manual of hygiene, taken over in 1896 and revised and enlarged by two of his successors, J. Lane Notter and R. H. Firth. It went on to become the standard work on military hygiene, passing through five more editions before 1905.[6]

---

[3] Patrick Manson, *Tropical Diseases: A Manual of the Diseases of Warm Climates* (London, 1898).

[4] (London, 1908).

[5] AMSR, 2:343–67 (1860).

[6] J. Lane Notter, and R. H. Firth, *The Theory and Practice of Hygiene*, 6th ed. (London, 1905).

French specialists published a parallel line of manuals, with a slightly different institutional base, since the French marine infantry did most of France's truly tropical fighting on land. Jean Baptiste Fosnagrive's *Traité d'hygiène navale*[7] covered preventive medicine at sea and on shore in the tropics. Alphonse Laveran published a number of manuals on military medicine, of which *Traité des maladies et épidémies des armées*[8] became a standard work based on experience in Algeria.

Besides specialized tropical manuals there was an explosion of hygienic works based on experience in Europe itself. In France, Jules Arnould's *Nouveaux élements d'hygiène* of 1881 already recognized the importance of microorganisms. By the third edition in 1895, it too had taken on new authors and expanded to more than 1,300 pages.[9]

The equivalent publication in Britain was Stevenson and Murphy's *Treatise on Hygiene and Public Health*. Its third edition, of 1894, consisted of three large volumes.[10] The first two contained twenty-five chapters by a variety of authorities and included 130 pages on meteorology and others on ventilation, water, food, meat inspection, baths, hospital hygiene, vital statistics, and the disposal of the dead. The third volume was a compendium of the substantial body of law and administrative regulation already in force in Britain.

By this time the subject matter of hygiene had so expanded that it contained the rudiments of what were soon to become separate disciplines – meteorology, for example, and sanitary engineering. At the same time, the clinical side of tropical medicine, which had been a large part of midcentury compendia, dropped out. Hygiene had become public health, and was no longer seriously concerned with the treatment of disease.

During the second half of the century, a variety of periodical publications became available to keep military physicians abreast of the latest developments in tropical and military medicine. Alongside the annual *Reports* of the British Army Medical Department, the French army had the *Receuil de mémoires de médecine militaire*, the principal medical publication for army doctors in France and Algeria since the early 1800s. In 1888, it was succeeded by the *Archives de médecine et de pharmacie militaire*. A parallel publication, *Archives de médecine navale*, served both naval surgeons and the doctors of the *infantrie de la marine*. It was later supplemented by the *Annales de médecine et de pharmacie coloniales*. Another periodical that appeared from 1903 onward was the *Journal of the Royal Army Medical Corps*, which had a strong interest in India's

[7] 2d ed. (Paris, 1877).
[8] (Paris, 1875).
[9] Jules Arnould, E. Arnould, and H. Surmont, *Nouveaux éléments d'hygiène*, 3d ed. (Paris, 1895).
[10] Thomas Stevenson and Shirley F. Murphy, *A Treatise on Hygiene and Public Health*, 3 vols. (London, 1892–4). (Originally published 1890–2)

medical practice. Both India and Algeria, for that matter, were served by a variety of medical journals for civilian and military doctors alike. By the 1860s, an international network existed by which any hygienic discovery or development rapidly became common knowledge within the broader fraternity of military medical men in the tropical world. More important still, by the 1890s the medical attitudes these publications formed and reinforced were closer to present-day medicine than they were to the traditional styles of medical thought still dominant in midcentury.

Hygienic Rules for Tropical Life

Meanwhile, parallel to the new growth of scientific knowledge, the old prescriptions for life in the tropics continued in force. They were individual and moral as much as medical. At base, they were the commonplace rules for good health at home – adjusted for increased rigor in the tropics. These rules urged moderation in all things, but more moderation than life in Europe required. Soldiers should have only light exercise, but they should be kept busy. Food should be light and taken in moderation, several small meals being better than a few large ones. Meat and poultry were to be avoided, as were local fruits. Clothing was to be light and loose-fitting, and preferably made of cotton but insulation against heat or cold was also important, especially at night and especially around the waist. A flannel wrapping or waist band was usually recommended.[11]

The proper liquid balance was also important. Even as the germ theory was gaining acceptance, humoral concepts still produced some echoes. In 1888, Georges Treille explained that the danger of tropical climates was water vapor in the air, not heat. Water vapor lowers the pressure of dry air and causes insufficient oxygen to be supplied to the blood. The lungs work less energetically, and evaporation from the skin decreases. The body retains heat and develops a tendency toward "pathological hyperthermia." All of this encourages the newcomer to seek an immoderate intake of liquids, which in turn cause liver malfunctions and a general lack of muscular energy.[12]

---

[11] Jean Pierre Ferdinand Thévenot, Traité des maladies des Européens dans les pays chauds, et spécialement au Sénégal, ou essai statistique, médicale et hygiènique sur le sol, le climat et les maladies de cette partie de l'Afrique (Paris, 1810), pp. 256–86; Alexandre M. Kermorgant and Gustave Reynaud, "Précautions hygiènique à prendre pour les expéditions et les explorations aux pays chauds," AHMC 3:346–56 (1900); M. Bonnafy, "Statistique Médicale de la Cochinchine (1861–88)," AMN, 67:182–3 (1897); Louis Joseph Garnier, Souvenirs médicaux du poste de Sédiou (Bordeaux, Thesis no. 43, 1888), pp. 83–7; W. Taylor, "Report of the Medical Transactions of the Ashanti Expeditionary Force during the Period from 14th December 1895 to 7th February 1896," AMSR, 38:305 (1896); Notter, Hygiene of the Tropics, pp. 25–32.

[12] Gustave A. Reyaud, L'armée coloniale au point de vue de l'hygiène pratique (Paris, 1892), p. 67; Georges Félix Treille, De l'acclimatation des européens dans les pays chauds (Paris, 1888), pp. 21–41, 64–7.

The usual recommendation was to drink as little as possible. As another authority explained it, drink brings on thirst, because it provokes perspiration. Perspiration is a debilitating loss of water, requiring still more drink, in a vicious circle. In the tropics one simply has to learn to put up with thirst just as one has to put up with heat. Many believed that trying to keep cool might lead to dangerous cooling of the stomach region and thus bring on hepatitis and fever. Cold was, indeed, the direct cause of dysentery.[13]

Léon Colin's association of malarial fevers and particular soils also lived on.[14] As late as 1903, when the mosquito vector for malaria was widely accepted, Gustave Reynaud, an important hygienist, still held that the real causes of malaria were *agents telluriques* arising from the soil. If climate alone were to blame, he argued, tropical climates in Tahiti and New Caledonia would be disastrous to the European constitution, which they were not. Although these climates were nearly identical with those of recognized danger, the soils were different. The difference must therefore be the cause of fevers. (In fact, islands in that part of the Pacific were and are malaria-free, because they have no anopheline mosquitos.)

Fear of upturning the soil therefore persisted. All work of that kind was best left to "natives," who were resistant to earth poisons. By 1903, dysentery, malaria, hepatitis, yellow fever, and cholera were all known to be caused by microorganisms, but Reynaud could still point out that these microbes themselves came from the soil and were closely related to its wealth of organic material.[15]

Fear of the native inhabitants was still another hygienic concern reinforced in the second half of the nineteenth century. Early in the century, European death rates were so much higher than those of the "natives" it was hard to blame them as a source of infection. The usual explanation was the claim they had some inborn source of immunity. By the 1870s, however, European health in the tropics had improved so much that death rates of Indian and European troops were nearly equal. It then became possible to switch sides and to blame "native filth and disease' for European illness. The bazaars were especially suspect, partly for contaminated food and water, partly for prostitution and the danger of venereal disease.[16] By the early twentieth century, an added fear was that food might be contaminated by "native

[13] Adolphe C. A. M. Nicholas, (ed.), *Manuel d'hygiène coloniale. Rédigé par une commission de la société* (Paris, 1894), pp. 63–4, 227–8.

[14] Adolphe C. A. M. Nicolas, *Hygiène industrielle et coloniale. Chantiers et terrassements en pays palundéen* (Paris, 1889).

[15] Jean Christan Marc François Boudin, *Traité de géographie et de statistique médicale et des maladies endémiques*, 2 vols. (Paris, 1857), pp. 65–85; Alphonse Laveran, *Paludism* (London, 1893), p. 135; Gustave A. Reynaud, *Hygiène coloniale*, 2 vols. (Paris, 1903), 1:9–15; Nicholas, *Manuel d'hygiène coloniale*, 51.

[16] AMSR, 32:165 (1891); AMSR, 29:149 (1893).

cooks".[17] In tropical Africa from the 1890s onward, sanitary segregation of European quarters from the "native town" became a major theme in town planning, and the idea spread.[18] No less an authority than Prof. W. J. R. Simpson of King's College noted in 1903 that pure water was hard to come by in the tropics "mainly due to the pollutions to which the water is subjected by the customs of the people."[19] Gustave Reynaud promoted the idea of sanitary segregation for the French colonies as well: "The ordinary filth of native villages, the contagious illness to which the natives are prey, and the frequency of malaria among the indigenous children who are a source of contagion demand that the European hold himself away from these unhealthy agglomerations. European quarters should be constructed at a distance upwind from industrial sites as well."[20]

Seasoning

These rules for tropical behavior and tropical hygiene were closely related to the idea that humans had to be acclimatized to tropical life through seasoning. By the 1870s, opinions were divided on this question, but many authorities came to believe that service in truly dangerous "climates" should be as short as possible. During the Anglo-Asante War of 1873–4, for example, the main British force had been kept on board ship until the moment of attack, had advanced successfully, and was then evacuated after only two months in Africa. French policy was similar for places like Mayotte or Madagascar, where malaria was a serious threat and the garrison was relieved each year. Alfonse Laveran believed that troops fresh from France could survive and fight better than the veterans of the Algerian climate, who tended to be more prone to dysentery with each passing year.[21]

J. Lane Notter also argued that true acclimatization is not possible. Soldiers might appear acclimatized because they had accustomed themselves to the local environment, but the seasoning was illusory; they were actually weakened in ways that would only emerge when they again moved to another environment. Acclimatization was thus only a statistical artifact; seasoned troops appeared to suffer less than the newly arrived, but only because the weakest were already weeded out by death, hospitalization, or invaliding. In military life, Notter argued, morbidity and mortality increase with age:

[17] AMSR, 46:245–8 (1902).
[18] Philip D. Curtin, "Medical Knowledge and Urban Planning in Tropical Africa," AHR, 90:594–613 (1985).
[19] W. J. Simpson, "Water Supplies," JTM, 6:132–8, 1723–74, 192–4 (1903).
[20] Reynaud, Hygiène coloniale, 1:171.
[21] Alphonse Laveran, Traité des maladies et épidémies des armées (Paris, 1875)1:145, 771.

The soldier ages much more rapidly than his fellow countrymen in civil life; the old soldier suffers from diseases of deterioration induced by climate, by night duties and fatigues, and to a large extent from his indifference in regard to his own health, and the latitude he takes in alcohol and sexual excess. A very large number contract syphilis, for which they are invalided; or, if they are permitted to serve on, they do so with an enfeebled constitution.[22]

Attempts to "season" troops were nevertheless recurrent in European military policy. For a time, the Spanish government used the Canary Islands as a tropical stepping-stone, where troops might pass a year of gentle seasoning before moving on to the Philippines or the Caribbean.[23] The French used Réunion as a similar stopover for troops bound for Madagascar. A French army doctor in Senegal made a somewhat different proposal. He suggested keeping newcomers on the coast at Saint Louis or Dakar for six months. At the end of that time, those who had resisted tropical infection would be chosen as most probable to survive expeditions into the more deadly interior.[24]

In India, the idea of a seasoning experience also had its following, despite the occasional evidence to the contrary. In 1889, the Madras medical authorities described their puzzlement at the high incidence of typhoid, especially among troops fresh from Britain, even where they believed the water supply was safe. They finally put it down to simple lack of seasoning. Meanwhile the statistics included with that same report showed that, though morbidity declined with time, the overall D + I index rose sharply in the second and third years of service in India.[25]

That was, as Notter had recognized, a recurrent pattern not only in Madras but in the rest of India. Table 5.1 gives the relevant data for Madras in 1891–94 and for all of India ten years later. In both samples, hospital admissions per thousand were highest during the first year, then lower in successive years. Deaths per thousand also fell after the first year, but the D + I index either rose (as in Madras, 1891–5) or remained comparatively level (as for India, 1901–5).

After about 1900, however, the very successes of the military doctors began to change their attitude toward the tropics, and the problem of acclimatization began to fade. In 1911, Aristide Le Dantec in France predicted that within a short time all tropical zones, even tropical Africa, would be habitable by colonists from Europe.[26]

[22] J. Lane Notter, "Hygiene of Troops in Peace and War," in Hygiene & Disease of Warm Climates, ed. Andrew Davidson, pp. 63–4.
[23] H. Poggio, "De la aclimatación en Canarias de las tropas destinadas al Ultramar," RGCMSM, 4:257–, 289–, 353–, 385–, 429–, 460–, 517–, 554–, 591– (1867).
[24] Edouard François Plouzané, Contribution à l'étude de l'hygiène pratique des troupes européenes dans les pays intertropicaux; Haut Sénégal et Haut Niger (Bordeaux, Thesis no. 89, 1887), pp. 12–14.
[25] AMSR, 30:155–7 (1889).
[26] Aristide Le Dantec, Précis de pathologie exotique (maladies des pays chauds et des pays froids), 3d ed. (Paris. 1911), pp. 44–5.

Table 5.1. *Length of Service as a Factor in Morbidity and Mortality in the British Army in India, 1891–94 and 1901–5*

Length of Service	Annual Average per Thousand			
	Admissions	Deaths	Invalided	D + I
Madras Seasoning 1891–94[a]				
Under 1 Year	1,437.4	13.38	15.25	28.63
1–2 years	1,468.1	11.25	29.26	40.51
2–3 years	1,243.9	8.70	38.24	46.94
3–4 years	1,437.7	10.06	33.10	43.16
4–5 years	1,167,9	10.75	33.47	44.22
5–10 years	1,150.9	14.33	38.08	52.41
10 years and more	594.8	14.71	22.74	37.44
Total	1,288.6	11.38	28.50	39.87
India seasoning 1901–5[b]				
Under 1 Year	1,131.9	16.23	18.54	34.77
1–2 years	1,033.4	10.67	27.09	37.77
2–3 years	979.1	9.08	24.95	34.03
3–4 years	1,003.2	8.48	25.40	33.88
4–5 years	893.0	8.75	25.15	33.90
5–10 years	1,124.1	17.22	43.40	60.62
10 years and more	743.4	13.71	40.12	53.83
Not stated				
Total	989.7	12.22	27.65	39.87

[a] Total sample size in 1894 was 13,407 men.
[b] Total sample size in 1901 was 60,838 men.
Source: AMSR for 1891, p. 164; for 1892, p. 118; for 1893, p. 124; for 1894, p. 136; for 1901, p. 146; for 1902, p. 190; for 1903, p. 210; for 1905, p. 118.

Sanitary Engineering: Sewage Disposal

The triumph of nineteenth-century medicine was prevention, not cure; and the key was the provision of clean water. A better water supply had been the most important single cause of the great mortality improvements over the midcentury. With the germ theory and other advances in Western science, people came to understand *why* earlier devices like the slow sand filter actually worked. It was then possible to build further and more securely on what had already been accomplished. By the early twentieth century sanitary engineers had learned how to deliver pure water and to carry away sewage – and were able to understand what went wrong if a particular project failed to work. Wealth from industrialization paid the cost for European and North American cities. The result shows in the declining death rates from typhoid fever and from the gastrointestinal group in Britain and France, and among European troops in the colonies overseas.

Industrialization, however, was a cause as well as a cure. It brought on intense urbanization, which made the safe removal of excrement all the more difficult. Crowding men together for military operations had done the same thing even earlier. Crowding was one of several reasons that barracks life had been more dangerous than civilian life, even in peacetime. As civilian overcrowding increased, civilian and military hygienic problems converged, and the solutions were to serve both.

The problem had been addressed early in the century, and the competing solutions of the water closet and the dry earth system were already at hand by midcentury. Looking back, the victory of the water closet and waterborne sewage may seem predictable, simply because it happened. At the time, it was less so. Raw sewage dumped into rivers simply passed the disease problem on to someone else downstream. For many parts of the Western world in the 1880s and 1890s, rising morbidity and mortality from typhoid fever has been traced directly to the new waterborne sewage systems.[27] Water supply and waste disposal were interrelated problems of great complexity, then as they are today. Alongside the technical problems for microbiology and engineering were political and administrative problems of finance and public policy.

The dry earth system continued beyond World War I, especially in northern England, France, Algeria, and India, but it met with increasing criticism. As early as 1880, health officers with the army in India asked whether "the continued presence of enteric fever at certain stations with conservancy arrangements apparently so perfect is alone sufficient to cause misgivings."[28] By the 1890s, doubts began to rise about the dry earth system in Britain itself. One investigation found that typhoid infection in Newcastle was about twice as common in homes with dry-earth "conservancy" as in those with water closets.[29]

In most colonies, however, the military problem was not a simple choice between waterborne removal and the dry earth system. None of the French colonial centers had waterborne sewage. The choice lay between fixed pit latrines and systematic night soil removal to a distant site for disposal. At first, the French military favored a variant of the Indian latrine system, and used local workers to remove the contents of "tinettes" every night, if only as the lesser of two evils. In time, however, the choice broadened as elaborations of the dry earth technique became available.[30]

In India, where the dry earth system was also dominant, the com-

[27] Joel A. Tarr, "Water and Wastes: A Retrospective Assessment of Wastewater Technology in the United States, 1800–1932," *Technology and Culture*, 25:226–63 (1984), p. 239.

[28] Anthony D. Home, AMSR, 22:147 (1880).

[29] J. Lane Notter, "Report on the Progress of Hygiene for the Year 1895," AMSR, 34:307–14 (1894), p. 313.

[30] A. Legrand, *L'hygiène des troupes européens aux colonies et dans les expéditions coloniales* (Paris, 1895), 77–86; Reynaud, *L'armée coloniale*, pp. 237–9.

plexity of the problem had become increasingly clear. By 1894, when Grant's *Indian Manual* appeared, sewage systems had become an issue far beyond the province of military medical authorities – even beyond that of the public health officials. Costs had to be borne by local governments, and they demanded a say. Farmers, as the potential final users of manure, were also involved. Grant tried to be even handed, keeping all these interests in mind, but the fact remained, as he saw it, that waste rainwater had to be removed from the cantonments in any case. Some form of drains or sewers was therefore required, whether or not they carried human waste. In his view, and that of many others, the simplest and least expensive solution was simply to add fecal matter to the other wastewater.[31]

It was always possible, however, that the dry system could be improved so as to provide its full potential benefits to agriculture. As late as 1899, some thought it was still the best system for India, as long as appropriate care was taken with the disinfection and handling of the waste matter.[32] A much-improved dry earth system was already in common use in France, introduced on agricultural, not medical initiative. It was devised in the 1860s by Pierre Nicholas Goux, a landowner near Paris. The "Goux system" spread rapidly in France and even to Halifax in England. By the 1870s, it had become the dominant method of sewage disposal for army barracks in both France and Algeria.

The system was simple. A container or tub lined with absorbent material was placed as a receptacle under the toilet seat. It was then removed every three to ten days and emptied into specially designed, horse-drawn wagons, which conveyed the waste matter to treatment centers. There, urine and other liquids were allowed to drain off during three or four days. The finished product was loaded into canal boats or railway wagons for transportation to the fields. The system's defenders claimed the odor was no more offensive than that of ordinary cow manure.

The tubs were then washed and repacked with the absorbent material – woolen shoddy or other refuse from textile manufacture – mixed with 5 parts per 100 of iron or calcium sulphate, and held in place with a mould until the renewed tub could be replaced under the toilet. In theory, the absorbent material took up more than 80 percent of the liquid content of the excreta and prevented its immediate oxidation. That, in turn, prevented abnormal fermentation, the deterioration of the product for agricultural use, and the formation of noxious gases.[33]

[31] Allen Ewing and Henry King, *The Indian Manual of Hygiene: Being King's Madras Manual of Hygiene, Revised, Rearranged, and in Great Part Rewritten* (Madras, 1894), pp. 133–47.
[32] Ernest Carrick Freeman, *The Sanitation of British Troops in India* (London, 1899), pp. 15–31.
[33] Legrand, *Hygiène des troupes*, pp. 78–82; R. J. Blackham, "The Goux System and Its Application to India," JRAMC. 6:662–7 (1906), pp. 664–7.

In spite of its numerous advocates, the Goux system never spread widely in the British colonial sphere.

From the 1890s onward, any and all forms of the dry system came under greater critical fire, partly because of the increased public intolerance of dirt and smells of all kinds, although in this respect the military lagged behind the civilian demand for conveniences. In the mid-1890s, for example, the usual urinal in British barracks was a wooden tub placed outside the dormitory room. The space around the urinal was unlighted at night, and spilled urine often dripped through the ceiling to the room below – at a time when flush-urinals were generally available in British railway rest rooms.[34]

British army tests of the dry earth system raised new medical doubts. In 1897, for example, tests showed that a dry earth privy could deodorize and apparently "purify," but it did nothing at all to lower the bacterial content of the excreta; although a 3 percent admixture of quicklime would kill cholera vibrios in four hours.[35] Studies of the typhoid bacillus showed that it lived much longer in dry soils than people had imagined. In India during the dry season, typhoid-bearing dust could be carried by the wind.[36]

By 1903, insect carriers entered the picture. L. O. Howard of the U.S. Department of Agriculture showed that more than half of the seventy-seven species of flies he examined bred on human excrement, including the species of housefly most common in India.[37] In 1902, Indian military authorities had begun once again trying to phase out dry earth latrines, and the new research reinforced the effort without producing wholesale change in the immediate future. The fly investigation also extended to fly-borne contamination of food.[38] Some recommended wire-gauze screening to protect kitchens and dining areas; but British authorities (unlike Americans) resisted screening as too expensive, and they feared that it would reduce all-important ventilation.

By 1910, flush toilets were still rare at British military establishments in India, although they were fully established as the goal for the future, at least for the military. As late as 1908, Professor W. J. R. Simpson's *Principles of Hygiene* took it for granted that Indian civilians would have to make do with night soil removal for the foreseeable future. Meanwhile, dry latrines were kept in use, but with the recommendation that a reagent, usually saponified cresol, be added to the feces. In the past, the excreta were disposed of in trenches, but incineration was now the

[34] G. J. H. Evatt, "The Sanitary Care of the Soldier by His Officer," JRAMC, 18:189–23 (1912), pp. 207–8.

[35] J. Lane Notter, "Report on the Progress of Hygiene for the Year 1897," AMSR, 38:323–41 (1896), p. 337.

[36] R. H. Firth, "Report of the Progress of Hygiene from the year 1901–02," AMSR, 43:345–68 (1901), pp. 358–9.

[37] AMSR, 46:240–3 (1904).

[38] AMSR, 46:245–8 (1904); AMSR, 49:98–102 (1907); AMSR, 50:77–82, 97 (1908).

preferred method. Liquid waste remained a problem, although one suggestion was to heat it to 180°F and then to bury it.[39]

Meanwhile, waterborne sewage systems were also changing. Bacterial purification of sewage – that is, the septic tank and associated processes – was first brought to notice by Meintz and Schloesing in France and by Warrington in Britain. The first practical, operating septic tank in Britain was installed at Exeter in 1896.[40] The principle was similar to the bacterial action of a slow sand filter. Sewage was first held in a closed tank, allowing time for bacteria to break down organic matter. It was then led to flow over filter beds of broken coke for further action by aerobic bacteria. Not all pathogenic organisms were destroyed, but their number was reduced enough for safe release in landspread fertilizer or into a stream for further natural purification. The possible application of this technology in the colonies was obvious, and an experimental septic tank was tested at Colombo in Ceylon shortly after 1900.[41]

But acceptance of sewage purification in Britain itself was not immediate. In 1900, a sharp debate on septic tanks took place at the annual meeting of the British Medical Association. Critics admitted that the process might work but claimed that no present septic tank held the sewage long enough for the process to reach completion. In the next few years, however, bacterial filtration of sewage came to be recognized as the cheapest and easiest way to purify sewage, whatever its remaining limitations. In 1908, a conference of military sanitary officers meeting in Poona adopted a formal resolution in favor of waterborne carriage of sewage from Indian military posts, followed by bacterial filtration.[42]

Even in Europe and North America, the recognition that sewage treatment would "work," was no guarantee that it would be used. A prolonged debate occurred between local medical officers and sanitary engineers; the engineers argued that it was easier and cheaper to dump raw sewage into the watercourses, where it would be cleaned naturally to some extent, and then to filter the polluted water when needed for urban water supplies. The debate began about 1905 and ran far into the 1920s, with the sanitary engineers generally in the ascendant.[43] It was not until the 1960s and later that pollution was

---

[39] AMSR, 51:74 (1909).

[40] J. Lane Notter, "Hygiene in 1897," AMSR, 38:323–41 (1896), p. 333.

[41] Freeman, British Troops, pp. 15–31. For technical description see R. Porter, "Bacterial Treatement of Sewage," JRAMC, 6:194–200 (1906).

[42] Firth, "Hygiene in 1900–01," AMSR, 43:345–68 (1901), pp. 389–90; AMSR, 50:97 (1908).

[43] Joel A. Tarr, James McCurley, and Terry F. Yosie, "The Development and Impact of Urban Wastewater Technology: Changing Concepts of Water Quality Control, 1850–1930," in Population and Reform in American Cities, 1870–1930, ed. Marton V. Melosi (Austin, 1980), pp. 72–7.

recognized and clean water in lakes and streams became a public issue in most of the advanced industrial countries.

The best sanitary systems known took time to install, particularly in the colonies and for the armed forces. By 1870, flush toilets had been furnished to the British military in Barbados and Trinidad, and to those stationed at Up-Park Camp in Kingston, Jamaica. At Newcastle and at Port Royal, however, the dry earth system continued, and Newcastle continued to be the principal locus of military typhoid fever on that island. During the 1870s, indeed, the dry earth system gained new supporters and earlier objections died down both in northern Britain and in India. The flush toilets at Up-Park Camp were reconverted to the dry earth system, and flush toilets returned only in 1904 – long after the dry earth system had fallen into general disrepute.[44] In India, the changeover to flush toilets was still under way at the beginning of the First World War.

Sanitary Engineering: The Search for Pure Water

The most significant new step in the search for pure water was the new attitude toward purity. With the acceptance of the germ theory and further research into waterborne disease, mere chemical purity was not enough, although it was, and continues to be, an important consideration. Gordon's *Army Hygiene* of 1866 pointed out that cholera, typhoid fever, and some parasites were all carried by impure water, and recommended a number of different ways to purify it. It could be passed over boards in a small stream (which would have helped); it could be boiled in order to drive off hydrogen sulphide and decomposed organic matter (which would have worked, but for other reasons); various percipitants like alum would help get rid of some of the vegetable organic matter (which might have improved the taste); Cody's solution of potassium permanganate could be added (which would have worked at appropriate strength); the water could be filtered through charcoal to draw oxygen from the organic matter and cause it to decompose (which again would have improved the taste). Even without a germ theory, only two of these four recommendations would have produced reasonably safe drinking water; but the evidence was still purely empirical. For troops on the march, Gordon recommended the wrong two – alum as a precipitant and charcoal filtration.[45]

Early in the century, researchers were conscious that water contained live "animalcules." By the 1870s, Ferdinand Cohn in Germany had found that dissolved organic matter in water was capable of put-

[44] Edmund Alexander Parkes, "Report on Hygiene for the Year 1874 and Part of 1875," AMSR, 15:181–205 (1873), p. 194; Henry King, *The Madras Manual of Hygiene* (Madras, 1875), pp. 226–8; AMSR, 16:75–7 (1874); AMSR, 43:111 (1901), AMSR 46:148 (1904).

[45] Charles Alexander Gordon, *Army Hygiene* (London, 1866), pp. 413ff., 431–3.

refication giving off "bacteria, zooglaea, vibriones, spirillae, monads," and the like. He thought these were dangerous impurities and associated some of them with cholera. The British Army knew about these discoveries, and about the work of Dr. Jean Champouillon at Val-de-Grâce, whose research on the waterborne character of dysentery was based on evidence from the French army.[46]

Meanwhile, all over Europe the more convenient water closet gradually won out over the dry earth system. This meant more raw sewage would be disposed of in watercourses and created a new sense of urgency about purification. Public piped water was rare enough until the 1880s, but sanitary engineers kept experimenting with different filtering systems – including the slow sand filter that could actually remove bacteria. Most were small units designed to filter the water within the house or at the point of delivery by straining the water through compressed sponge or woolen waste material.

The breakthrough came in the 1880s, when Robert Koch and his colleagues in Germany worked on the water supply for Hamburg and Altona, at the mouth of the Elbe. Koch showed that the slow sand filter serving Altona removed bacteria, even though the river had already received the sewage from a city of 800,000 people higher up. He also showed that the effective filter was the slimy deposit on the surface of the fine sand layer, not the sand itself, and he established the desirable standards for the thickness of sand and other filter components, and for the proper speed of filtration. A few years later, W. J. Simpson described the basic process as follows:

On the surface of a sand filter there is a slimy deposit, composed of finely-divided clay with strong absorbent properties, and a gelatinous mass of intercepted bacilli and streptococci, micrococci, algae and other bodies, and immediately below this film is a layer of nitrifying organisms.

It is this slimy layer on the sand which is the important factor in removing micro-organisms and the organic matter from the water. By the film the pathogenic micro-organisms are intercepted and destroyed, the organic matter is broken up into carbonic acid and ammonia, while by the nitrifying organisms the ammonia is resolved into nitrous and nitric acid.[47]

Most important, Koch showed that gelatine plates could be prepared to act as cultures for bacteria that might have passed through the filter – making microscopic examination of water reasonably effective for the first time.[48]

[46] Edmund Alexander Parkes, "Report on Hygiene for 1871," AMSR, 12:226–59 (1870), pp. 231–2; "Report on Hygiene for 1870," AMSR, 11:205–28 (1869), pp. 232–3.
[47] W. J. Simpson, "Water Supplies," JTMH, 6:192–3 (1903).
[48] J. Lane Notter, "Report on the Progress of Hygiene for the Year 1893," AMSR, 33:281–300 (1892), pp. 286–7.

In 1885, Dr. Percy Frankland examined British water filtration with these principles in mind. He began by testing the London water supply, and further tests from 1886 through 1888 showed that the existing slow sand filtration eliminated all the most serious microbes then known.[49] (It would not have taken care of some viruses, like hepatitis A and B, but viruses had not yet been discovered.) In 1888, British Army researchers using the same techniques concluded that "there does not appear to be any connexion between the goodness or badness of a water from a chemical aspect, and the presence of bacterial growth or liquefaction; neither the chlorine, nor the free ammonia, nor the albuminoid ammonia seem to bear any relation to the bacterial characters of the water."[50] The principal Army medical authorities accepted that conclusion. By 1892, research by R. H. Firth at the army's research establishment at Netley, supported by similar research in France, had shown that a complete examination for all possible microorganisms was not required. The detection of Bacillus coli communis (now Escherichia coli) was enough to indicate fecal pollution and to condemn the medium in which it was found. This test is still recognized by the World Health Organization and other sanitary authorities, although other tests are necessary to ensure complete safety.[51]

By 1890, slow sand filtration was applied in many European municipal water systems. France had lagged somewhat behind Britain and Germany in the use of central, slow sand filtration in urban water systems (which may account for the higher French rate of typhoid deaths among soldiers in France). In the 1890s, however, France also began slow sand filtration. From the 1890s through the first third of the twentieth century, the dominant system there was the Peuch-Chabal multiple filter and aerators, followed by slow sand filtration as a final stage.[52]

Once the Europeans had accepted efficient central water filtration, they began installing it in their colonies overseas. By 1894, slow sand

[49] Percy and Grace Frankland, *Micro-Organisms in Water: Their Significance, Identification, and Removal, together with an Account of the Bateriological Methods Employed in Their Investigation* (London, 1894); J. C. Thresh, *The Examination of Water and Water Supplies*, 2d ed. (London, 1913), p. 225ff.

[50] A. M. Davis, "Report on Bacterial Cultivations from Drinking Water," AMSR, 29:307–66 (1887), p. 309.

[51] J. Lane Notter, "Report on the Progress of Hygiene for the Year 1892," AMSR, 33:339–49 (1891), pp. 316–47; Notter, "Hygiene for 1893," pp. 296–97; Thresh, *Water and Water Supplies*, p. 145; W. H. Horrocks, "Report on the Progress of Hygiene for the Year 1900," AMSR, 41:349–72 (1899), pp. 356, 358–9. See also John Pickford, "Water Treatment in Developing Countries," in Richard Feachem, Michael McGarry, and Duncan Mara, *Water, Wastes, and Health in Hot Climates* (London, 1977), p. 164.

[52] M. N. Baker and M. J. Taras, *The Quest for Pure Water*, 2 vols. (n.p., 1981), 1:63, 259–62. The United States, however, tended to use rapid sand filtration more frequently than other countries did. An equivalent degree of purification could be obtained by combining physical filtration and chemical action (Baker and Taras, *Quest for Pure Water*, 1:179–247).

filtration was the standard that Grant's manual recommended for Indian hygiene. Cairo, Egypt, had a slow sand filter in operation even earlier, and it already met Koch's output standard of no more than 100 microbes per cubic centimeter. By 1903, Calcutta, too, had a slow sand filter capable of reducing the microorganisms in water from 250,000 per cubic centimeters of input water to 15 per cubic centimeters at the output.[53]

Field Filters: Pure Water for the Military

The water problem was far from solved for the military, however. Soldiers might live most of the year in urban barracks, but their purpose was to fight in the countryside, where piped water and large-scale slow sand filtration were unheard of. The search for a field filter began before the germ theory came into fashion – at a time when pure water meant clean-looking, chemically pure water. The most common filter elements were sand (to remove suspended solids) and charcoal (to reduce unpleasant odors and remove dissolved organic matter). By the 1860s, several filters were available commercially. In Britain, the Silicated Carbon Filter Company made some filters of vegetable and others of animal charcoal. Spence's filter of sand and magnetic iron oxide was said to reduce the organic content of water by 30 to 40 percent. Lind's filter was a larger contraption based on two casks and a thick layer of sand, but filtration was rapid, not slow.[54] The French had a similar variety of portable filters, some of them pocket filters for the individual soldier. In the late 1860s, the dominant type of nonportable filter for field use in Algeria was essentially a rapid sand filter with layers of charcoal to remove unpleasant tastes.[55]

Through the 1870s and well into the 1880s, new filters appeared, which were based on similar principles. Macnamara's filter became the standard for the British army. It was constructed in layers – first coarse sand, then fine sand with charcoal below it, and finally another layer of coarse sand. By the early 1880s, the Maignen filter, for larger quantities of water, came into use in both the French and British service. The filter substances in this case were asbestos, charcoal, chalk, animal charcoal, and hydrochloric acid. A single filter, the load of a pack animal, could process 40 litres an hour.

By the early 1890s, however, it was discovered that Macnamara's

[53] Grant, *Indian Manual*, facing p. 54; J. B. Piot Bey, "L'eau d'alimentation dans les villes du Caire et d'Alexandre," AMPM, 33(3d ser):487–96 (1895), pp. 489–92; Simpson, *Water Supply*, pp. 192–3. The recent WHO standard is zero *Escherichia coli* per cubic centimeter of water, and this is now attainable in municipal water systems that combine filtration with chemical purification (Pickford, *Water Treatment*, p. 164).

[54] Charles Alexander Gordon, *Army Hygiene* (London, 1866), p. 432.

[55] Pinchard, "Filtre destiné à la purification de l'eau," RMMM, 18(3d ser.):504–7 (1867).

filter could not stop microorganisms. After continuous use, the filter itself could begin to act as a culture, catching microbes and letting them multiply before passing them on. In 1889, experimenters at Netley showed the Meignen filter to be ineffective as well, although it still had its followers up to 1900 and even later. The Macnamara and Meignen filters were nevertheless gradually phased out.[56]

The next generation of filtration technology developed in the wake of the germ theory and at a time when microscopic examination of water was possible. By the mid-1880s, two competing filters had gained widespread attention: the Pasteur–Chamberland, first demonstrated in France in 1884, and the Berkeland filter developed by the British Army medical facility at Netley. The filtering device of the Chamberland consisted of a porcelain cylinder about an inch and a half in diameter and 1–2 feet long, called a candle or bougie because of its shape – the size and number of these cylinders varied greatly in the large assortment of machines that were produced. The porcelain was so dense that it could physically stop the passage of microorganisms, but the density also meant that water had to be forced through the candles from one end to the other. The Berkeland device was similar, but its filter was made of diatomaceous earth – that is, earth containing many fossil diatoms, still widely used as a filter element.[57]

After some initial resistance, both the Berkeland and the Chamberland filters were proven effective, but they also had problems. Both were fragile, expensive, and hard to clean and keep working.[58] They were heavy, and they were liable to clog up if the input water carried suspended matter – so that a prefilter was needed. They also required a force pump to achieve a reasonable quantity of output. Both were found wanting on actual military expeditions, but both played a valuable role in barracks where slow sand filters were not available.

By the mid-1890s, researchers turned their attention to possible chemical purification. Potassium permanganate had been used in India and elsewhere even before the germ theory was proposed. Properly used, it could be an effective germicide. In 1895, Dr. Bassenge of the German Navy announced a way to purify water using calcium chloride to release free chlorine – the actual disinfectant. Experiments with bromide followed. In 1902 in France, Dr. Vaillard surveyed the field purification methods of all major European and North American armies for the Technical Committee on the Health of the Army and concluded that many systems worked, but that chemical purification

---

[56] Grant, *Indian Manual*, to fact p. 93; Reynaud, *L'armée coloniale*, p. 149ff.; Notter, "*Hygiene for 1893*," p. 297; Thresh, *Water and Water Supplies*, p. 253ff.; M. Bonnafy, "Les moyens d'assurer la salubrité de l'eau au point de vue de l'hygiène coloniale," ICHD, 10:667–78 (1900), pp. 675–77.

[57] Grant, *Indian Manual*, p. 92; Legrand, *Hygiène des troupes européenes*, pp. 207–35; Reynaud, *L'armée coloniale*, pp. 147–54.

[58] Firth, "Hygiene in 1900–01," pp. 384–6; Simpson, *Water Supply*, p. 194.

held the greatest promise. Of various methods using bromium, potassium permanganate, chlorine, or iodine, he preferred iodine.[59] Vaillard in France and V. B. Nesfield in India developed the iodine purification system independently, but newer and more complex systems of chemical purification appeared almost every year.[60]

In the mid-1890s, heat sterilization also began to be explored. Distillation and boiling had been known for decades, but both were regarded as too troublesome for field use and too expensive in terms of the fuel used. One solution was to use a closed vessel, and the French developed two such methods by 1895. The breakthrough came with the Forbes–Waterhouse heat-transfer apparatus, first developed in the United States and used in the Philippine campaign. The principle was to use the hot output water to help heat the input, while the cool input water simultaneously helped to cool the finished product for drinking. Researchers in several countries began looking for a simple, light, and effective apparatus that could yield a large output of cooled water ready for use. The British used the Maiche system in the Anglo-Boer War. It could turn out a thousand gallons a day, but it was too large for field use, requiring permanently fixed tanks to receive the purified water.[61]

In 1905, Dr. D. P. Griffith came up with a machine based on the premise that water did not need to reach the boiling point for full purification. His experiments suggested that 80°C was enough to kill all germs. The result was a water-purification apparatus that fitted into two boxes that weighed only about 80 pounds each, yet were capable of providing 60 gallons of pure water each hour – and that with only three-quarters of a pint of fuel oil for each 100 gallons of sterile water.[62]

Other alternatives combined physical and chemical methods mounted on water carts that could both sterilize water and have it ready for use. One type used candle filters alone. Another combined pre-filters using asbestos cloth and charcoal with a final-stage Berkeland sterilizing filter. Still another cart from France used a clarifying filter followed by a heat-exchange sterilizer. New types proliferated year by year, although many authorities agreed that the best combination of size, capacity, and convenience had not yet been reached.[63] All

---

[59] Vaillard, "L'épuration de l'eau potable en campagne," AMPM, 40:1–37 (1902).

[60] Notter, "Hygiene in 1895," p. 311; Notter, "Hygiene in 1898," pp. 366–7; Horrocks, "Hygiene in 1900," pp. 370–1; Pottier, "Epuration de l'eau potable en campagne," AHMC, 5:599–605 (1902), pp. 599–603; V. B. Nesfield, "The Rapid Chemical Sterilization of Water," JRAMC, 24:146–54 (1915); Gabriel Lambert, "De la purification des eaux de boisson et nouveau procédé chimique de purification totale et rapide des eaux destinées à l'alimentation," AHMC, 9:266–97 (1906).

[61] Simpson, Water Supplies, p. 192.

[62] R. H. Firth, "The Griffith Water Steriliser," JRAMC, 7:218–25 (1906), pp. 218–20.

[63] Anon., "Sterilisation of Drinking Water for Troops in the Field," JRAMC, 4:349–52 (1905), pp. 350–2; T. McCulloch, "The Field Service Filter Water Cart," JRAMC, 6:449–54 (1906), pp. 449–52; R. H. Firth, "On the Application of Heat for the Purification of Water, with Troops in the Field," JRAMC, 11:570–81 (1908), pp. 570–3.

would work under certain circumstances, but each had its own place in a battery of different purification techniques varying from ultraviolet light through chemical and mechanical to biological filtration.[64] The goal was to supply every soldier with readily available pure water, both in the field and in the barracks. After the mid-1890s, that goal was technically attainable, but theory and reality are not always the same.

Sanitary Engineering Applied: West Indies, India, Algeria

Conditions in the colonies necessarily posed special problems. In the West Indies, the pure-water problem in the Windward and Leeward Command was solved by the 1860s. Jamaica was another matter. Newcastle, high in the mountains, had no malaria, but it had a much higher incidence of typhoid deaths than any other post in the West Indies. Its water from mountain springs was assumed to be "good." It was not until 1891 that new and better springs were tapped and the water was passed through charcoal and sand filter beds. Two years later, a new filter of a similar type was installed at Up-Park Camp near Kingston, but the local medical officers did not trust it. In 1893, they added a Pasteur–Chamberland as the final stage before drinking, but it could only yield 250 gallons every twenty-four hours.[65] Until the beginning of the First World War, the post limped along with badly filtered water from the river sources for bathing, with Chamberland-filtered water for drinking. Medical officers suspected that the men were not careful about the distinction. By 1909–13, the reported relocation cost in deaths from typhoid was nevertheless lower in the West Indies than it was in Algeria or India.

Water supply to Indian military posts in the 1870s was still a mixture of older methods. Some posts drew water from wells. Others used the tanks or reservoirs of nearby Indian urban areas. Medical authorities, however, treated these with suspicion. From the 1870s into the 1890s, reports from Bangalore amounted to a chorus of complaint about drawing water from a particular tank, known to receive sewage from the Indian town. Burmese barracks drew some water from the moats surrounding fortifications and some from the Irriwaddy River. In India as a whole, more posts got piped water with each decade, but, into the 1890s and beyond, many used the traditional leather sack, thrown across the back of a bullock or carried by men – in spite of efforts to substitute water carts when piped water was not available.[66]

Water from all sources was filtered before use, but the filter was not

---

[64] C. F. Wanhill, "Water Supply in the Field," JRAMC, 17:157–64 (1911), pp. 157–59; V. B. Nesfield, "The Chemical Sterilization of Water for Military Purposes," JRAMC, 12:513–22 (1919), pp. 520–2; Nesfield, "Rapid Chemical Sterilization."

[65] AMSR, 33:89 (1891); AMSR, 34:58 (1892); AMSR, 37:96 (1896); AMSR 39:126 (1907).

[66] AMSR, 30:168 (1889); AMSR, 34:124–30 (1892).

always the most effective type available. From the 1860s, the filter consisted of some combination of sand and charcoal, and whatever else, it would have strained out suspended particles and improved the taste. From the early 1880s up to 1900, Macnamara's filter was standard issue at all Indian military posts, even though many recognized that it could not remove bacteria. By the 1880s, many posts (perhaps most) began to boil as well as filter drinking water. Whether this was done systematically at a rolling boil for a full half-hour depended on the efficiency of the Indian servants who did the work.

Outside the barracks, a similar pattern of boiling and filtering was used in Anglo-Indian households. The usual filter was a set of three chatties or pots, one above the other on a bamboo stand. The top chatty contained powdered charcoal; a small hole in the bottom allowed it to drain slowly into the second, which contained powdered sand and drained into the third, which held the filtered water. The highest chatty was filled daily with boiled water, and the whole apparatus was cleaned and renewed every two weeks or so. As with the barracks filters, its effectiveness depended on the efficiency of the servants. For travelers, a small bottle filter was sold widely throughout India and Burma. The filter itself was stoneware, simply a way of removing suspended matter, but the instructions called for adding potassium permanganate and boiling as well, so that the product was probably safe.[67]

In the early twentieth century, iodine and chlorine purification began as well, at least on an experimental basis, and Griffith heat purifiers began to arrive in 1909. Boiling, however, was still the main form of purification, and it continued to be used in Anglo-Indian homes until after independence, although chemical purification, especially for chlorinization, was increasingly promoted after 1913.[68] By 1915, one of the principal British military hygienists could announce the dawn of the new era: "Now that iodine, chlorine, and permanganate of potash have been definitely proved to be reliable for the sterilization of water, surely the unpracticable and cumbersome methods of boiling and filtration for troops on the march will be discarded, and in future military expeditions water-borne epidemics will be a thing of the past."[69]

The search for pure water was international, and the French were among the leaders. The French military in North Africa was an intregal part of the French Army, not a separate command like the presidency armies in India or the French Colonial Army elsewhere. In barracks, it used the water supply available to civilians, but with its own point-of-delivery filtration. In the field, from the 1860s into the

[67] Grant, *Indian Manual*, pp. 94, 96.
[68] AMSR, 51:82 (1909); F. H. Treherne and J. J. H. Nelson, "Sterilization of Infected Water in Camp and on the March in India," JRAMC, 21:443–51 (1913).
[69] Nesfield, "Rapid Chemical Sterilization."

1880s, it used variants of the common filter materials – cloth, sponge, and charcoal, in varying combinations. The important difference from the British usage was less insistence on boiling water, whatever the filtration. The French knew that boiling killed microbes, but they thought it was impractical in field conditions.

In the early 1880s, both the British in Egypt and the French in Algeria began using the Maignen, with reputed success, although it could not, in fact, remove bacteria. It continued in use even after the French research had produced the Pasteur–Chamberland filter, which *did* remove bacteria.

By the early 1890s, high morbidity and mortality from typhoid fever prompted a new investigation, which underlined the effectiveness of the Chamberland. The French government ordered 200,000 units to be installed in barracks, including 15,000 in Algeria. Between 1886–8 (before the filters came into general use) and 1891, total hospital admissions in the French Army dropped by more than half. Total mortality dropped by 38 percent.[70] The filters were still unpopular for field use, because of fragility, low yield, and the need for a pre-filter; as late as 1895, charcoal-based pocket filters were still recommended, although some authorities were afraid they would give the men a false sense of security about bad water.[71]

During the early decades of the twentieth century, the French, like the British, moved to more and more elaborate systems for the field delivery of pure water.[72] By 1913, in the Moroccan campaign, French troops had Lefebvre heat-exchange water purifiers mounted on two-wheeled carts. The sterilizers burned either wood or charcoal briquettes, could turn out 195 gallons of water every four hours, and could go virtually anywhere the troops could go. As a final refinement, the French also introduced a few field ice machines, which could also follow the troops on two-wheeled carts.[73]

The process of sanitary engineering was all very well, but the final stage depended on the soldiers themselves. In ignorance of bacteriology, they went by taste; many turned down "doctored" water that tasted of chlorine or potassium permanganate. Really thirsty soldiers would drink any water they could find. Military doctors knew this – hence the elaborate devices for making pure water available at the point of action.

Wash water was another matter. All European armies insisted on parade-ground spit and polish; what went on in the barracks was another matter, and the odor of a "well-turned-out" soldier was still

---

[70] Legrand, *Hygiène des troupes*, pp. 207–35; Notter, "Hygiene in 1892," 342–3.

[71] Legrand, *Hygiène des troupes*, pp. 112–35; Bonnafy, "Eaux potables," pp. 675–77.

[72] Pottier, "Epuration," pp. 599–603; Lambert, "Purification des eaux," pp. 168–9.

[73] C. E. P., "Water sterilizers and Ice Machines with the Troops in Morocco," JRAMC, 22:380–1 (1914).

another. In Britain of the mid-1890s, the official space in barracks was still 600 cubic feet per man, as it had been since midcentury; and regulations required a change of air twice an hour. At the same time, the official allowance of bathtubs was one for each 100 soldiers, plus twelve basins and four footbaths. If spare time allowed the bathtub to be used ten times a day, each soldier had potential access to a bath every ten days. In fact, the army provided only cold water, which meant that the tub was hardly used at all between October and May.[74]

Barracks bedding in Britain was straw, issued at the rate of 24 pounds per man each quarter. The straw was covered by heavy canvass sheets that were washed once a month. Underpants were issued only to mounted troops, and they normally slept in them; while the infantry slept in the flannel shirts they had worn all day. The issue of linen was more generous in the tropics, but personal sanitation was still appalling by present-day standards.[75]

Nutrition

Good nutrition is essential to good health, yet the possible relationship between nutrition and falling military mortality – either at home or abroad – is hard to determine. The ration for British soldiers in the first part of the nineteenth century followed an old tradition, going back to the sixteenth century, when the English soldier in wartime was supposed to receive daily, 2 pounds of meat, 1 pound of bread, and 1 pint of wine. The total would have yielded over 4,000 calories, with far more protein than present-day nutritionists would advise, and less carbohydrates.[76] At least it was generous, and this tradition persisted. Another tradition was slipshod food preparation. The food provided by regulation was not always provided; when provided, it was not always edible.

At the beginning of the 1840s, the daily ration of the British services was established at a pound of bread and a pound of meat a day (Table 5.2). Sailors got a little more, plus supplementary rations of vegetables, flour, or dried peas. For soldiers, the basic ration of meat and bread was considered to be their "free" ration, which was to be supplemented as they saw fit from their pay. This makes it especially hard to find out what the men actually ate, but the basic ration seems to have provided enough in calories to sustain a man at hard labor. It was certainly far more than most British civilians could afford at the time. Soldiers on tropical duty had an extra allowance of sugar, cocoa, peas, and rice, although their meat ration was reduced to 1½ pounds per

[74] Evatt, "Sanitary Care," pp. 208–9.
[75] Evatt, "Sanitary Care," pp. 211–15.
[76] National Academy of Sciences (NAS), Food and Nutrition Board, Recommended Daily Allowances (Washington, D.C., 1974), pp. 1–10.

Table 5.2. *Daily Ration in the British Armed Services, 1840*

Sailor's Daily Ration		Soldier's Daily Ration	

| 1½ lbs | bread, or |
| 1 lb. | biscuit |

| 1 lb. | bread, or |
| ¾ lb. | biscuit |

1 lb.	fresh meat, and
½ lb.	vegetables
	or
¾ lb.	salt beef, and
¾ lb.	flour
	or
¾ lb.	salt pork, and
½ pt.	peas

| 1 lb. | fresh or salt beef or pork |

In tropical service, the salt pork was reduced to 12 oz. two days a week, in return for which the soldier received the following issue daily:

1 gal.	beer, or
1 pt.	wine, or
¼ pt.	spirits

1²⁄₇ oz.	sugar
5⁄₇ oz.	cocoa
¼ lb.	rice
½ pt.	peas.

| ¼ oz. | tea |

| 1½ oz. | sugar |

| 1 oz. | cocoa |

In addition, weekly
½ pt. oatmeal
½ pt. vinegar

Source: A. M. Tulloch, "Comparison of Sickness among Seamen and Soldiers," USSL, 4:11 (1841).

week. If the meat was well prepared and of good quality, that would have been an adequate quantity of protein. The sugar allowance of 29 pounds a year for the soldier on tropical duty was nearly double the average home consumption of only 15 pounds. On the other hand, occasional reports of scurvy suggest that the unmeasured additional fruits and vegetables probably failed to provide the necessary vitamins and minerals.[77]

Nor was the ration served in the most healthful way. Until 1845, soldiers in Britain were fed only twice a day, at eight in the morning and one in the afternoon, leaving a long gap to be filled by what the individual could afford to purchase on his own. After 1845, the principal meal was still at midday, but a "tea" was added after "evening parade."[78]

[77] See Kenneth J. Carpenter, *The History of Scurvy and Vitamin C* (Cambridge, 1986), esp. pp. 98–102.

[78] Alexander Tulloch, "Comparison of the Sickness, Mortality and Prevailing Diseases among Seamen and Soldiers, As Shown by the Naval and Military Statistical Reports," JSSL, 4:1–16 (1841), pp. 10–11; James Burnett, *Plenty and Want: A Social History of Diet in England from 1815 to the Present* (London, 1966), p. 9; Gordon, *Army Hygiene*, p. 38.

The English working class certainly ate less well. Urban workers ate better than farm workers, who rarely got any meat at all other than a little pork or bacon they could raise themselves. Urban workers got by on about a half-pound of bread each day, supplemented by potatoes and a little meat. Tea with sugar, however, had become standard working-class fare by this time.[79]

The French soldier's ration in midcentury was not far different from the British. Soldiers in Algeria about 1850 were supposed to receive 643 grams of biscuit, 300 grams of meat, 60 grams of rice, 12 grams each of coffee and sugar. The diet contained about twice the English bread ration, barely half the meat, and half the sugar.[80] Without more information about supplements, both diets appear adequate in energy, although the French balance between protein and carbohydrates appears closer to recent recommendations.

By the early 1860s, medical studies of nutritional needs and norms began to appear. Dr. Edward Smith conducted an inquiry on behalf of the Medical Officer of the Privy Council. He found that the most common food in Britain was bread, at about 1¾ pounds per day per person, followed by potatoes at nearly a pound per day. That was more carbohydrate than the military standard, but each adult farm worker got less than a pound of meat a *week*. By that time, some nutritionists had begun to complain that the British Army's meat ration was too high, and some feared that the common hepatitis of the tropics came from overeating; but Madras army authorities stuck with a pound of meat a day as a reasonable standard for men serving in the tropics.[81]

Also in the 1860s, E. A. Parkes, the Professor of Military Medicine, recommended diets suited to the climate for soldiers in Britain and in India. He reduced the protein requirements sharply and increased the carbohydrates. For tropical service, however, the total was slightly less than for Britain, with protein slightly more and carbohydrates slightly less.[82] Recent nutrition doctrine holds that energy requirements need

[79] Burnett, *Plenty and Want*, pp. 23–32.
[80] Auguste Haspel, *Maladies de l'Algérie; des causes, de la symptomatologie, de la nature et du traitement des maladies endémo-épidémique de la province d'Oran*, 2 vols. (Paris, 1850–2) 1:47–8. A decade later, French field rations were 750 grams bread, 32 grams coffee, 42 grams sugar, 120 grams rice, 100 grams bacon or salt pork, 16.66 grams salt, plus 500 grams fresh meat, issued daily – a little meat and a little less bread, but still not up to the British standard (Joshua Paynter, "Report upon the Sanitary Condition of French Troops Serving in Algeria," AMSR, 7:437–51 (1865), p. 442).
[81] Burnett, *Plenty and Want*, p. 121; Gordon, *Army Hygiene*, p. 40; AMSR, 7:381 (1863).
[82] Dietary elements (ounces):

	Home	India
Water	38.33	30.07
Nitrogenous substances	3.86	4.36
Fats	1.30	1.38
Carbohydrates	17.35	14.47
Salts	0.80	1.54

Source: Gordon, *Army Hygiene*, p. 41.

to be increased slightly for work in heat above 30°C, or cold below 20°C.[83]

The British service continued its higher rations for service in India than in Britain. At the end of the century, the "free ration" in Britain was still 12 ounces of meat daily and 1 pound of bread. The additional "grocery ration" was paid for by a sum (usually 3½ pence per day in Britain) deducted from each soldier's pay and spent for extras at the discretion of the regimental authorities. In India, the meat ration was increased to 1 pound, while the bread ration was reduced to 1 pound.[84] After 1900, British Army rations increased still more. The army entered the South African war with a recommended 3,900 calories a day for field service, later raised to 4,500 to 5,000.[85] The standard or metropolitan French ration followed its earlier trend, with slightly less food, by weight, but with a little more bread and a little less meat.[86] Like the British, the French tried to match diet to climate: They had a Saigon and a Madagascar diet, just as the British had their Egyptian and Indian diets.

Meanwhile, nutrition began to emerge as a separate field of medical science. I. Burney Yeo's manual, *Food in Health and Disease*, first appeared in 1889, passed through a second major revision in 1896, with many reprintings in the early twentieth century. As a text for this developing field, it drew on research from all over Europe and North America, summarizing the findings about each particular food, and including sections on cooking for maximum nutritional value, and the diets appropriate for particular medical conditions such as tuberculosis, cardiac problems, and obesity.[87]

In the new century, nutritional concern in both armies shifted from the adequacy of the basic diet to the delivery of that diet to troops in the field – parallel to the new concern about getting pure water to the front. Field kitchens were designed to follow the troops closely. Army dietitians planned for greater variety in rations and worked on ways to preserve food until it was ready to be eaten. Meat at the beginning of the South African war, for example, had been packed in 9-pound tins. This meant that a unit's full-day allotment had to be eaten at one sitting or thrown away for fear of spoilage.

The new goal was nutritious, attractive food, packed in small containers for troops out of touch with the field kitchens. One was a mixture of meat, potatoes, vegetables, and gravy that provided 960

---

[83] NAS, *Recommended Dietary Allowances*, p. 25.

[84] Notter and Firth, *Military Hygiene*, pp. 944–97.

[85] W. W. O. Beveridge, "Some Essential Factors in the Construction of Field Service and Expeditionary Rations," JRAMC, 23:377–96 (1914), p. 383.

[86] Notter and Firth, *Military Hygiene*, pp. 946–9; G. Reynaud, *L'armée coloniale*, pp. 66–77.

[87] I. Burney Yeo, *Food in Health and Disease* (London, 1889 and later editions).

calories and weighed 22 ounces. Polar expeditions were an additional source of experience and experimentation.[88] Nutritionists by this time knew a good deal about the importance of minerals, as well as the balance of protein, carbohydrates, and fats, and they were beginning to learn about vitamins as well. Food for the armies became steadily more appetizing as well as more nutritious.

In retrospect, despite the lack of specific nutritional information in many areas, it is clear that both the British and the French Army tried to pay serious attention to the feeding of their troops. It is nevertheless almost impossible to know precisely what the troops ate, as opposed to what was assigned them. Both armies reported some scurvy and some beriberi, the clear result of dietary deficiencies; yet in peacetime, the army ate at least as well as the civilian population. Vitamin deficiency diseases appeared principally on campaign, when fresh food could not easily be found. Aside from these diseases, it is impossible to associate presumed improvements in nutrition with falling death rates from specific diseases, in the way a new water supply can be shown to lead directly to decreased death rates from waterborne diseases. Yet nutrition must have played some role in the gradual fall of death rates, though that role was certainly less than that of improved water supply or sewage disposal. From the 1890s on, moreover, growing knowledge of particular diseases and their prevention also became more important than ever before.

---

[88] G. Fahey, "Rations on Active Service," JRAMC, 19:714–29 (1912), pp. 724–9; Beveridge, "Field Service Rations," pp. 377–96 (1914); Carpenter, Scurvy and Vitamin C, pp. 133–57.

CHAPTER 6

THE PURSUIT OF DISEASE, 1870–1914

Even though specific therapy made slow progress until after 1914, in the period between the 1890s and the beginning of the war, the combination of general hygienic measures and better ways to fight particular diseases brought the steepest percentage decline of the whole century in the death rate of soldiers at home or abroad. The best of medical knowledge was not automatically translated into practice, but the information network available to military doctors steadily narrowed the time gap between discovery and implementation of practical preventive measures.

Yellow Fever

Yellow fever was a special case – unknown in Asia, only rarely seen in Europe. Like other epidemic disease, it varied through time. From the 1870s to the 1890s, however, it accounted for a quarter of all deaths from disease among British troops in the West Indies. Only typhoid fever was a serious rival, and typhoid caused more deaths than yellow fever only in the sample period, 1886–94.

Down to 1900, medical men could only suspect the cause, and they had no cure. Yet the trend in mortality for European troops was slightly downward, both in deaths per thousand and the proportion of total deaths (Table 6.1). A peak for this half-century occurred in the late 1870s and early 1880s, but still higher peaks must have occurred before the 1860s, although British army records failed to distinguish yellow fever from malaria at that time. The Jamaican death rate from "fevers," for example, was more than 100 per thousand for 1817–36 (Table 1.6) – a figure that certainly hid some very high yellow fever death rates in particular years.

Medical authorities made progress by following empirical leads – even though some were false leads. In the 1840s, escape to a hill station like Newcastle on Jamaica seemed to work, but it actually only worked for malaria. In the 1850s, yellow fever appeared at Newcastle. It reappeared in late 1860s and in 1877, and the authorities had to fall

130

Table 6.1. *Deaths from Yellow Fever, European Troops in the British West Indies*

Date	Deaths per Thousand	Percentage of All Deaths from Disease
1859–67	3.43	21.63
1869–77	2.20	28.65
1879–84	8.12	45.29
1886–94	0.68	8.56
1895–1904	1.52	20.46
1909–13	0.00	0.00

Source: See Table 6.2.

back on the old alternative of flight. This time, they evacuated Newcastle completely, moving the troops back to sea level posts near Kingston. In 1878, even these came under attack. Yellow fever broke out at Port Royal, and the troops were moved once more, across the harbor mouth to a battery on the opposite shore.[1] In retrospect, what probably made Newcastle relatively safe was its isolation from civilian populations, not its elevation. Port Royal was, in fact, a point of special danger – because it was a port, not because it was at sea level.

Yellow fever gave its victims lifelong immunity; an epidemic stopped when it ran out of victims, or when so few victims remained that "herd immunity" set in. On most West Indian islands, residual yellow fever among primates in the forest was insufficient to keep the disease going. It could only return when it was reintroduced from abroad, and all strangers arrived by sea. The typical epidemic began with a few cases in the port towns, then traveled to wherever it could find victims.

A new epidemic on Barbados in 1880–1 was especially alarming, and it illustrates a failure to use the preventive measures that had worked earlier in the century. The disease appeared among the civilian population late in 1880, but with some uncertainty about the diagnosis. By April 1881, Bridgetown, the chief port as well as the capital, was clearly suffering from epidemic yellow fever, but the troops were allowed to stay in the barracks just outside the city. Only when the fever reached these troops in late July, were they ordered to safety on Gun Hill, as they had been so often in the past. This time, the disease went with them. By late October, the death rate became so alarming that all European units were ordered to embark for England. Even then, several men died on the way home. All told, yellow fever admissions were 138 per thousand; deaths were 57 per thousand. In retrospect,

[1] AMSR, 19:54–5 (1877); AMSR, 20:64 (1878).

it is clear that flight saved lives – in Jamaica and in Barbados as well
– but more timely flight might have saved more lives.[2]

Through the middle decades of the century, yellow fever had been
one of several battlegrounds between contagionists and anticontagionists. Several commentators suspected an infective agent of some kind –
just as cholera was known to be carried by water. In 1881, Dr. Carlos
Finlay of Havana not only suggested a mosquito vector; he correctly
pinpointed *Aëdes Aegypti* (then called *Stegomya fasciata*) as the species
involved. It was impossible at the time to follow up with further steps,
like Laveran's discovery of plasmodia in the blood of a malaria victim.
Whereas a plasmodium, a protozoa, was easily visible with the micro-
scopes then available, the filtrable virus responsible for yellow fever
was too small to be detected at that time.

It was not until 1900 that the American Yellow Fever Commission
under Walter Reed (including Finlay as one of the members) began a
concerted attack on the problem. By 1901, *Aëdes Aegypti* was implicated
clearly enough to justify an experimental mosquito eradication program in Havana, then under American occupation. Because of *A. Aegypti's* "domestic" habits, systematic eradication was reasonably easy. In
the first year, yellow fever deaths in Havana dropped by 90 percent.
Over the period 1902–11, the total number of yellow fever deaths in
Havana dropped to an annual average of 4 per year in a population of
about 300,000.[3] Similar methods were tried again in Panama and New
Orleans and were quickly adopted by other Caribbean countries. The
British on Jamaica brought in their own antimosquito measures, with
similar success. In 1904, the last case of yellow fever was recorded
among the European troops at Port Royal.[4] The yellow fever problem
was far from solved everywhere, but it had become negligible as a
cause of death in the British West Indies. With the yellow fever danger
gone, Jamaica began to encourage tourism to exploit the comfort of its
winter climate and its new reputation for healthfulness.[5]

Malaria

From the 1840s on, with the introduction of quinine, malaria began
to decline as a killing disease. Yet that achievement, like many other
advances against malaria still to come, raised false hopes. (Malaria
remains the principal cause of death in the tropical world today.) In

---

[2] AMSR, 23:47 (1881); Edmond Hoile, "Report of the Epidemic of Yellow Fever at
Barbados in 1881," AMSR: 22:331–9 (1881), p. 331.
[3] Great Britain, Colonial Office Confidential Prints, Africa 975, CO 879/108.
[4] AMSR, 44:103, 113 (1902).
[5] F. M. Mangin, "Causation and Prevention of the Spread of Yellow Fever, JRAMC,
7:369–71 (1906), p. 371. The relocation cost for British troops to Jamaica in 1909–13
was, nevertheless, still higher than 200 percent. See Table 1.2.

Madras, for example, military death rates per thousand dropped by 60 percent between the 1840s and 1860s (probably because of the use of quinine) – only to level off afterward in the range of 0.35 to 0.62 deaths per thousand. As a result, its importance as a cause of death rose steadily as other causes of death declined (Table 6.2). The only spectacular achievement after the 1860s was a drop of 44 percent in India's malaria death rate between 1895–1904 and 1909–13 (probably because of antimosquito measures).

A similar pattern prevailed in the West Indies. Malaria deaths per thousand dropped slowly and irregularly, but malaria deaths as a percentage of all deaths were higher in 1909–13 than at any period back to the 1860s. Only Algeria showed regular progress against malaria from one decade to the next – for a total drop in the malaria death rate of 87 percent between the 1860s and 1909–13. The difference in Algeria was almost certainly its vectors, which were more easily controlled there than elsewhere. By the late twentieth century, malaria had virtually disappeared from North Africa and was greatly weakened in the West Indies, but still it flourished in India and in tropical Africa.[6]

By the 1870s, long before the mosquito vector was known, European medicine distinguished different types of malaria by their patterns of intermission – tertian returned the third day after an attack (actually about forty-eight hours elapsed, since the reckoning counted the initial day); quartan returned in the fourth. Tertian was subdivided into "benign tertian," the present-day *Plasmodium vivax*, and "malignant tertian," the present *P. falciparum*. These two were the most serious strains for the European military in the tropical world. Other nineteenth-century fever classifications, like "typhomalarial fever" were more ephemeral disease classifications, and they are hard to identify in retrospect.

For centuries, Europeans had associated all kinds of remittent fevers with marshes and the "malarious" vapors arising from them. Studies in medical topography sharpened the European appreciation of where malaria occurred and where it did not. By the 1870s, however, many authorities accepted Léon Colin's argument that dry soils should also be incriminated.[7] In 1875, Alphonse Laveran drew a synthesis from the malaria literature, showing that malaria was not a purely tropical dis-

---

[6] William Cohen has argued that the French military death rates from malaria continued to be high up to the end of the nineteenth century, but his evidence came principally from tropical Africa, where malaria death rates were high for everyone. French imperialism could nevertheless take encouragement from the victory over malaria in Algeria, which had the largest French force by far in any part of Africa in the second half of the nineteenth century (Cohen, "Malaria and French Imperialism," JAH, 24:23–36 [1983]).

[7] Edmond Alexander Parkes, "Report on Hygiene for 1870," AMSR, 11:205–28 (1869), pp. 238–40; Hamet, "Malaria and Military Medicine during the Conquest of Algeria," MS, 4:24–33 (1932); Léon Colin, *Traité des fièvres intermittentes* (Paris, 1870), pp. 1–24.

Table 6.2. *Deaths from Malaria, 1860s to 1913*

	Deaths per Thousand				Percentage of All Deaths from Disease			
	France	Algeria	India	British West Indies		France	Algeria	India	British West Indies
1860s	0.22	2.69	0.70	3.21		2.25	19.13	3.52	20.23
1870s	0.10	2.33	0.35	0.97		1.07	18.39	1.99	12.63
1880s	0.03	0.95	0.28	3.02		0.39	9.84	2.55	16.84
1890s	0.00	0.75	0.74	0.97		0.00	8.78	5.56	12.22
1900s	0.01	0.58	0.62	1.48		0.27	8.84	4.68	19.94
1909–13	0.00	0.34	0.18	1.52		0.00	7.16	4.76	20.99

Source: For France and Algeria, *Statistiques médicales*, annual series, as aggregated in appendix tables. For Britain, Army Medical Service, annual reports, as aggregated in appendix tables. West Indian data are for both commands – Barbados and Jamaica – except for 1909–13 Jamaica alone, the Barbados Command having been discontinued. The dates of all British samples are 1859–67, 1869–77, 1879–84, 1885–94, 1895–1904, because the years were aggregated in this way in the reports. They therefore represent the indicated decades only approximately. The Indian data are for Madras Presidency alone through 1884. Thereafter, for all British troops in India.

ease. It occurred in some cold countries. It had once been common in northern Europe. It was absent in some tropical countries like New Caledonia and Tahiti, but it was generally more prevalent in warm countries than in cold. It tended to occur in wet and humid plains, but some such plains were malaria-free and some dry and mountainous regions had malaria.[8]

Laveran's authoritative manual of military medicine was written from an Algerian background, but it summarized the standard advice of the period. Virtually all authorities prescribed quinine to cure malaria. Prevention was another matter. Lavernon put greatest emphasis on draining the soil and planting crops. He was conscious of the claims of prophylactic quinine, especially those based on the experience of the British navy and lessons of the American Civil War, but he doubted that its wholesale use was required in Algeria. He thought prophylactic quinine should be reserved for military units at especially malarious posts, or for epidemics.[9] Other authorities expressed different reservations. Quinine was known to have side effects. In high dosages it was a recognized poison. Some authorities also feared that, taken prophylactically, it would wear out its influence and become less effective when the disease actually occurred. Ronald Ross, whose research confirmed the hypothesis of a mosquito vector, argued at one point that routine use of preventive quinine would weaken its curative power.[10]

---

[8] Alphonse Laveran, *Traité des maladies et épidémies des armées* (Paris, 1875), pp. 101–2.

[9] Laveran, *Maladies des armées*, pp. 193–203.

[10] Ronald Ross, *Malarial Fever: Its Cause, Prevention, and Treatment* (London, 1902), pp. 36–47. William Cohen has argued that: "On the whole French medical authorities did not believe in the prophylactic qualities of quinine." But he cited only four opinions of French doctors commenting on particular times and places (Cohen, "Malaria and French Imperialism," p. 26). A survey of the manuals of tropical medicine, both in French and in English, gives the impression that most authorities favored prophylactic quinine, but with a strong dissenting element among the French and British alike.

The following recommended regular quinine prophylaxis: Auguste Frédéric Dutroulau, *Traité des maladies des Européens dans les pays chauds*, 2d ed. (Paris, 1868) p. 254; Charles Alexander Gordon, *Army Hygiene* (London, 1866), p. 290; Laveran, *Maladies des armées*, pp. 196–7; Jean Baptiste Fosnagrive, *Traité d'hygiène navale*, 2d ed. (Paris, 1877), pp. 50–5; Adolphe C. A. M. Nicolas (ed.), *Guide hygiènique et médicale du voyageur dans l'Afrique centrale*, 2d ed. (Paris, 1885), pp. 333–9; Andrew Davidson (ed.), *Hygiene & Diseases of Warm Climates* (Edinburgh, 1893), pp. 103–6; Paul Edward Villedary, *Guide sanitaire des troupes et du colon aux colonies. Hygiène coloniale, prophylaxie et traitement des principals maladies des pays chauds* (Paris, 1893), pp. 107–29; Fernand Burot and Maximilien Albert Legrand, "Maladies des marins, épidémies nautiques," RC, 130:17–81 (1897), pp. 130, 457; A. Legrand, *L'hygiéne des troupes européens aux colonies et dans les expéditions coloniales* (Paris, 1895), pp. 309–18; Gustave A. Reynaud, *Considerations sanitaires sur l'expédition de Madagascar et quelques autres expéditions coloniales, françaises et anglaises* (Paris, 1898) p. 461; Patrick Manson, *Tropical Diseases: A Manual of the Diseases of Warm Climates* (London, 1898), p. 125; Devaux, "Suite aux quelques conseils de médecine pratique à l'usage des officiers en campagne," RTC, 3(2):175–82 (1904); H. A. Caille, *Considerations sanitaires sur les expéditions coloniales* (Bordeaux, Thesis no. 64, 1904), p. 73; Alexandre Marie Kermorgant and Gustave Reynaud, "Précautions hygiènique à prendre pour les expéditions et les explorations

Investigators going back at least to some early Roman physicians had suspected that mosquitos were somehow involved. Africans of the Usambara highlands in Tanzania also associated malaria with mosquitos – and had done so for such a long time that their word for the disease, *mbu*, was the same as their word for the insect.[11]

Transmission by mosquitos and transmission by bad air fitted the known facts equally well until 1880, when Laveran discovered the plasmodia itself in the blood of a malaria victim. In 1879, Patrick Manson had shown that the embryos of *Wuchereria bancrofti* were transmitted by culex mosquitos. Other investigators added other filaria to the insect-borne category – some with human hosts, others with animal hosts. By the 1890s, several researchers had begun to implicate mosquitos in the spread of disease, and Laveran suggested them as the vector for malaria. Patrick Manson and others showed that filiariasis could be found in the digestive tract of mosquitos which had bitten human victims. The breakthrough came in 1897–8, when Ronald Ross showed that bird malaria in India was transmitted by culex mosquitos, while Italian scientists showed the connection between malaria and anopheles mosquitos. In 1898, Ross finally worked out the complex life cycle of the plasmodia as they moved back and forth between people and mosquitos, parasitizing both.[12]

These discoveries suggested new forms of prevention. Ross's work led to the organization of antimosquito brigades throughout the tropical British Empire. The French Academy of Medicine appointed a blue-ribbon committee of tropical medical specialists, with Laveran as rapporteur. In 1901, its report called first, for the eradication of dan-

---

au pays chauds," AHMC 3:305–414 (1900), pp. 397–402; Vallin, Kelsch, Raillet, Blanchard, and Laveran, "Instruction pour le prophylaxie du paudisme," AMPM, 39:160–7 (1901), pp. 160–7; A. M. Kermorgant, "Prophylaxie du paudisme," AHMC, 9:18–46 (1906); J. Rieux and Paul Hormus, "Note sur le paludisme dans le Maroc occidental," AMPM, 62:1–32 (1913).

But the following either disapproved of or failed to mention the possibility: Colin, *Fièvre Intermittents*; Achille Louis Félix Kelsch and Paul Louis Keiner, *Traité des maladies des pays chauds, région prétropicale* (Paris, 1889), pp. 877–2; Pierre Navarre, *Manuel d'hygiène coloniale* (Paris, 1895), p. 430; J. Lane Notter. "The Hygiene of the Tropics," in *Hygiene & Diseases of Warm Climates*, ed. Davidson, p. 67; F. H. Treherne, "Quinine in Malarial Fever," JRAMC, 9:276–81 (1907), pp. 76–81; J. B. Anderson, "Malaria in India," JRAMC, 14:50–60 (1910), pp. 50–7; P. S. Lelean, "Quinine as a Malarial Prophylactic: A Criticism," JRAMC, 17:463–80 (1911), p. 480; H. N. Thompson, "The Prophylactic Use of Quinine," JRAMC, 21:587–9 (1913); W. E. Huddleston, "An Analysis of Our Present Position with Regard to the Prevention and Cure of Malarial Infections," JRAMC, 21:320–38 (1913), pp. 320–38.

[11] David F. Clyde, *History of the Medical Services of Tanganyika* (Dar-es-Salaam, 1962), p. 20.

[12] Alphonse Laveran, *Du paludisme et de son hémotozaire* (Paris, 1891); J. Lane Notter, "Report on the Progress of Hygiene for the Year 1897," AMSR, 38:323–41 (1896), p. 336; Henry Harold Scott, *A History of Tropical Medicine*, 2 vols. (London, 1939), pp. 159–69. For the history of malariology in general, see Gordon Harrison, *Mosquitos, Malaria, and Man* (New York, 1978).

gerous mosquitos, and then for the the isolation of infected persons from any possible contact with mosquitos, so as to break the chain of infection through the parasitized human. The committee also restated and reinforced common antimalarial practices of recent decades – especially those that would work just as well against mosquitos as against miasma – drainage, cultivation, and clearing of undergrowth. For personal prophylaxis, it recommended mosquito nets, screening, care in choosing mosquito-free sleeping quarters, the use of punkahs and other aids to ventilation, and, for European visitors to malarious regions, 20 centigrams of sulphate of quinine every day, or 40 centigrams every other day.[13] The telluric theory nevertheless lived on. The committee's final recommendation was that Europeans should not be employed in agriculture or in digging that involved the upturning of the earth. "Nègres," who alone were thought to have a degree of immunity, should be assigned this work in their place.[14]

European medical opinion soon settled on four points that became dominant in malaria prevention in the first decades of this century – mosquito eradication, prophylactic quinine, segregation of victims, and personal protection from mosquitos. The success of the anti–yellow fever campaigns in the American tropics reinforced the importance of eradicating mosquitos, but without the same success. The anopheline genus was large and diverse; not all species carried malaria, in any case; some were comparatively easy to control; others have so far proved to be uncontrollable.

The use of prophylactic quinine also grew. Studies made in the 1890s showed the actual effect of the drug on plasmodia in human blood. Robert Koch investigated malaria in the Dutch East Indies and in East Africa and placed his personal prestige behind a recommendation for the prophylactic quininization of whole colonial populations, European and non-European alike, as the first line of defense against malaria.[15]

Mosquito nets for personal protection had been common for decades, but were far from universal in the tropical world. Americans in the United States had long since been using metal gauze door and window screens against flies and mosquitoes, although Europeans had almost never used them at home, and rarely in the tropics. Americans carried their habit of screening to Cuba and Panama, and their success in eradicating yellow fever and reducing malaria gave this form of personal protection a new popularity elsewhere.

[13] Vallin and others, *Prophylaxie de Paludisme*, pp. 160–7.

[14] "Dans des pays où l'endémie palustre règne avec beaucoup d'intensité, les Européens ne doivent pas être employés aux travaux agricoles ni aux travaux de terrassement; les nègres, qui jouissent d'une immunité réelle, quoique incomplète, pour le paludisme, seront employés de préférence pour ces travaux" (Vallin and others, *Prophylaxie du paludisme*, p. 167).

[15] P. D. Curtin, "Medical Knowledge and Urban Planning in Tropical Africa," AHR, 90:594–613 (1985).

One purpose of screening was segregation, and segregation took two forms – to screen the mosquitos away from malaria victims, and to protect non-victims from infected mosquitos. It was relatively simple to provide antimosquito protection for men in hospital, in an effort to prevent a new generation of mosquitos from acquiring the disease and passing it on. The problem came with malaria victims who were not in the hospital. Medical authorities had once believed that non-Europeans were more or less immune to malaria, so that only European victims would need that kind of protection. It soon became clear, however, that local populations in the tropics were far from immune. On the contrary, they were often infested with the parasite from childhood, even though they rarely showed clinical symptoms as adults. With the new knowledge about sources of infection, local children, who *did* show clinical symptoms, were considered especially dangerous. The result was a spate of projects for the sanitary segregation of European troops and officials away from the "native quarters" of African and Asian towns.

In theory, any one of these major lines of antimalaria action, even sanitary segregation, might have worked. If any one of them had been perfectly successful, the others would have been redundant. In the dozen years before the First World War, the military medical journals were full of articles favoring one over the others. Quinine was, by this time, almost universally accepted, but the *Journal of the Royal Army Medical Corps* nevertheless published a number of articles by military doctors with Indian or Chinese experience who opposed quinine and favored one of the other lines of attack.[16]

In the West Indies, mosquito control was the front line of antimalarial defense. It began even before the discovery of the mosquito vector. In 1898, the chief military medical officer on Jamaica reported that malaria had declined sharply at Up-Park Camp once the nearby brush had been cleared away. But the telluric theory was also current; the same officer reported the deleterious consequences of upturning the earth to build the Kingston sewage system and a new barracks on St. Lucia.[17]

From 1901 onward, as the mosquito theory became known, West Indian explanations changed slightly, often accommodating the old and the new. Upturning the earth could still be blamed – as on Barbados – for the breeding opportunities that uneven soil presented after heavy rains. Officials on St. Lucia began to worry about the "native town," and "native troops" – now presumed to be infected

---

[16] Treherne, "Quinine in Malarial Fever," pp. 76–81; Anderson, "Malaria in India," pp. 50–7; Lelean, "Quinine," p. 480; Thompson, "Prophylactic Quinine," pp. 587–9; Huddleston, "Prevention and Cure of Malarial Fevers," pp. 320–38.
[17] AMSR, 39:111 (1898).

Table 6.3. *Health Indicators for Malaria, European Troops in India and the British West Indies, 1886–1914*

| | Rates per Thousand Mean Strength | | | |
Date and Location	Admitted	Died	Invalided/ Discharged	Constantly Sick
1886–94				
India	361.90	0.74	1.75	11.13
West Indies	42.70	0.97	0.58	1.86
1895–1904				
India	291.40	0.62	3.96	10.81
Jamaica	84.9	0.84	0.84	3.98
1909–13				
India	126.60	0.18	0.04	4.29
West Indies	89.5	1.52	0	4.73

Source: Appendix tables.

rather than immune, and the West African precedent for sanitary segregation had a hearing. Some authorities began to recommend antimosquito screening for barracks and hospitals, but little or nothing was done. After the bulk of the troops were concentrated on Jamaica, screening was installed only at selected barracks where brush clearing was impractical. By 1902, the Army response at Port Royal was to move all European troops away in the warm season – either to the Newcastle or to a second high-altitude establishment at Greenwich Ridge. Prophylactic quinine may also have been used, but the annual reports said little or nothing about it.[18]

In India, malaria was a far less serious cause of death than it was in the Caribbean. The principal Indian plasmodium was *P. vivax* – which was far less fatal than the *P. Falciparum* more common in the West Indies. In the early twentieth century, surveys in India showed two hospital admissions with *vivax* for each admission with *falciparum*.[19] The difference appears in the full set of health indicators over the period from 1886 to 1914 (Table 6.3). India had more admissions, more men invalided, and more men in hospital per thousand, but the West Indies had more deaths. Much of India was comparatively safe in any event. In 1894, only three districts of Madras Presidency reported any malaria deaths – Rangoon, Mandalay, and Madras District itself. In

[18] AMSR, 43:97 (1901); AMSR, 44:103 (1902); AMSR, 45:101 (1903); AMSR, 46:132, 138 (1904); AMSR, 42:80 (1912).
[19] AMSR, 51:79–81 (1909); AMSR, 46:286–97 (1904).

1913, only five of the eleven divisions of the Indian Army reported any malaria deaths.[20]

As in the West Indies, the Indian authorities had a wide choice of antimalarial methods. After 1904, all stations were supposed to administer prophylactic quinine at the rate of 15 grains a week, but some units did so more methodically than others.[21] Some medical officers were still suspicious of quinine – afraid that it could reawaken dormant cases, that it would destroy white corpuscles, and much more – and simply refused to use it prophylactically.[22]

The favorite antimalarial measure was mosquito eradication, which was tried everywhere. The least favorite was screening – either fixed screening for barracks or mosquito nets over individual beds. The British may have resisted screening because it was uncommon in Britain, or perhaps because of deep-seated beliefs about bathing, body odor, and ventilation. As one medical officer wrote of screening; "It would be very expensive, it would gravely interfere with ventilation, it would render the atmospheric temperature in the rooms, already oppressive enough, during the rains almost unbearable. It would render necessary that abomination the spring door, which invariably gets broken."[23]

In spite of the considerable investment in mosquito brigades, the Indian army refused until 1912 to issue mosquito nets to all soldiers – on grounds of expense – although individual regiments sometimes found funds to do so, and individuals who could afford a net could always buy their own.[24] It seems fair to say that the sharp drop in European death from malaria in 1909–13 was due to a combination of prophylactic quinine and mosquito control – not nets and screening.

Without annual local reports like those of the British Army Medical Department, it is impossible to know what antimalarial measures the French Army actually took in Algeria, as opposed to those recommended. Whatever they were, they worked. In the 1860s, malaria accounted for a fifth of all deaths among French troops in Algeria – as it did in the West Indies. In the years 1909–13, it still accounted for a fifth of all deaths among British troops in the West Indies, but only 7 percent of deaths among French troops in Algeria.

Tuberculosis

The largely unexplained rise and fall of tuberculosis in Europe is clearly reflected in the military statistics. The disease was epidemic in Europe

[20] AMSR 36:139 (1894); AMSR, 49:89–90 (1907); AMSR, 55:45–7 (1913).
[21] AMSR, 46:286–97 (1904).
[22] Treherne, "Quinine in Malarial Fever," pp. 76–81; Thompson, "Prophylactic Quinine," pp. 587–9.
[23] Huddleston, "Malarial Infections," pp. 336–7.
[24] Anderson, "Malaria in India," pp. 50–7; AMSR, 55:45–7 (1913).

from the seventeenth century, and rose to become the single largest killer in many European countries by the early nineteenth. After 1850, it began a gradual decline with no known cause; it was not until the 1950s that the new antibiotics made some cases curable.[25]

For European troops overseas, tuberculosis tended to be a relocation benefit, but the level of benefit diminished statistically through time – simply because European death rates from tuberculosis also fell, and they declined more rapidly than the death rates of Europeans abroad. They dropped more rapidly in France than they did in Algeria; and they dropped more rapidly in Britain than they did in either the British West Indies or India. By 1909-13, relocation benefits were either absent or insignificant (see Tables 4.7 and 6.4).

When men served only about three years overseas – as they did in this period – the interaction of certain diseases and place of death may be uncertain. The tubercular bacillus is usually fairly inactive and slow to make serious inroads on its adult victim – though one variety common among children can lead to a rapid death. The infection was mainly spread by droplets injected into the air by coughing or spitting. Crowding and general lack of cleanliness at the home and workplace encouraged its spread. The victim's general level of health, including nutrition from childhood onward, made him more or less vulnerable. Soldiers whose tuberculin condition was first identified on tropical duty may well have been infected months or years before. By the same token, infection acquired on tropical duty might not appear until the victims returned home. The general openness of tropical life with more time outdoors and a greater flow of air through barracks should explain part of the relocation benefit. These conditions should certainly have reduced the rate of initial infection, and they may have made the disease more benign, once acquired. Medical people by the nineteenth century had long accorded some therapeutic value to sunshine, warm climates, and rest – especially rest in sanatoria located high in the mountains.[26]

The advantages of the tropics were not lost on the European and North American medical practitioners. As early as steamship transportation became available, a few tuberculosis sufferers began to find their way to the American tropics, often seeking to combine the advantages of the tropical climate with those of high altitudes – like those of European sanatoria. By the 1880s, some North Americans with lung problems went to the West Indies for the winter, especially to Cuba, but also to Jamaica, the Danish West Indies, and the Bahamas. In 1889, the advantages of highland Mexico were publicized by a team from

[25] Selman A. Waksman, *The Conquest of Tuberculosis* (Berkeley, 1966). For a summary account, see Marfarlane Burnet and David O. White, *Natural History of Infectious Disease*, 4th ed. (Cambridge, 1972), pp. 213–24; Roderick E. McGrew, *Encyclopedia of Medical History* (New York, 1985), pp. 336–50.

[26] Waksman, *Conquest of Tuberculosis*, pp. 48–64.

Table 6.4. *Deaths from Tuberculosis, 1860s to 1913*

Date	Deaths per Thousand					Percentage of All Deaths from Disease				
	France	Britain	Algeria	India	British West Indies	France	Britain	Algeria	India	British West Indies
1860s	2.09	3.16	1.51	2.23	1.62	21.85	37.62	10.81	11.23	10.18
1870s	1.25	2.55	1.57	1.63	1.76	13.67	33.17	12.37	9.25	22.92
1880s	0.81	2.08	0.69	0.90	0.94	9.97	34.61	7.17	8.19	5.24
1890s	0.85	0.93	0.86	0.83	0.19	19.78	21.58	10.14	6.23	2.39
1900s	0.84	0.59	0.83	0.77	0.71	23.82	16.76	12.63	5.82	9.62
1909–13	0.76	0.25	0.73	0.24	0.52	26.06	12.82	15.22	6.35	7.19

Source: As for Table 6.2. In the period 1862–6, the French recorded some pthisis as chronic bronchitis. The data here for the 1860s therefore combine totals for *bronchite* and *phthsie pulmonaire*, for France and Algeria. For Britain, India, and the British West Indies, as of 1903, the Army Medical Department introduced the practice of invaliding all confirmed tuberculosis patients from the service. Many deaths after that date were therefore counted as civilian deaths (Simpson, "Tuberculosis," JRAMC, 12:21 [1909]).

Heidelberg University. At least one sufferer from tuberculosis moved to Senegal and recovered, although, for Europeans in general, Senegal in the 1880s was one of the most dangerous places on earth.[27]

For civilians in Europe in the second half of the nineteenth century, tuberculosis was more serious for men than for women; it was most serious for postadolescents between fifteen and thirty-four years of age, especially for those in the twenty to twenty-four age group. It was therefore worst of all for men of military age. Early in the century, barracks life was recognized to be more deadly than civilian life for the same age group, yet in Britain after the 1860s the deaths from tuberculosis were greater among civilians aged fifteen to thirty-four than they were among the military stationed at home.[28] This was, in turn, part of a broader trend, as the military death rate dropped more rapidly than that of civilians of the same age.

Pulmonary Diseases

Diseases of the respiratory system are a more problematical category – in the early century, this was little more than a catchall phrase for lung disease. By the 1860s, pulmonary pthisis, or tuberculosis of the lung, was listed separately, leaving pneumonia as the most serious disease in the group, accounting for about three-quarters of respiratory deaths in 1909–13. But pneumonia is not really a disease. It is a condition of pulmonary infection caused by a variety of different agents. Medical men in the nineteenth century sometimes distinguished pneumonia, bronchial pneumonia, and bronchitis, but separation into these subcategories must have been extremely uncertain. So, too, was the distinction between any of these and influenza in periods when influenza was listed separately. Pneumonia was also sometimes listed separately, but not often enough to make separate tabulation useful. All of this calls for a wider-than-usual margin for error.

Pulmonary death rates dropped substantially in all five of the samples, both in Europe and abroad (Table 6.5), but with more improvement in Europe than overseas – and they lagged behind the falling death rates from other causes.[29] The stability of these death rates is less

---

[27] Daniel Henry Culimore, *The Book of Climates: Acclimatization, Climatic Diseases, Health Resorts and Mineral Springs, Sea Sickness, Sea Voyages, and Sea Bathing* (London, 1890), pp. 236–7; Georges Félix Treille, *Principles d'hygiène coloniale* (Paris, 1899), pp. 34–7.

[28] Tuberculosis deaths as a percentage of all deaths:

	1860s	1870s	1880s	1890s	1900s
Troops stationed in Britain	37.62	33.17	34.61	21.58	16.76
Civilian males aged 14–34	43.3	40.6	40.2	37.5	38.2

Source: Table 6.4; Gillian Cronjé, "Tuberculosis and Mortality Decline in England and Wales, 1851–1910," in *Urban Disease and Mortality in Nineteenth-Century England*, ed. Robert Woods and John Woodward (New York, 1984), p. 84.

[29] The slight rise in deaths from this cause reported for Jamaica in 1909–13 runs counter to the trend, but the Jamaican evidence is less reliable than most.

Table 6.5. *Deaths from Diseases of the Respiratory System, 1860s to 1913*

Date	Deaths per Thousand					Percentage of All Deaths from Disease				
	France	Britain	Algeria	India	British West Indies	France	Britain	Algeria	India	British West Indies
1860s	1.07	1.32	1.18	0.67	0.44	11.19	15.71	8.40	3.59	2.75
1870s	1.43	1.32	1.35	0.57	0.27	15.64	17.19	10.69	2.80	3.52
1880s	0.95	1.30	0.75	0.47	1.13	11.78	21.63	7.77	4.28	6.30
1890s	0.80	1.31	1.01	0.89	0.68	18.47	30.39	11.84	6.23	8.56
1900s	0.84	0.99	0.83	0.76	0.28	23.82	28.13	12.63	5.74	3.79
1909–13	0.65	0.41	0.77	0.37	0.52	22.27	21.15	16.14	9.79	7.18

Source: As for Table 6.2. Included pneumonia, bronchitis, bronchopneumonia, etc., when listed separately.

Table 6.6. *Deaths from Cholera, 1860s to 1900s*

Date	Deaths per Thousand			Percentage of All Deaths from Disease		
	France	India	Algeria	France	Algeria	India
1860s	0.53	2.76	0.50	5.49	3.59	13.90
1870s	0.09	1.58	0.02	1.01	0.16	8.97
1880s	0.09	1.12	0.21	1.07	2.16	10.19
1890s	0.03	1.42	0.10	0.79	1.17	10.66
1900s	0.00	0.55	0.00	0.00	0.00	4.15
1909–13	0.00	0.13	0.00	0.00	0.00	3.44

Source: See Table 6.2.

of a puzzle than the decline of tuberculosis. The pneumococcus, the bacterium that most often caused pneumonia, was isolated in 1882, and a variety of subtypes were soon identified; but no effective treatment was introduced until the sulfonamides came along in the late 1930s. Nor could improvements in drinking water and sewage disposal be expected to have any effect on a disease mainly transmitted by contact or through the air.[30] The quality of nutrition is thought to play an important role in the outcome of most respiratory infections,[31] and improved nutrition may possibly account for what change did take place.

Climate, however, seems to have played a larger role. These infections were associated epidemiologically with winter weather in northern Europe. It is hardly surprising that respiratory diseases were among the relocation benefits overseas (second only to tuberculosis), or that the incidence varied with the coolness of the cool season – lowest in the West Indies, a little higher in India, and still higher in Algeria. By 1909–13, however, Europe's improved record in pulmonary health tended to wipe out the colonial advantage.

Cholera

Although the earlier and worst of the cholera pandemics had disappeared in Europe, North Africa, and the West Indies by the mid 1870s, the fifth and sixth were still to come. The fifth pandemic began in 1881 and carried on until 1896, hitting Europe in 1884 to 1887, especially southern Europe. It missed Britain, and failed to make the

[30] Roberick E. McGrew, *Encyclopedia of Medical History*, pp. 268–72.
[31] Robert I. Rotberg and Theodore K. Rabb (eds.), *Hunger and History: The Impact of Changing Food Production and Consumption Patterns on Society* (New York, 1985), pp. 305–8.

Atlantic crossing, but it did sweep across all of North Africa in 1893; and it reached across the Sahara to both Western and Nilotic Sudans in 1894.[32] Table 6.6 is therefore limited to Algeria, France, and India, although the fifth pandemic made little mark on either France or Algeria.

The usual numbering of pandemics includes a sixth beginning about 1899 and extending into the 1920s, but it was confined to South Asia.[33] Cholera deaths among British soldiers, even in India, remained at an annual average of less than 1 per thousand. Cholera's contribution to relocation costs slipped below the combination of gastrointestinal diseases plus typhoid. In 1909–13, it even dropped behind malaria (see Chapter 4).

It would be convenient to associate this improvement with the progress of sanitary engineering outlined in Chapter 5, but dysentery and typhoid were equally waterborne, and they declined less dramatically. Part of the difference may be that cholera's frightening symptoms and case-fatality rate spurred investigation. Cholera was the first disease to be identified as being water borne; by the early 1870s, investigators had begun a microscopic search for cholera "germs" in water and in the victims' blood, intestines, and stools. When Robert Koch isolated the *Vibrio cholerae* in 1883, it was one of the earliest microorganisms to be identified as the cause of a major disease.[34]

Until well into the 1880s, some scientists still denied that cholera could be carried by water. In the absence of solid knowledge as to what "good" water was, it was always possible to claim that an afflicted location *had* "good" water and that the disease must therefore have some other cause. Where nothing could be demonstrated scientifically, one opinion was as good as another, and the range of medical opinion in the 1870s was as broad as it had been in the 1840s. As late as 1873, in the Ninth Annual Report of the Sanitary Commission for India, Dr. Cunningham claimed it was then "known" that cholera could not be transmitted by contact, by food, by water, or through the air. But the widespread belief in transmission by water held up, and it was confirmed by Cornish's careful detective work in his survey of cholera and its transmission in southern India.[35]

[32] R. Pollitzer, *Cholera* (Geneva, 1959), pp. 38–40.

[33] Pollitzer, *Cholera*, pp. 41–8.

[34] Edmund A. Parkes, "Report on Hygiene for 1871," AMSR, 12:226–59 (1870), pp. 231–2; E. A. Parkes, "Report on Hygiene for the Year 1873," AMSR, 15:220–56 (1872), pp. 252–5.

[35] AMSR, 13:212–13 (1871); E. A. Parkes, "Report on Hygiene for the Year 1872," AMSR, 13:174–201 (1871), pp. 182–8; E. A. Parkes, "Report on Hygiene for the Year 1873," AMSR, 15:220–56 (1872), pp. 252–5; W. R. Cornish, *A Record of the Progress of Cholera in 1870, and Resumé of the Records of Former Epidemic Invasions of the Madras Presidency* (Madras, 1871).

The British in India still had two lines of preventive action – pure water and flight. In 1881 and again in 1883, the main force of infantry and artillery at Kamptee in Madras Presidency was moved under canvas. In the first instance, cholera persisted, and the force moved once more. In the second, the move worked; cholera continued at the old barracks site but died out at the camp.[36]

By 1913, preventive water purification was so successful that only five European soldiers were admitted to hospital with cholera in all of India. It was still impossible to attack the vibrio itself, but doctors had a new source of direct therapy. Cholera victims die from dehydration, not from the microbe's damage to the body. In India in 1913, cholera victims began to be treated with intravenous injections of "Rogers' hypertonic saline solution" to combat dehydration. As a result, the case-fatality rate fell from 55 percent in 1911 – the usual rate up to then – to 20 percent in 1913.[37]

Intestinal Diseases

"Diseases of the digestive system" formed another confusing nineteenth-century category. In British army usage, it came to include any disorder of the entire gastrointestinal tract, from dental caries to hemorrhoids, which makes it useless for analyzing morbidity. On the other hand, few people died of caries or hemorrhoids; most of the deaths were caused by one or another of the common waterborne intestinal infections. Both the French- and British-published statistics listed cholera and typhoid fever separately. They also sometimes distinguished dysentery from diarrhea, but in practice the distinction came down to loose stools with bleeding as against loose stools without bleeding. Both can be merged into a general gastrointestinal category, although it would exclude cholera and typhoid fever (Table 6.7).

Under this large category, army reports listed several different causes of death. In Madras over 1886–94, the heading covered twenty-one separate diseases, but the six most numerous accounted for 94 percent of all deaths in the category as a whole.[38] Of these, "diarrhea" serious enough to cause death was probably a form of dysentery. "Liver abscesses" were most likely amoebic dysentery. Lumped together with "dysentery," they would bring the total of various dysenteries up to 69 percent of the total, and part of the category, "hepatitis," may well have been a form of dysentery rather than viral

---

[36] AMSR, 23:82 (1881); AMSR, 25:98 (1883).

[37] AMSR, 53:45–6 (1911); AMSR, 55:48 (1913).

[38] In order of importance in deaths per thousand per year, these were abscess of the liver 1.13, dysentery 1.07, hepatitis 0.68, peritonitis 0.09, diarrhea 0.08, and intestinal inflamation 0.06. Total deaths per thousand from gastrointestinal diseases as a whole were 3.3 per thousand.

Table 6.7. Deaths from Diseases of the Digestive System, 1860s to 1900s

| Date | Deaths per Thousand | | | | | Percentage of All Deaths from Disease | | | | |
	France	Britain	Algeria	India	British West Indies	France	Britain	Algeria	India	British West Indies
1860s	1.14	0.77	2.68	7.03	1.28	11.91	9.21	19.06	35.40	8.08
1870s	1.09	0.55	1.49	6.74	0.70	8.63	7.16	10.90	38.25	7.00
1880s	0.76	0.49	1.23	3.23	1.51	9.38	8.15	12.78	29.39	8.42
1890s	0.28	0.37	0.71	2.52	0.78	6.43	8.58	8.29	18.92	9.82
1900s	0.32	0.32	0.58	2.69	0.64	9.22	9.09	8.76	20.30	8.68
1909–13	0.19	0.28	0.50	1.01	0.52	6.61	14.36	10.33	26.72	7.18

Source: As for Table 6.2. Total includes diseases of the digestive system plus diarrhea and dysentery when listed separately. Includes diseases of the liver and spleen when listed separately.

hepatitis B. This leaves only "peritonitis" and "intestinal inflammation" of uncertain origin, but most of the category was certainly some
form of dysentery.

Medical investigators had already begun to identify the responsible
agents. Living amoeba were discovered in the stools of victims as early
as 1859. In 1875, Frederick Lösch identified *Entamoeba histolica* and
showed its role in transmitting the disease from one person to another.
In 1898, Kiyoshi Shigu of Japan isolated one of the bacilli responsible
for bacillary dysentery, the first known representative of the genus
now called shigella. None of these manifestations was, or is, peculiarly
tropical, although transmission through fecal contamination made
them dangerous where water supplies were contaminated, or in
crowded conditions like those of a military camp.[39]

Several of these dysenteries could be treated with the drug ipecac,
derived from the root of the Brazilian plant, *Cephaëlis ipecacuanha*. It had
been known from the seventeenth century. By the 1830s, the effective
agent had been isolated and was used in a variety of medicines, often
combined with calomel and opium. These drugs no doubt reduced the
death rate, but improved water supply was more important still.[40]

Water supply improved in some places faster than others. Gastrointestinal death rates in France, Britain, Algeria, and the British West
Indies in the 1860s were at a similar level – about 1 per thousand (Table
6.7) – and they fell regularly from one decade to the next with the
gradual improvement of sanitary engineering. In Britain after 1900,
military and civilian death rates from this cause were nearly the
same.[41] Gastrointestinal death rates were a little higher for French
troops in Algeria than in France itself, but in the British West Indies
they never accounted for more than 9 percent of annual average relocation costs (Table 4.9). On the whole, deaths from this cause dropped at
about the same rate as mortality in general.

Gastrointestinal deaths in India were at another level altogether. In
the 1860s, 1870s, and 1880s, they were about a third of all deaths and
accounted for more than half of the relocation cost. With the 1890s and
improved water supply, even the Indian death rate began to drop, but
it was still higher there than elsewhere.

---

[39] Acherknecht, *History and Geography, of the most Important Diseases* (New York, 1965),
pp. 47–50; McGrew, *Encyclopedia*, pp. 104–5;

[40] R. J. C. Hoeppli, *Parasitic Disease in Africa and the Western Hemisphere: Early Documentation and Transmission by the Slave Trade* (Basel, 1969), pp. 62–3; Pluchon, *Médecins de
marine*, pp. 155–6.

[41] Samuel H. Preston, Nathan Keyfitz, and Robert Schoen, in *Causes of Death: Life Tables
of National Populations* (New York and London, 1972), pp. 224–47 assembled cause-of-
death data for the population of England and Wales over these same decades. Deaths
from their category of "diarrheal disease" correspond to those reported here for the
military. Other categories of disease, however, are too different from military usage to
make a comparison useful.

New drugs made some difference. In India, amoeba accounted for about two-thirds of all dysentery. In the early twentieth century, when hydrochloride of emetine (a derivative of ipecacuanha) became available, direct therapy came to the aid of prevention. In 1913, British medical authorities in India believed that emetine made possible a 50 percent decrease in deaths from amoebic dysentery and liver abscesses.[42]

Typhoid Fever

Typhoid fever poses another diagnostic problem. In the early nineteenth century it was listed under continued fevers – as distinct from the paroxysmal fevers like malaria. The "continued" category also included typhus, typhoid, and "fever of unknown origin." Some doctors in the 1850s began to distinguish typhus from typhoid, and typhoid fever appears on the French military medical records from their beginning in 1862. British records, however, made no distinction between "enteric" and other "continued fevers" until the late 1870s.[43] Typhoid fever is, in any event, hard to diagnose accurately; its symptoms can resemble a range of other diseases from yellow fever and malaria to infectious hepatitis.

In spite of diagnostic problems, the military medical records are fairly consistent between countries and over the decades, and therefore suggest some trends and comparisons, if not complete reliability by present-day medical standards (Table 6.8). Military doctors consistently reported typhoid fever as several times more fatal in France than in Britain. This may suggest that French military doctors tended to file uncertain cases under the typhoid label. If so, they did it consistently decade after decade.

The typhoid death rate was markedly higher in Algeria and India than it was in the West Indies, although its contribution to total relocation costs was about the same (Table 4.9). The West Indian advantage was probably the safe water supply and waterborne sewage of the Barbados Command. The most serious West Indian outbreaks all occurred at Newcastle in Jamaica, where the dry earth system persisted longest, and the mountain location made it hard to dispose of excreta far from the post.[44] Its altitude may thus have saved deaths from malaria, but it cost deaths from typhoid.

Typhoid deaths declined with a different timing in Algeria and in

[42] AMSR, 55:50–1 (1913). Although it was effective at the time, emetine is no longer used because of the danger of adverse side effects and the availability of better drugs.
[43] British records used "enteric" in preference to the French use of "typhoid" through the nineteenth century. When paratyphoid was distinguished in the early twentieth, enteric became a cover term for typhoid and paratyphoid together.
[44] AMSR, 15:75–6 (1873); AMSR, 21:40 (1879).

Table 6.8. Deaths from Typhoid Fever, 1860s to 1900s

Date	Deaths per Thousand					Percentage of All Deaths from Disease				
	France	Britain	Algeria	India	British West Indies	France	Britain	Algeria	India	British West Indies
1860s	1.93	—	2.16	—	—	20.23	—	18.50	—	—
1870s	3.40	—	3.50	—	—	37.28	—	27.68	—	—
1880s	4.34	0.18	4.10	1.51	1.32	53.66	3.00	42.63	13.37	7.36
1890s	0.98	0.27	3.66	5.11	3.01	22.80	6.26	43.05	38.36	35.39
1900s	0.59	0.21	2.74	5.62	0.88	16.77	5.97	41.79	42.42	11.79
1909–13	0.27	0.06	1.50	0.62	1.03	9.08	3.08	31.12	16.40	14.23

— Not distinguished from other continued fevers in British records until 1880s.
Source: As in Table 4.3.

India. The French death rate reached a peak in 1880 – 1881 for Algeria and Tunisia. These rates then fell steeply over the next decade to less than a third of the peak rate in each of the three territories. This success was widely associated with the general introduction of the Pasteur–Chamberland water filters in army posts at home and in North Africa.[45] In British India, on the other hand, 1881 was a low point – both for mortality and morbidity. After that, hospital admissions and deaths both rose steeply over exactly the same years they were declining in France. In 1898, the Indian typhoid death rate reached its peak at 10 per thousand, as against only 2 per thousand in 1881; although it dropped again to 3 per thousand by 1901.[46]

In general, typhoid deaths in this period began to fall sooner or later, but only after rising. This poses a problem. Death rates from cholera and the gastrointestinal group fell systematically in Britain, France, and the three overseas sample territories (see Tables 6.6 and 6.7). The obvious explanation is the steady improvement of water supply and sewage disposal. Why was typhoid fever different?

Many medical people had suspected for some time that typhoid fever was also waterborne, as was confirmed after the identification of *Bacillus typhosus* by Karl Joseph Eberth in 1880 and further studies by Georg Gaffky later in the decade. The medical authorities in India were therefore especially puzzled and alarmed in the 1890s, as death rates continued to rise in spite of what they regarded as their success in providing clean water. They suspected that the typhoid bacillus could live in the soil and then be blown by the wind as dust. Investigation proved that it could not live long in the soil, but it *could* travel as blown dust if it were fresh enough.

The main line of investigation, however, implicated sewage systems. Experiments in the 1890s showed a positive correlation between the dry earth system and morbidity rates from enteric fever. The problem was transmission by insects. Before the end of the century, Edward B. Vedder of the U.S. Army argued that flies were capable of carrying cholera from the feces of one victim to the food of the next, and he suggested the same for typhoid as well. L. O. Howard, the American entomologist, followed up with still more detailed studies. G. H. F. Nuttall in Britain then published a general survey of insect-borne diseases, which drew new attention to the problem of flies – especially to flies that had access to latrines and latrine trenches in proximity to food preparation. By 1902, most authorities in India had come to

[45] Schneider, "Prophylaxie de la fièvre typhoïde dans l'armée française," TSICHD, 8:101–3 (1891); Ministère de Guerre, *Statistiques Médicales*, 1900, p. 31; J. C. Thresh, *The Examination of Water and Water Supplies*, 2d ed. (London, 1913) p. 249.
[46] AMSR, 46:255 (1904).

believe that typhoid affecting the troops was no longer a water problem but a sewage problem.[47]

From about 1904 onward, they launched a serious effort to block these sources of infection. The long-term goal was to move fully to the wet system. In the short run, they mounted a two-pronged attack. One was against flies – with special care to protect food storage, preparation, and eating places by screening. The second was to protect excrement from flies. Instead of taking it straight to the "filth trenches," feces were treated with chemical agents like saponified cresol or, preferably, incinerated. Wet excrement was still a problem; one solution was to heat it to 280° before burial.[48]

Drastic segregation of those who were infected was another kind of preventive action. New drafts of troops arriving in India were sent to separate parts of the camp, with their own latrine and cooking facilities, for a quarantine period of twenty-eight days. If any came down with typhoid, the period was extended. Individuals who became infected, especially convalescents, were sent to separate quarters – and anything they had worn or used was rigorously disinfected.[49]

After 1905, the Army Medical Department's Research Institute at Kasauli was especially concerned with the "carrier" problem. Recent research in Europe had shown that typhoid victims could discharge bacilli for long periods after an attack – even indefinitely. One German study estimated that up to 1 percent of the population might be long-term typhoid carriers.[50] Other studies showed that as many as 3 percent of all typhoid victims became carriers, if only for a short time. In India, one solution was to set up convalescent depôts in the hills, where all convalescents were held until tests established that they were no longer infectious. Genuine long-term carriers were treated to make them less harmful and discharged from the service.[51]

[47] J. Lane Notter, "Report on the Progress of Hygiene for the Year 1895," AMSR, 34:307–14 (1894), p. 313; Notter, "Report on the Progress of Hygiene for the Year 1896," AMSR, 37:279–90 (1895), p. 288–9; G. H. F. Nuttall, The Rôle of Insects, Archnids, and Myriapods as Carriers in the Spread of Bacterial and Parasitic Diseases of Man and Animals: A Critical and Historical Study (Baltimore,1899), pp. 30–1. AMSR, 54:104 (1907); R. H., Firth, "Report of the Progress of Hygiene from the year 1900–01," AMSR, 42:369–98 (1900), pp. 357–60; Notter, Spread and Distribution of Infectious Diseases; Spread of Typhoid Fever, Dysentery, and Allied Diseases among Large Communities, with Special Reference to Military Life in Tropical and Sub-Tropical Countries (London and Manchester, 1904) pp. 6–7; AMSR, 46:240–3 (1904). The French in Algeria also tended to suspect some source other than water (Granjux, "Etiologie de la fièvre jaune typhoïde dans l'armée d'Afrique," RHPS, 23:245–58 [1910], pp. 246–8). For a recent analysis, see James C. Riley, "Insects and European Mortality Decline," AHR, 91:833–58 (1986), p. 845.
[48] AMSR, 51:68–71, 74 (1909).
[49] AMSR, 46:248–51 (1904).
[50] AMSR, 49:96–8 (1907); AMSR, 50:76–7 (1908).
[51] AMSR, 51:70–1 (1909); AMSR, 52:43–5 (1910); AMSR, 55:41–2 (1913).

In the first decade of the century, immunization also entered the picture. Typhoid inoculation was used on a small, experimental scale from the late 1890s. It was made available on a voluntary basis to British troops leaving for service in the Anglo-Boer War. Results were uncertain at first. By 1905, however, improved vaccines and appropriate dosages showed a positive advantage. The army then made vaccination available on a voluntary basis to all troops leaving Britain for foreign stations. It was not until 1909, however, that as many as half of the British troops in India had actually been vaccinated with the two shots then required. By 1913, 93 percent of the troops in India had been vaccinated, along with most of the Indian food handlers and cooks.

By that time, other preventive measures were also showing signs of effectiveness. The annual average death rate from typhoid fever dropped from 3.1 per thousand in 1904–8 to 0.62 per thousand in 1909–14. Even the death rate of the noninoculated was down to 1.76 per thousand. For the inoculated, it was even lower, 0.15 per thousand, from paratyphoid and typhoid together.[52] The triumph was genuine, but, even in 1909–13, typhoid still accounted for 65 percent of the relocation cost of movement from France to Algeria, and for 31 percent of the cost of movement from Britain to India.

Diseases of the Central Nervous System

"Diseases of the nervous system" as a category was rarely among the four or five principal causes of death among the military, but the category was important both in India and in the West Indies (Table 6.9). It also poses a problem for retrospective analysis. None of the conditions that doctors then described or assigned to this group could be expected to produce death rates as high as 2 per thousand among men of military age. British authorities mentioned apoplexy and sunstroke, and delerium tremens. The French statistics of the 1860s carry a more detailed breakdown of "diseases of the brain and spinal cord," under which encephalitis, meningitis, cerebrospinal meningitis, and apoplexy were the principal killers. After 1875, the French renamed the category "nervous and cerebrospinal diseases."[53]

None of these possibilities, however, is a sufficient explanation. Sunstroke is no longer a recognized disease, although heatstroke is. It has a high case-fatality rate, but 2.2 *cases* (not deaths) per thousand

---

[52] W. B. Leishman, "The Progress of Anti-Typhoid Inoculation in the Army," JRAMC, 8:463–71 (1907); AMSR, 51:75–7 (1909); AMSR, 55:40–1 (1913).

[53] See, for example, France, Ministère de Guerre, *Statistiques médicales*, volume for 1865, p. 276; volume for 1875, p. 158.

Table 6.9. *Deaths from Diseases of the Brain and Nervous System, 1860s to 1913*

Date	Deaths per Thousand					Percentage of All Deaths from Disease				
	France	Britain	Algeria	India	British West Indies	France	Britain	Algeria	India	British West Indies
1860s	0.40	0.72	0.27	1.54	1.74	4.19	8.57	1.94	7.75	10.99
1870s	0.43	0.57	0.50	1.99	0.97	1.82	7.42	4.76	11.31	11.29
1880s	0.35	0.46	0.28	1.32	0.57	4.35	7.65	2.87	12.01	3.18
1890s	0.21	0.34	0.23	0.38	0.18	4.98	7.89	2.67	2.85	4.91
1900s	0.18	0.26	0.21	0.33	0.14	5.15	7.39	3.31	2.49	1.91
1909–13	0.19	0.16	0.20	0.19	0.00	6.38	8.21	4.11	5.03	0.00

Note: French classification changed in 1875. From that date the separate listings for encephalitis, meningitis, and cerebrospinal meningitis are aggregated as diseases of the nervous system.
Source: As for Table 6.2.

would be high in extreme conditions.[54] In 1886, in any event, the British army medical records removed "sunstroke" from the category of mental disease and placed it under injuries.[55] The change made little difference to the number of deaths from "diseases of the brain" although twenty-six of the thirty-eight deaths from injuries in Madras in 1886 were put down as either heatstroke or sunstroke. The other forms of stroke associated with blockage of cerebral blood supply are curiously missing from most of these records, although high levels of morbidity or mortality would not be expected from men of military age.

The French records mention cerebrospinal meningitis, which reached epidemic levels among European troops in Europe, but it was rare in England and unreported by name in either India or the West Indies. The most prominent epidemics struck soldiers in Algeria in 1901, and troops in France itself in 1909–11.[56] Even in epidemic years, the mortality rates per thousand were only 0.14 in Algeria and 0.16 in 1909 in France. In other years, the usual rate was about 0.06 per thousand in both France and Algeria.

This leaves a number of possibilities that were *not* mentioned at the time. Cerebral malaria could be added, along with the possibility of widespread lead poisoning. Some forms of beriberi also include a symptomatic loss of control over bodily motions, which might have been put down as a disease of the nervous system – especially in India where beriberi was likely to occur but rarely reported as such. The uncertainty is so great, however, that this category may properly belong to the heading "other and unknown," along with "debility" and "pyrexia of unknown origin." In any event, deaths per thousand from this cause dropped steeply after the 1880s, although it kept its relative ranking as a killing disease in Britain, France, and Algeria.

Venereal Disease

Venereal disease is an obvious component of mortality, but virtually impossible to take into account accurately. Death rates for acute early infections of gonorrhea and syphilis are low. Those who died at later stages of these diseases would already have been discharged from the service. Venereal disease was, nevertheless, the most important single cause of hospitalization in most nineteenth-century armies – at home or overseas.

There were, however, marked differences between morbidity rates in Europe and among European forces overseas, although they varied by

[54] G. Thomas Strickland (ed.), *Hunter's Tropical Medicine*, 6th ed. (Philadelphia, 1984), p. 875.
[55] AMSR, 37:131 (1886).
[56] France, Ministère de Guerre, *Statistiques médicale*, volume for 1914, facing p. 171.

disease. Between 1879 and 1913, the annual morbidity rate for syphilis among French soldiers in France was a nearly lineal curve with little variance – from a range of 8 to 10 hospital entries per thousand in the years centered on 1880, to 4 to 5 per thousand on the eve of the First World War. Morbidity in Algeria began at nearly the same level, but it rose steadily and systematically to about 20 per thousand. The relocation cost in morbidity from gonorrhea also increased, but, in this case, the hospital entries in North Africa were relatively constant at about 40 per thousand, while those in France dropped from that same level to only 11.7 in 1913.

British experience was quite different, although the difference could be in the mode of reporting. In the British service in all regions, admissions for venereal disease rose steadily to a peak in the 1880s or 1890s, then declined. The admission rate in India was not remarkably different from that in Britain itself, but the rate of infection in the West Indies was about three-quarters of the British and Indian rate up to 1909–13, when it fell less rapidly than the others.

Soldiers and Civilians

The record of the military doctors in France, Britain, and in their colonies was remarkable, not only in lowering death rates over the decades, but also in lowering military death rates compared with those of civilians. In the 1820s and 1830s, the death rate for soldiers in Britain was about 50 percent higher than it was for male civilians in the same age range. In France of the early nineteenth century, the contrast between military and civilians was similar, although death rates in the unhealthiest towns in either country were about the same as those of the military, and often twice those of the healthiest country districts.[57] Civilian mortality in England and Wales dropped by 22 percent between 1848–54 and 1901. Military mortality for British soldiers serving in the United Kingdom dropped by more than 80 percent over that same period, with equivalent changes in France.[58]

In the decade before the First World War, British military doctors published a number of articles calling attention to this achievement and to the reduced mortality overseas.[59] They and their French colleagues

---

[57] 1839, xvi [C.166], "Statistical Reports of the Sickness, Mortality, and Invaliding among Troops in the United Kingdom, Mediterranean, and British North America," by Major Alexander M. Tulloch, pp. 6–7, 21; Jean Chrisitan Marc François Joseph Boudin, *Statistique de l'état sanitaire des armées de terre et de mer* (Paris, 1846), p. 135; Great Britain, *Report of the Commissioners Appointed to Inquire into the Sanitary State of the Army in India*, p. x.

[58] See Woods and Woodward, *Urban Disease*, pp. 29–30 for the civilian rate; appendix tables for the military.

[59] C. H. Melville, "The Place of Sanitation as a Factor in Strategy," JRAMC, 11:64–9 (1908); Alfred Keogh, "The Results of Sanitation on the Efficiency of Armies in Peace

had every right to take pride in it,but it was as much an achievement of medical hygiene in general. The military statistics apply to a select, though large, segment of the population, but they also reflect the broader victory against infectious disease in Europe as well as the European ability to deal successfully with tropical conditions.

Military statistics over the long run from the early nineteenth to the early twentieth century need, however, to be read with some care as to interpretation. By the early twentieth century, civilians were somewhat more likely to die of disease than soldiers of the same age, and this pattern continued at least into the 1970s.[60] Both medical knowledge and military policy account for the change. Recruits were subject to medical examination, and medical knowledge and instruments in this century make it possible to detect problems that were hidden in the past. Countries with compulsory national service call up more men than the armies could possibly use. It is therefore common to reject men for trivial causes. Once in the service, free medical attention and frequent medical examinations kept the military healthier than their civilian counterparts. Those who were chronically unhealthy were discharged on medical grounds.

While these factors create a bias in military medical records, other factors give them a special value. Just as the soldiers received better care than civilians, military doctors took more care with statistical reporting, if only because their superior officers used these records for medical purposes. Civilian doctors also reported the cause of death, but the accuracy of their reports made little practical difference to their own practices.

Most of the victory over infectious disease in this period was the result of better preventive medicine, growing out of the scientific breakthrough following the discovery of the germ theory. The first decade and a half of the new century, however, brought with it two new factors. The first was the beginning of a new kind of immunization, represented here by the typhoid inoculation, but to be continued with a host of new measures over the next half-century and more. The second was the beginning of effective direct therapeutic intervention, illustrated here by new drugs against amoebic dysentery and new measures against dehydration for cholera victims. The effectiveness of either measure was only a beginning, but it forehadowed the direction of medical progress in the decades to come.

and War," JRAMC, 12:357–785 (1909); M. W. Russell, "Recent Tendencies in the Development of Army Medical Services," JRAMC, 4:178–86 (1905); R. H. Firth, "Fifty Years of Sanitary Effort," JRAMC, 21:654–9 (1913); E. Blake Knox, "Some Medical Notes on War," JRAMC, 4:440–6, 580–6 (1905), 5:230–9, 616–22 (1906), 7:703–14 (1907).

[60] Jacques Houdaille, "La mortalité (hors combat) des militaires français à la fin du XVIIIe et au debut du XIXe siècle," *Population*, numéro special: 481–97 (1977), esp. p. 482.

CONCLUSION

The real conclusions of this study are in the text itself – in the quantitative tables, the explanations that go with them, and the surveys of hygienic ideas and practices. It is not really necessary to sum up these findings, but one way to highlight the potentially important ones is to take a retrospective look at what was expected at the beginning of the study – as opposed to what was actually found. People who are well informed about the main currents of historical epidemiology might not be surprised, but my own surprise may illustrate some common perceptions that need to be modified.

The sheer size of the drop in mortality for men of military age was itself unexpected. Annual average death rates dropped by 85 to 95 percent between the earliest surveys of the 1820s and 1830s and the eve of the First World War. The ordinary view of the mortality revolution suggests a much more gradual process, beginning far back in the eighteenth century and continuing into the twentieth. This was no doubt true for the population as a whole; but the male population of military age was not typical of the whole, and that fact makes it more significant, not less. Raw mortality figures reflect the fact that everyone has to die sometime. In the absence of infective disease, few men between twenty and thirty years of age are likely to die. Few do today. What the military doctors and their civilian colleagues achieved in this period was to put an end to the vast majority of unnecessary deaths among the young – whether in Europe or in the tropics. It was simply the first and largest step toward a world in which infectious disease has ceased to be the main cause of death for this age group. Accidents, both unintentional and self-inflicted, have taken the place of disease, although at a much lower level of deaths per thousand.

A second source of surprise was the distribution of these changes through time. The normal expectation would have been a gradual decrease in death rates until perhaps the 1880s or 1890s, when scientific medicine and sanitary engineering began to be common in Europe and North America. Before that time, only smallpox inoculation and quinine for malarial regions brought a significant drop in death rates. Instead, the greatest drop in absolute death rates – in deaths per

159

thousand men – came over the mid nineteenth century both in Europe and overseas. The main cause was neither quinine nor smallpox inoculation, although both played some role. The improvement came instead from empirical measures, like moving troops into the highlands to escape malaria, moving them under canvas away from barracks and cities to escape cholera and yellow fever, or improving the water supply – even at a time when no one yet knew how safe and unsafe water could be identified. The size of this change between the 1840s and the 1860s was a drop of 59 deaths per thousand in Algeria, 51 deaths per thousand in the Windward and Leeward Command, 45 deaths per thousand in Jamaica, 22 deaths per thousand in Madras, and 11 deaths per thousand in Great Britain (Table 1.4). The sheer size of this change even in Great Britain – and its clear association with particular causes of death – tends to reduce the probable role of less demonstrable causes of mortality change, like nutrition.

Even relocation costs provided some surprises. The phenomenon in general had been known for some time. Historians of the United States have long been familiar with the high death rates in the early settlements. For the tropical world, the "white man's grave" of West Africa had been famous through the eighteenth century. In the early nineteenth, it was the recognition of relocation costs – though not under that name – that prompted military doctors to make the first statistical studies.

The popular view of historical epidemiology was that relocation costs were universal. It stood to reason that the human immune system worked best combating the parasites it had dealt with from childhood onward – although nineteenth-century doctors would not have phrased their knowledge in those terms. Perhaps for that reason, it was known but not widely recognized that mortality from tuberculosis and respiratory infections among Europeans decreased as they moved overseas. Nor was the existence of a Pacific region of relocation benefits widely publicized in the historical literature. It was known, of course, that the South and Central Pacific was generally free of malaria for lack of anophelines, but that was all. Curiously enough, the relocation benefits from tuberculosis and pneumonia tended to weaken and disappear in the later nineteenth century simply because death rates from these causes declined so steeply in Europe itself.

The relative stability of relocation costs was also unexpected. The obvious and dramatic drop in European deaths overseas suggests a convergence in age-specific death rates toward some point where the difference between European and overseas rates become negligible. Instead, the relative relocation costs remained stable in most cases, right down to the First World War. Further investigation of soldiers and travelers during the interwar years may show a convergence of death rates at a slightly later time, but the persistence of malaria and the recalcitrance of other disease, even in the face of modern medicine, may mean that relocation costs still exist at some level.

In human and political terms, these costs were staggering, and the role of disease in human history was clearly greater than is generally recognized. It was known that the overseas empire was expensive in human life, but historians have too seldom been conscious of that cost. Even this study can be faulted for expressing in gross statistical terms what must have been a terrible weight of individual human tragedy.

APPENDIX

STATISTICAL TABLES

The military medical records of the nineteenth century are a rich source, particularly because they were often collected following international agreements as to what should be included. One might therefore hope to compare the data by disease, territory, and territorial subdivisions – but this is not always possible. Medical reporting was carried out for conventional military units. Sometimes these units were too small to be statistically viable for a single year or a short period of years. The solution is to use an annual average for a series of years, but disease terminology has changed with time, and it is hard to create multiyear aggregates when the original compilers of the records changed the names of categories.

Military medical records are also different from many other archival records – at least in England and France. The official manuscript sources for political and military history, and for many kinds of social history, are carefully preserved in the Public Record Office and the Archives Nationales. Medical records were either collected and printed, or else they were destroyed. Neither the French nor the British archives kept the manuscript reports or the intermediate calculations that led to the published statistics. This makes it impossible to disaggregate data that were once aggregated for publication, or to search for records that seem valuable in retrospect but were not printed at the time.[1]

As a result, one often has to accept the aggregates that are offered.

[1] It is conceivable, of course, that some of these records were not destroyed – that their continued existence is simply not recorded. I have pursued the French records through the National Archives in all branches, including naval and army records at Vincennes, the headquarters of the Troupes Coloniales in Versailles, and the archive and library of the Hôpital de Val-de-Grâce (which does still have a small collection of unaggregated individual records from the Mexican intervention of the 1850s). In Britain they are not recorded by the Royal Manuscripts Commission at the Public Record Office, British Library, Wellcome Institute, or the Royal Army Medical Corps training center in London. They might be found, however, at Netley, the logical place for preparing the nineteenth-century reports, or at the headquarters of the Royal Army Medical Corps at Aldershot.

From the 1880s onward, the British published medical indicators for the current year alongside those for the preceding five or ten years. Earlier, however, the compilers followed less systematic policies. They began with the period 1817–36, or as close to that as possible, followed by 1837–46, and 1847–56. With the resumption of regular publication in 1859, they adopted a new and complex nosology, which they carried through to 1868. They therefore aggregated for the years 1859–67, and again under the new system for 1869–77, and again for 1879–84, and 1886–94. These and the decade 1895–1904 are therefore used as sample periods. After another interruption, the period 1909–13 was aggregated in the British records and can serve as a measure for the final quinquennium before the First World War.

The French followed a different policy. After publishing only occasional data in the first half of the century, they began a new annual series from 1862, publishing the data one year at a time. For purposes of this study, I have aggregated the French data into five-year samples to represent each decade – 1862–6, and so on – on the assumption that five years will yield a large enough sample, yet cover a period short enough to catch the pattern of disease at approximately the middle of each decade.

The British published totals for their troops in Europe for the United Kingdom and for its major parts. The French published general mortality figures for the entire country, but published mortality by disease separately for each military district in France – and for the three provinces of Algeria, as well as Tunisia and Morocco once they fell under French control. For this study, the three Algerian provinces are aggregated into a sample of about 50,000 troops stationed in North Africa. On the metropolitan side, the Gouvernement de Paris was taken as the sample unit, about the same size as the Algerian sample and located in a central region of French population distribution.

The French and British records differ in still another way. The British always distinguished between British troops and "native troops," recruited overseas and serving under British officers and noncoms. The French Army records for Algeria (but not those of the *troupes de la marine* serving elsewhere) do not always distinguish between metropolitan French recruits and others. French and non-French sometimes served in the same unit. Within the margin for error expected in a study of this kind, however, the French Army in Algeria can be taken as a single unit. Samples from units that were clearly non-French, like *tirailleurs algériens* or *légion etrangère*, are not necessarily or systematically either higher or lower than the great majority of French soldiers that actually made up the French Army in Algeria, although some error from this source is possible.

The French and British also reported morbidity differently. In most periods, the British measured illness by hospital entries. The French, on the other hand, recorded illness or injury on a scale of relative seriousness. A French soldier might be treated in quarters (*à la chambre*), in a *salle de convalescents*, in a regimental infirmary, or in hospital. Of those who reported sick in 1862, only 26 percent in France and 30 percent in Algeria were actually in hospital. The rest were in one of the other categories. Both the French and British treated each new admission as a "case," which meant that chronic illnesses like vivax malaria or venereal disease were likely to be double-counted. With the French system, furthermore, a soldier transferred from one place of treatment to another appears as a new admission. Thus, a soldier whose condition worsened steadily might pass through three tiers of possible treatment and appear on the records three times. For these and other reasons, morbidity data are much less valuable than mortality figures – especially for comparisons through time or between the two armies. They are therefore used sparingly, although they are reported for the British units represented in Tables A.1–A.52.

The French, furthermore, counted the mean strength of a unit in two ways. *Hommes effectifs* included all the men assigned to the unit, whether they were present or not. *Hommes présent au corps*, those actually on duty at any moment, could be considerably less. In 1862, for example, the force was 326,817 *effectifs*, but only 85 percent, or 276,161 were actually present. In Algeria that same year, only 88 percent of the *effectif* force was present. But the army tried to keep track of those who had died on leave or detached duty, and each unit reported separately on men temporarily attached, but who appeared on the strength of some other unit.[2] The unit could therefore find out about the cause of death of a soldier who was absent, even on leave. It was much more difficult to find out about the illness of the absent. Mortality was therefore calculated on the basis of men listed on the strength of the unit (the *effectifs*), while morbidity was calculated on the basis of men actually present. British reporting policy was not quite so clear on this issue until the 1880s, after which deaths and discharged included men detached, while illness included only those present. For purposes of this study, mortality data refer to deaths per thousand *effectifs*, or the official strength of the unit, whereas morbidity data, where used, can be assumed to be illness per soldier present with the unit.

The Indian data were originally presented for each of the three presidencies – Bengal, Madras, and Bombay. For reasons outlined in Chapter 1, the Madras data seem most nearly to represent normal peacetime conditions, although troops from this command sometimes served in Burma or the Straits Settlements, as well as in India itself. Units so serving, however, were not a large part of the total.

---

[2] Statistiques médicales for 1862, pp. 6–7; AMSR, 3:151–4 (1962).

As the century progressed, ocean transportation improved and military doctors had more of a choice between treating a patient on the spot or sending him home ("invaliding"). This option opens a potential source of uncertainty. At some periods, soldiers with a long-lasting chronic disease like tuberculosis or syphilis were likely to be sent home and given a medical discharge. Their deaths from a disease incurred on foreign service would thus appear on the record as civilian deaths in Britain on France. Invaliding varied with time, place, and disease. Few cases of yellow fever or cholera were ever invalided, simply because the victim either died or recovered before he could be shipped off. It is sometimes possible to get around the invaliding problem by using a separate index of dead plus invalided per thousand (the D + I index). French army data, however, do not record repatriation on a disease-by-disease basis. It is therefore impossible to compare French and British D + I indices.

In the tables that follow, the British data at first pertain only to hospital entries and deaths, but in later periods they take in a four-part set of health indicators – admissions, deaths, invalided or discharged, and "constantly sick" (the proportion per thousand in hospital).

For a listing of all of the Appendix Tables, see pp. vii-xi.

Table A.1. *Causes of Death and Hospital Admissions among Dragoons and Dragoon Guards Serving in Great Britain, 1830–6*

Disease	Per Thousand Mean Strength		Percentage of Total	
	Admissions	Deaths	Admissions	Deaths
Fevers	75	1.40	9.43	10.00
Eruptive fevers	3	0.10	0.38	0.71
Diseases of the lungs	148	7.70	18.62	55.00
Diseases of the liver	8	0.40	1.01	2.86
Stomach and bowels	94	0.80	11.82	5.71
Epidemic cholera	4	1.20	0.50	8.57
Diseases of the brain	6	0.70	0.75	5.00
Dropsies	1	0.30	0.13	2.14
Rheumatic	50	0.00	6.29	0.00
Venereal	181	0.00	22.77	0.00
Abscesses and ulcers	133	0.00	16.73	0.00
Diseases of the eye	19	0.00	2.39	0.00
Diseases of the skin	29	0.00	3.65	0.00
Other	44	1.40	5.53	10.00
Total disease	795	14.00	100.00	100.00
Wounds and injuries	126			
Punishment	8			
Other disease and accidents		1.30		
Grand total	929	15.30		

N = 5,950 annually.
Source: PP, 1839, xvi [C.1661], p. 7.

Table A.2. *Causes of Death and Hospital Admissions among Foot Guards Serving in Great Britain, 1837–47*

Disease	Per Thousand Mean Strength		Percentage of all Deaths from Disease	
	Admissions	Deaths	Admissions	Deaths
Zymotic				
Eruptive fevers	7.90	0.32	0.98	1.63
Intermittent fevers	0.52	0.00	0.07	0.00
Continued fevers	77.72	2.44	9.65	12.31
Dysentery/diarrhea	54.04	0.02	6.71	0.12
Cholera	2.84	0.07	0.35	0.37
Ophthalmia	15.00	0.00	1.86	0.00
Rheumatism	39.43	0.00	4.90	0.00
Enthetic diseases	250.30	0.02	31.09	0.10
Dietic diseases	0.10	0.02	0.01	0.10
Parasitic disease	0.10	0.00	0.01	0.00
Constitutional				
Diathetic	2.30	0.09	0.29	0.45
Tubercular	27.80	12.58	3.45	63.38
Local diseases				
Nervous system	8.20	0.59	1.02	2.97
Circulatory system	2.90	0.62	0.36	3.12
Respiratory system	137.10	1.62	17.03	8.16
Digestive system	24.60	0.64	3.06	3.22
Urinary system	0.80	0.04	0.10	0.20
Reproductive system	1.10	0.00	0.14	0.00
Integumentary system	0.40	0.04	0.05	0.20
Other or not specified	151.94	0.73	18.87	3.66
Total from disease	805.10	19.85	100.00	100.00
Accidents	56.30	0.58		
Punishment	1.00	0.00		
Total	862.40	20.43		

N = 4,012 annually.
Source: AMSR for 1859, p. 11; PP, 1852–3, lix, p. 60.

Table A.3. *Causes of Death and Hospital Admissions among Troops Serving in the United Kingdom, 1860–7*

Disease	Rate per Thousand		Percentage of Total	
	Admissions	Deaths	Admissions	Deaths
Zymotic diseases				
Myasmatic Diseases				
Eruptive fevers	8.28	0.31	0.89	3.72
Paroxysmal fevers	3.08	0.00	0.33	0.00
Continued fevers	28.02	0.42	3.02	5.04
Yellow fever	0.00	0.00	0.00	0.00
Dysentery/Diarrhea	25.54	0.23	2.76	2.76
Sore throat/influenza	70.23	0.04	7.58	0.48
Ophthalmia	14.12	0.00	1.52	0.00
Rheumatism	47.04	0.08	5.08	0.96
Enthetic diseases	314.10	0.11	33.89	1.32
Dietic diseases	8.20	0.07	0.88	0.84
Parasitic diseases	38.70	0.00	4.18	0.00
Constitutional diseases				
Diathetic	3.50	0.13	0.38	1.56
Tubercular	17.20	3.16	1.86	37.94
Local diseases				
Nervous system	19.10	0.72	2.06	8.64
Circulatory system	8.80	1.00	0.95	12.00
Respiratory system	88.50	1.32	9.55	15.85
Digestive system	37.00	0.54	3.99	6.48
Urinary system	3.00	0.16	0.32	1.92
Reproductive system	10.20	0.00	1.10	0.00
Locomotive system	4.10	0.02	0.44	0.24
Integumentary system	125.30	0.05	13.52	0.60
Other or not specified	3.39	0.04	0.37	0.48
Total disease	877.40	8.40	94.67	100.83
Accidents	84.00	0.61		
Homicide	0.20	0.02		
Suicide	0.00	0.30		
Punishment	1.80	0.01		
Grand Total	963.40	9.34		

N = 70,000 to 78,000 annually.

Note: The category "myasmatic diseases" is disaggregated in proportion to the annual data for household troops stationed in London and Windsor. 1860–4.

Source: AMSR for 1868, pp. 2–3; 1864, p. 6; for 1860, p. 11; for 1861, p. 10; for 1862, p. 11; for 1863, p. 10.

Table A.4. *Causes of Death and Hospital Admissions among Troops Serving in the United Kingdom, 1869–77*

Disease	Per Thousand Mean Strength		Percentage of Total	
	Admissions	Deaths	Admissions	Deaths
General diseases				
Febrile group				
Eruptive fevers	10.90	0.24	1.56	3.11
Continued fevers	38.54	0.34	5.50	4.44
Yellow fever	0.00	0.00	0.00	0.00
Paroxysmal fevers	1.56	0.00	0.22	0.00
Constitutional group				
Rheumatism	23.61	0.04	3.37	0.55
Syphilis	115.40	0.21	16.48	2.74
Scrofula, phthisis	8.39	2.55	1.20	33.17
Local diseases				
Nervous system	12.00	0.57	1.71	7.42
Ear/eye/nose/circulation	34.40	1.39	4.91	18.10
Respiratory system	86.10	1.32	12.30	17.19
Digestive system	105.40	0.55	15.05	7.16
Urinary/reproductive system	109.20	0.26	15.60	3.39
Locomotive system	5.10	0.05	0.73	0.65
Cellular tissue/cutaneous	122.70	0.03	17.52	0.39
Conditions				
Debility	8.40	0.01	1.20	0.13
Other or not specified	18.50	0.12	2.64	1.56
Total from disease	700.20	7.68	100.00	100.00
Injuries				
Battle	0.00			
Accidents	106.20	0.81		
Grand total	806.40	8.49		

N = 78,000 to 101,000 annually.

Note: The categories "febrile" and "constitutional" are disaggregated in proportion to the annual data for household troops stationed in London and Windsor in the years 1869–73.

Source: AMSR for 1878, p. 4; AMSR for 1874, p. 3; for 1869, p. 9; for 1870, p. 7; for 1871, p. 6; for 1872, p. 6; for 1873, p. 7.

Table A.5. *Health Indicators for British Troops Serving in the United Kingdom, 1879–84*

Disease	Rates per Thousand Mean Strength			
	Admitted	Died	Invalided/ Discharged	Constantly Sick
Febrile group				
Smallpox	0.1	0.01	0.00	0.01
Other eruptive fevers	5.6	0.05	0.00	0.29
Enteric fever	1.3	0.18	0.00	0.15
Other continued fevers	13.7	0.12	0.00	0.43
Paroxysmal fevers	12.3	0.01	0.04	0.41
Constitutional group				
Rheumatism	40.3	0.07	1.28	2.45
Syphilis	130.3	0.02	0.59	2.31
Tubercular diseases	9.7	2.08	3.80	1.33
Local disease				
Nervous system	11.9	0.46	2.78	1.19
Circulatory system	13.8	0.66	4.37	1.29
Respiratory system	72.1	1.30	1.14	3.64
Digestive system	111.2	0.49	2.03	3.77
Gonorrhea urinary	123.8	0.15	0.47	0.60
Other	210	0.41	5.53	24.33
Total diseases	756.2	6.01	22.03	42.2
Injuries	106.9	0.72	0.95	4.33
Grand total	863.1	6.73	22.98	46.53

N = 78,000 to 87,000 annually.
Source: AMSR for 1885, pp. 154–5.

Table A.6. *Health Indicators for British Troops Serving in the United Kingdom, 1886–94*

Disease	Per Thousand Mean Strength			
	Admitted	Died	Invalided/ Discharged	Constantly Sick
Other eruptive fevers[a]	8.00	0.05	0.00	0.56
Enteric fever	1.30	0.27	0.00	0.21
Other continued fevers	4.90	0.01	0.00	0.18
Dysentery	0.70	0.02	0.04	0.07
Yellow Fever	0.00	0.00	0.00	0.00
Malaria	6.00	0.01	0.01	0.21
Septic diseases	2.10	0.08	0.01	0.14
Rheumatism	36.50	0.05	0.66	2.28
Tuberculosis	3.50	0.93	1.71	0.56
Syphilis	102.00	0.05	0.77	9.55
Gonorrhea	92.30	0.00	0.05	6.15
Parasitic diseases	0.50	0.00	0.00	0.01
Alcoholism	2.50	0.04	0.00	0.08
Local diseases				
Eye	11.80	0.00	0.69	0.71
Nervous system	8.80	0.34	2.10	0.74
Circulatory	9.60	0.40	3.28	0.92
Respiratory	64.60	1.31	0.91	3.24
Digestive	106.60	0.35	0.92	3.19
Lymphatic	16.90	0.01	0.10	1.77
Urinary	2.30	0.16	0.26	0.20
Generative	37.40	0.01	0.29	2.36
Locomotive	7.60	0.03	0.92	0.61
Connective tissue	23.10	0.01	0.09	1.05
Skin	74.70	0.00	0.20	2.77
Other disease	35.60	0.18	2.06	1.80
Total disease	659.30	4.31	15.07	39.36
Injuries/poisons	101.50	0.74	0.76	4.15
Grand total	760.80	5.05	15.83	43.51

N = c.100,000 annually.
Note: Data on deaths and discharged include men detached.
[a] Other than smallpox.
Source: AMSR for 1901, pp. 240–1.

Table A.7. *Health Indicators for British Troops Serving in the United Kingdom, 1895–1904*

| | Per Thousand Mean Strength | | | |
Disease	Admitted	Died	Invalided/ Discharged	Constantly Sick
Other eruptive fevers[a]	9.10	0.06	0.00	0.75
Influenza	19.20	0.04	0.01	0.68
Diphtheria	1.10	0.02	0.00	0.09
Enteric fever	1.20	0.21	0.01	0.20
Other continued fevers	2.20	0.02	0.00	0.10
Dysentery	0.90	0.02	0.08	0.07
Yellow fever	0.00	0.00	0.00	0.00
Malaria	7.10	0.02	0.09	0.29
Septic diseases	1.00	0.05	0.00	0.07
Tuberculosis	3.20	0.59	1.72	0.44
Syphilis	—	—	—	—
Gonorrhea	61.80	0.00	0.10	4.46
Parasitic diseases	27.10	0.00	0.09	0.93
Alcoholism	2.20	0.06	0.01	0.08
Rheumatism	26.30	0.06	0.99	1.80
Local diseases				
Eye	12.10	0.00	1.42	0.72
Nervous system	9.50	0.26	2.63	0.77
Circulatory	14.20	0.41	5.21	1.28
Respiratory	48.50	0.99	0.96	2.48
Digestive	99.50	0.30	2.64	3.57
Lymphatic	8.40	0.00	0.13	0.83
Urinary	2.90	0.11	0.53	0.25
Other	194.60	0.30	7.30	13.33
Total disease	552.10	3.52	23.92	33.19
Injuries	96.50	0.68	1.88	4.23
Grand total	648.60	4.20	25.80	37.42

— No data.
N = c.100,000 annually.
[a] Other than smallpox.
Source: AMSR for 1905, pp. 274–5.
Data on deaths and discharged include men detached.

Table A.8. *Health Indicators for British Troops Serving in the United Kingdom, 1909–13*

Disease	Per Thousand Mean Strength			
	Admitted	Died	Invalided/ Discharged	Constantly Sick
Cerebrospinal fever	0.0	0.01	0.00	0.00
Enteric fever	0.4	0.06	0.01	0.09
Influenza	13.7	0.01	0.00	0.41
Dysentery	0.2	0.00	0.02	0.02
Malaria	2.5	0.00	0.02	0.09
Septic diseases	33.2	0.08	0.06	0.07
Pneumonia	2.8	0.29	0.00	0.25
Tonsilitis	25.9	0.00	0.00	0.69
Rheumatic fever	5.7	0.02	0.18	0.54
Tuberculosis	2.1	0.25	1.46	0.29
Venereal disease	59.9	0.01	0.32	5.79
Diabetes	0.1	0.02	0.04	0.01
Carcinoma/sarcoma	0.2	0.06	0.05	0.05
Nervous and mental	5.2	0.16	0.55	0.09
Diseases of the ear	6.1	0.02	0.91	0.38
Circulatory system	6.5	0.29	1.52	0.55
Respiratory system	15.9	0.12	0.21	0.70
Digestive system	28.1	0.28	0.71	1.53
Urinary system	2.3	0.12	0.34	0.22
Generative system	6.8	0.00	0.07	0.37
Locomotive system	14.1	0.01	0.61	0.74
Other diseases	68	0.14	2.3	4.59
Total disease	299.7	1.95	9.38	17.47
Injuries/poisons	55.3	0.6	0.67	2.72
Grand total	355	2.55	10.05	20.19

N = c.110,000 annually.
Source: AMSR for 1914, pp. 144–57.

Table A.9. *Causes of Death and Hospital Admissions among European Troops Serving in the Windward and Leeward Command, 1817–36*

Disease	Per Thousand Mean Strength		Percentage of Total	
	Admitted	Died	Admitted	Died
Fevers	717.00	36.90	41.59	48.81
Eruptive fevers	0.20	0.00	0.01	0.00
Diseases of the lungs	115.00	10.40	6.67	13.76
Diseases of the liver	22.00	1.80	1.28	2.38
Stomach and bowels	421.00	20.70	24.42	27.38
Diseases of the brain	28.00	3.70	1.62	4.89
Dropsies	7.80	2.10	0.45	2.78
Rheumatic	49.00	0.00	2.84	0.00
Venereal	35.00	0.00	2.03	0.00

172

Abscesses and ulcers	204.00	0.00	11.83	0.00
Diseases of the eye	89.00	0.00	5.16	0.00
Diseases of the skin	6.00	0.00	0.35	0.00
Other	30.00	0.00	1.74	0.00
Total disease	1,724.00	75.60	100.00	100.00
Wounds and injuries	129.00			
Punishment	50.00			
Other disease and accidents		2.90		
Grand total	1,903.00	78.50		

N = c.3,000 annually.
Source: PP, 1837–8, xl(136), p. 7.

Table A.10. *Causes of Death and Hospital Admissions among British Troops Serving in the Windward and Leeward Command, 1836–47*

Disease	Per Thousand Mean Strength		Percentage of Total	
	Admissions	Deaths	Admissions	Deaths
Zymotic				
Miasmatic diseases				
Eruptive fevers	0.7	0.03	0.04	0.04
Paroxysmal fevers	553.8	34.66	30.46	50.01
Continued fevers	159.0	5.24	8.75	7.56
Dysentery/diarrhea	326.5	13.65	17.96	19.69
Cholera	0.0	0.00	0.00	0.00
Ophthalmia	169.4	0.03	9.32	0.04
Rheumatism	52.8	0.17	2.90	0.25
Enthetic diseases	62.5	0.06	3.44	0.09
Dietic diseases	2.4	0.06	0.13	0.09
Parasitic disease	1.4		0.08	0.00
Constitutional				
Diathetic	5.8	0.73	0.32	1.05
Tubercular	16.0	5.22	0.88	7.53
Local diseases				
Nervous system	34.0	3.88	1.87	5.60
Circulatory system	1.7	0.14	0.09	0.20
Respiratory system	106.2	3.33	5.84	4.80
Digestive system	117.4	1.65	6.46	2.38
Urinary system	2.5	0.01	0.14	0.01
Reproductive system	1.3		0.07	0.00
Integumentary system	191.1	0.26	10.51	0.38
Other or not specified	13.4	0.19	0.74	0.27
Total from disease	1,817.9	69.31	100.00	100.00
Accidents	106.0	0.23		
Punishment	11.9			
Total	1,935.8	69.54		

N = 1,950 annually.
Source: AMSR for 1859, pp. 70–1, 74–5.

Table A.11. *Causes of Death and Hospital Admissions among European Troops Serving in the British West Indies, 1859–67 (per thousand mean strength)*

Disease	Windward/Leeward Command[a]		Jamaica Command[b]	
	Admissions	Deaths	Admissions	Deaths
Zymotic diseases				
Miasmatic diseases				
Eruptive fevers	1.10	0.00	0.60	0.00
Paroxysmal fevers	253.20	3.28	141.30	3.10
Continued fevers	48.70	0.54	106.80	3.10
Yellow fever	2.80	1.55	15.00	6.37
Dysentery/diarrhea	55.80	0.27	50.80	0.32
Sore throat/influenza	11.80	0.09	19.80	0.00
Ophthalmia	72.50	0.00	58.50	0.00
Rheumatism	21.60	0.00	32.70	0.16
Enthetic diseases	173.70	0.00	121.20	0.00
Dietic diseases	33.60	0.50	32.80	0.49
Parasitic diseases	5.50	0.00	10.90	0.00
Constitutional diseases				
Diathetic	7.00	0.00	2.90	0.16
Tubercular	10.70	1.60	9.60	1.64
Local diseases				
Nervous system	33.90	1.81	22.20	1.64
Circulatory system	7.40	0.90	5.90	1.80
Respiratory system	33.70	0.30	44.60	0.65
Digestive system	67.70	0.90	69.80	0.14
Urinary system	1.20	0.00	2.60	0.16
Reproductive system	17.10	0.00	6.40	0.00
Locomotive system	3.50	0.00	4.20	0.16
Integumentary system	164.60	0.00	148.70	0.00
Other or not specified	65.20	0.69	32.20	0.34
Total disease	1,092.30	12.43	939.50	21.23
Accidents	100.30	0.70	140.00	1.47
Homicide	0.00	0.00		
Suicide	0.40	0.50		
Punishment	2.20	0.00		
Grand total	1,195.20	13.63	1,079.50	22.70

[a] N = 806 in 1868.
[b] N = 778 in 1868.
Source: AMSR, 10:76 (1868).

Table A.12. *Causes of Death and Hospital Admissions among European Troops Serving the British West Indies Command, 1869–77*

Disease	Per Thousand Mean Strength		Percentage of Total	
	Admissions	Deaths	Admissions	Deaths
General diseases				
Febrile group				
Eruptive fevers	0.90	0.00	0.12	0.00
Continued fevers	126.00	1.76	16.16	17.09
Yellow fever	4.40	2.20	0.56	21.36
Paroxysmal fevers	52.80	0.97	6.77	9.42
Constitutional group				
Rheumatism	22.10	0.00	2.83	0.00
Syphilis	67.30	0.00	8.63	0.00
Scrofula, phthisis	8.50	1.76	1.09	17.09
Local diseases				
Nervous system	11.10	0.97	1.42	9.42
Ear/eye/nose/circulatory	30.50	0.97	3.91	9.42
Respiratory system	32.70	0.27	4.19	2.60
Digestive system	127.40	0.70	16.34	6.80
Urinary system/reproductive	109.60	0.09	14.06	0.87
Locomotive system	5.60	0.00	0.72	0.00
Cellular Tissue/cutaneous	113.20	0.00	14.52	0.00
Conditions				
Debility	12.90	0.17	1.65	1.65
Other or not specified	54.60	0.44	7.00	4.27
Total from disease	779.60	10.30	100.00	100.00
Injuries				
Battle	0.00	0.00		
Accidents	122.10	0.97		
Grand total	901.70	11.27		

N = 1,119 to 1,709 annually.
Source: AMSR for 1874, pp. 74–5.

Table A.13. *Health Indicators for European Troops Serving in the British West Indies, 1879–84*

Disease	Rate per Thousand Mean Strength			
	Admitted	Died	Invalided/ Discharged	Constantly Sick
Febrile group				
Smallpox	0.00	0.00	0.00	0.00
Other eruptive fevers	0.40	0.00	0.00	0.02
Enteric fever	4.00	1.32	0.00	0.35
Other continued fevers	135.70	0.00	3.02	4.53
Yellow fever	12.90	8.12	0.00	0.33
Paroxysmal fevers	41.50	3.02	1.13	1.93
Constitutional group				
Rheumatism	37.20	0.00	0.75	1.88
Syphilis	66.60	0.00	0.57	5.02
Tubercular diseases	7.40	0.94	4.53	1.82
Local diseases				
Nervous system	16.20	0.57	5.28	1.69
Circulatory system	14.70	0.75	3.77	1.38
Respiratory system	23.80	1.13	0.57	1.60
Digestive system	119.70	1.51	1.51	3.90
Gonorrhea/urinary	84.80	0.19	3.80	4.50
Other	185.90	0.38	8.47	9.77
Total diseases	750.80	17.93	33.40	38.72
Injuries	124.20	1.51	0.94	4.41
Grand total	875.00	19.44	34.34	43.13

N = 970 in 1884.
Source: AMSR for 1885, pp. 201–2.

Table A.14. *Health Indicators for European Troops Serving in the British West Indies, 1886–94*

	Rates per Thousand Mean Strength			
Disease	Admitted	Died	Invalided/ Discharged	Constantly Sick
Other eruptive fevers[a]	4.80	0.00	0.00	0.14
Enteric fever	10.60	2.81	0.10	1.46
Other continued fevers	109.50	0.19	0.00	3.55
Dysentery	6.60	0.49	0.29	0.39
Yellow fever	1.20	0.68	0.00	0.04
Malaria	42.70	0.97	0.58	1.86
Septic diseases	0.50	0.00	0.00	0.03
Rheumatism	35.10	0.10	0.97	2.05
Tuberculosis	1.80	0.19	1.45	0.37
Syphilis	79.50	0.19	2.04	7.39
Gonorrhea	151.70	0.00	0.19	11.06
Parasitic diseases	1.50	0.00	0.00	0.04
Alcoholism	8.00	0.00	0.00	0.20
Local diseases				
Eye	13.00	0.00	1.07	0.80
Nervous system	14.50	0.39	2.62	1.17
Circulatory	10.50	0.49	2.13	0.91
Respiratory	29.60	0.68	0.49	1.53
Digestive	103.40	0.29	1.65	3.10
Lymphatic	43.20	0.00	0.39	4.67
Urinary	1.80	0.29	0.10	0.11
Generative	113.30	0.00	0.19	7.79
Locomotive	8.20	0.10	1.16	0.66
Connective tissue	39.80	0.00	0.00	1.57
Skin	77.80	0.00	0.39	2.97
Other disease	68.40	0.08	3.40	3.20
Total disease	977.00	7.94	19.21	·57.06
Injuries/poisons	144.80	1.08	0.78	5.00
Grand total	1,121.80	9.02	19.99	62.06

N = 1,061 to 1,261 annually.
[a] Other than smallpox.
Source: AMSR for 1895, pp. 286–7.

Table A.15. *Health Indicators for European Troops Serving in the Barbados and Jamaica Commands, 1895–1904*

Disease	Jamaica[a]	Barbados[b]	Deaths per Thousand		Invalided per Thousand		Constantly Sick per Thousand	
			Jamaica	Barbados	Jamaica	Barbados	Jamaica	Barbados
Other eruptive fevers[c]	0.7	6.8	0.00	0.00	0.00	0.00	0.03	0.35
Influenza	6.4	5.7	0.00	0.00	0.00	0.00	0.26	0.18
Diphtheria	0.0	0.1	0.00	0.12	0.00	0.00	0.00	0.00
Enteric fever	5.0	1.1	1.51	0.37	0.34	0.12	0.72	0.27
Other continued fevers	28.1	52.3	0.00	0.00	0.00	0.25	1.10	1.95
Dysentery	9.5	1.7	0.17	0.12	0.17	0.00	0.56	0.10
Yellow fever	4.5	2.0	2.02	1.12	0.00	0.00	0.30	0.09
Malaria	84.9	123.4	0.84	1.99	0.84	0.99	3.98	4.10
Septic diseases	0.3	0.1	0.00	0.00	0.00	0.00	0.01	0.00
Tuberculosis	4.2	2.7	0.67	0.75	3.03	1.86	0.83	0.51
Syphilis	—	—	—	—	—	—	—	—
Gonorrhea[d]	97.9	147.3	0.00	0.00	0.34	0.12	6.93	10.75
Parasitic diseases	18.2	40.9	0.00	0.00	0.00	0.00	1.56	1.11
Alcoholism	3.5	14.5	0.17	0.25	0.00		0.13	0.36
Rheumatism	20.0	36.3	0.00	0.12	0.84	0.99	1.42	2.00

Local diseases								
Eye	11.1	8.1	0.00	0.00	1.01	0.37	0.80	0.38
Nervous system	6.9	8.6	0.17	0.12	2.52	2.36	0.62	0.76
Circulatory	8.9	11.6	0.34	0.5	4.54	4.22	1.03	1.26
Respiratory	20.0	16.0	0.17	0.37	0.00	0.62	1.06	1.13
Digestive	64.4	82.6	0.67	0.37	2.69	1.49	2.65	2.90
Lymphatic	29.8	51.3	0.00	0.00	0.17	0.62	4.18	6.27
Urinary	1.9	2.6	0.34	0.25	0.00	0.62	0.15	0.24
Generative	33.8	36.8	0.00	0.00	0.5	0.12	2.59	7.18
Organs of locomotion	15.6	00.0	0.00	0.00	2.35	0.00	1.25	1.46
Other	173.8	392.3	0.16	1.13	9.08	9.47	13.09	24.41
Total disease	649.4	1044.8	7.23	7.58	28.42	24.22	45.25	67.76
Injuries	105.9	112.1	3.37	1.49	2.19	0.75	4.87	4.27
Grand total	755.3	1156.9	10.6	9.07	30.61	24.97	50.12	72.03

— No data.

[a] N = 602 Jamaica in 1904 admissions.

[b] N = 744 Barbados in 1904 per Thousand.

[c] Other than smallpox.

[d] Includes soft chancre.

Source: AMSR for 1905, pp. 302–3, 306–7.

Table A.16. *Health Indicators for European Troops Serving in Jamaica,*
1909–13

| | Rates per thousand per year | | | |
Disease	Admitted	Died	Invalided/ Discharged	Constantly Sick
Cerebrospinal fever	0.5	0.52	0.00	0.01
Enteric fever	2.1	1.03	0.52	0.33
Influenza	2.6	0.00	0.00	0.09
Dysentery	2.1	0.00	0.00	0.09
Malaria	89.5	1.52	0.00	4.73
Septic diseases	51.2	0.00	0.00	4.64
Pneumonia	0.5	0.52	0.00	0.01
Tonsilitis	15.5	0.00	0.00	0.38
Rheumatic fever	3.1	0.00	0.00	0.71
Tuberculosis	2.6	0.52	2.59	0.28
Venereal disease	101.3	0.52	0.52	10.95
Diabetes	1.0	0.52	0.52	0.08
Carcinoma/sarcoma	0.5	0.52	0.00	0.02
Nervous and mental	3.7	0.00	2.59	0.48
Diseases of the ear	5.2	0.00	1.55	0.24
Circulatory system	8.3	1.03	2.07	0.63
Respiratory system	9.8	0.00	0.52	0.56
Digestive system	29.5	0.52	0.00	1.70
Urinary system	2.1	0.00	0.52	0.11
Generative system	6.2	0.00	0.00	0.50
Locomotive system	14.5	0.00	0.00	1.10
Other diseases	114.1	0.02	7.21	5.09
Total disease	465.9	7.24	18.61	32.73
Injuries/poisons	46.5	0.52	0.00	2.51
Grand total	512.4	7.76	18.61	35.24

N = 375 in 1912.
Note: Addition in the original corrected.
Source: AMSR for 1914, pp. 144–57.

Table A.17. *Causes of Death and Hospital Admissions among European*
Troops Serving in Madras Presidency, 1827–38

| | Rate per thousand Mean Strength | | Percentage of Total | |
Disease[a]	Admissions	Deaths	Admissions	Deaths
Fever, continued	156.00	2.04	9.24	4.24
Fever, intermittent	132.00	1.41	7.82	2.93
Fever, remittent	59.00	2.12	3.49	4.41
Pulmonary disease	4.00	0.80	0.24	1.66
Thoracic Inflammation	34.00	1.55	2.01	3.23

Table A.17. *(cont.)*

Disease[a]	Rate per thousand Mean Strength		Percentage of Total	
	Admissions	Deaths	Admissions	Deaths
Hepatic disease	116.00	5.62	6.87	11.69
Colic	26.00	0.08	1.54	0.17
Diarrhea	78.00	1.55	4.62	3.23
Dysentery	188.00	15.03	11.13	31.27
Abdominal inflammation	22.00	0.93	1.30	1.94
Cholera	27.00	7.60	1.60	15.81
Apoplexy	2.00	1.33	0.12	2.77
Cephalic inflammation	8.00	0.18	0.47	0.37
Insanity	3.00	0.19	0.18	0.40
Dropsies	5.00	1.08	0.30	2.25
Rheumatism	102.00	0.95	6.04	1.98
Syphilis, etc.	192.00	0.57	11.37	1.19
Ulcers	74.00	0.22	4.38	0.46
Diseases of the eye	72.00	0.06	4.26	0.12
Other	389.00	4.75	23.03	9.88
Total disease	1,689.00	48.06	100.00	100.00
Wounds and accidents	149.00	0.57		
Grand total	1,838.00	48.63		

N = 10,660 annually.
[a] Classification of Madras medical returns.
Source: "Report of a Committee of the Statistical Society of London," JSSL, 3:127 (1840).

Table A.18. *Causes of Death and Hospital Admissions among British Troops Serving in Madras Presidency, 1837–46*

Disease	Rate per thousand Mean Strength		Percentage of Total	
	Admissions	Deaths	Admissions	Deaths
Fever	293	3.80	16.83	9.16
Eruptive fevers	2	0.20	0.11	0.48
Diseases of the lungs	106	2.90	6.09	6.99
Diseases of the liver	88	4.50	5.05	10.84
Diseases of the stomach and bowels	367	12.70	21.08	30.60
Epidemic cholera	17	8.30	0.98	20.00
Diseases of the brain	31	2.60	1.78	6.27
Dropsies	3	0.60	0.17	1.45
Other diseases, wounds (not including killed in action)	834	5.90	47.90	14.22
Total	1,741	41.50	100.00	100.00

N = c.11,000 annually.
Source: AMSR, 1860, pp. 134, 137.

Table A.19. *Causes of Death and Hospital Admissions among British Troops Serving in Madras Presidency, 1860–67*

Disease	Rate per Thousand Mean Strength		Percentage of Total	
	Admissions	Deaths	Admissions	Deaths
Zymotic diseases				
Miasmatic disease				
Eruptive fevers	0.9	0.80	0.06	3.63
Paroxysmal fevers	166.7	0.70	11.95	3.18
Continued fevers	78.3	1.23	5.61	5.59
Dysentery/diarrhea	174.5	3.07	12.51	13.95
Spasmodic cholera	5.6	2.76	0.40	12.54
Sore throat/influenza	16.7	0.00	1.20	0.00
Ophthalmia	34.4	0.00	2.47	0.00
Rheumatism	61.5	0.04	4.41	0.18
Enthetic diseases	252.3	0.36	18.08	1.64
Dietic diseases	21.4	0.17	1.53	0.77
Parasitic diseases	12.6	0.00	0.90	0.00
Constitutional diseases				
Diathetic	6.5	0.22	0.47	1.00
Tubercular	16.9	2.23	1.21	10.13
Local diseases				
Nervous system	36.6	1.54	2.62	7.00
Circulatory system	17.2	1.31	1.23	5.95
Respiratory system	52.7	0.63	3.78	2.86
Digestive system	148.0	3.96	10.61	17.99
Urinary system	3.2	0.17	0.23	0.77
Reproductive system	17.3	0.00	1.24	0.00
Locomotive system	4.9	0.03	0.35	0.14
Integumentary system	125.0	0.08	8.96	0.36
Other or not specified	28.9	0.56	2.07	2.54
Total disease	1,282.1	19.86	91.90	90.23
Accidents	110.6	1.85	7.93	8.41
Homicide	0.0	0.00	0.00	0.00
Suicide	0.0	0.30	0.00 ·	1.36
Punishment	2.4	0.00	0.17	0.00
Grand total	1,395.1	22.01	100.00	100.00

N = c.10,000 annually.
Source: AMSR for 1868, pp. 155–6.

Table A.20. *Causes of Death and Hospital Admissions among British Troops Serving in Madras Presidency, 1869–77*

Disease	Rate per Thousand Mean Strength		Percentage of Total	
	Admissions	Deaths	Admissions	Deaths
General diseases				
Febrile group				
Eruptive fevers	1.20	0.08	0.11	0.45
Continued fevers	122.70	1.60	11.23	9.08
Yellow fever	0.00	0.00	0.00	0.00
Paroxysmal fevers	99.10	0.35	9.07	1.99
Cholera	3.00	1.58	0.27	8.97
Constitutional group				
Rheumatism	38.20	0.02	3.49	0.11
Syphilis	101.00	0.19	9.24	1.08
Scrofula, phthisis	11.90	1.63	1.09	9.25
Local diseases				
Nervous system/ear/eye	48.30	1.99	4.42	11.29
Circulatory system	18.40	1.86	1.68	10.56
Respiratory system	42.80	0.51	3.92	2.89
Digestive system	335.00	6.74	30.65	38.25
Urinary/reproductive system	84.40	0.16	7.72	0.91
Locomotive system	4.60	0.03	0.42	0.17
Cellular tissue	16.90	0.02	1.55	0.11
Conditions				
Debility	35.30	0.06	3.23	0.34
Other or not specified	130.20	0.80	11.91	4.54
Total from disease	1,093.00	17.62	100.00	100.00
Injuries				
Battle and accidents	108.90	1.78		
Grand total	1,201.90	19.40		

N = 10,900 annually.
Source: AMSR for 1874, pp. 74–5.

Table A.21. *Health Indicators for European Troops Serving in Madras Presidency, 1879–84*

	Rates per Thousand Mean Strength			
Disease	Admitted	Died	Invalided/ Discharged	Constantly Sick
Febrile group				
Smallpox	0.70	0.05	0.00	0.06
Other eruptive fevers	0.60	0.00	0.00	0.02
Enteric fever	5.00	1.51	0.02	0.62
Other continued fevers	78.80	0.17	0.00	2.46
Paroxysmal fevers	183.10	0.28	0.00	4.99
Cholera	1.90	1.12	0.41	0.03
Constitutional group				
Rheumatism	29.90	0.02	1.04	1.57
Syphilis	128.70	0.05	1.37	2.16
Tubercular diseases	6.30	0.90	2.19	0.97
Local diseases				
Nervous system	15.30	1.32	3.14	1.08
Circulatory system	17.90	0.68	4.56	1.47
Respiratory system	31.10	0.41	0.91	1.56
Digestive system	238.10	3.23	7.24	11.61
Gonorrhea/urinary	126.90	0.24	0.61	8.01
Other	229.10	1.01	10.04	20.56
Total diseases	1,093.40	10.99	31.53	57.17
Injuries	102.10	1.44	1.01	3.85
Grand total	1,195.50	12.43	32.54	61.02

N = c.10,400 annually.
Source: AMSR for 1885, pp. 201–2.

Table A.22. *Health Indicators for European Troops Serving in India, 1886–94*

Disease	Rates per Thousand Mean Strength			
	Admitted	Died	Invalided/ Discharged	Constantly Sick
Other eruptive fevers[a]	1.80	0.00	0.00	0.04
Enteric fever	18.80	5.11	0.22	2.64
Other continued fevers	60.20	0.04	0.03	2.38
Dysentery	28.80	0.70	1.07	2.28
Cholera	2.00	1.42	0.00	0.03
Malaria	361.90	0.74	1.75	11.13
Septic diseases	1.60	0.09	0.00	0.09
Rheumatism	30.00	0.07	0.97	2.06
Tuberculosis	3.30	0.83	1.39	0.65
Syphilis	178.30	0.10	2.58	14.92
Gonorrhea	169.50	0.00	0.13	12.10
Parasitic diseases	3.50	0.00	0.10	0.09
Alcoholism	8.90	0.07	0.01	0.28
Local diseases				
Eye	13.30	0.00	0.58	0.81
Nervous system	11.80	0.38	2.34	0.52
Circulatory	10.90	0.38	2.79	1.11
Respiratory	34.30	0.96	0.70	1.95
Digestive	133.60	1.82	2.04	5.61
Lymphatic	32.10	0.03	0.41	3.18
Urinary	2.10	0.16	0.36	0.21
Generative	88.30	0.02	0.29	3.98
Locomotive	7.40	0.03	0.72	0.57
Connective tissue	21.30	0.01	0.10	1.01
Skin	69.30	0.00	0.16	2.86
Other disease	52.90	0.36	5.64	8.79
Total disease	1,345.90	13.32	24.38	79.29
Injuries/poisons	106.80	2.34	0.14	2.42
Grand total	1,452.70	15.66	24.52	81.71

N = c.68,300 annually.
[a] Other than smallpox.
Source: AMSR for 1895, pp. 286–87.

Table A.23. *Health Indicators for European Troops Serving in India,*
1895–1904

Disease	Rates per Thousand Mean Strength			
	Admitted	Died	Invalided/ Discharged	Constantly Sick
Smallpox	0.60	0.06	0.00	0.06
Other eruptive fevers	2.60	0.02	0.00	0.11
Influenza	6.50	0.02	0.01	0.28
Diphtheria	0.00	0.00	0.00	0.00
Enteric fever	22.30	5.62	0.76	3.31
Other continued fevers	27.60	0.03	0.06	1.27
Dysentery	24.00	0.79	1.15	1.74
Cholera	0.70	0.55	0.00	0.01
Malaria	291.40	0.62	3.96	10.81
Septic diseases	1.20	0.11	0.01	0.08
Tuberculosis	4.20	0.771	1.32	0.76
Syphilis	—	—	—	—
Gonorrhea	141.50	0.00	0.38	11.07
Parasitic diseases	11.60	0.00	0.36	0.52
Alcoholism	3.80	0.09	0.03	0.15
Rheumatism/rheumatic fever	24.00	0.03	0.92	1.74
Local diseases				
Eye	10.50	0.00	0.65	0.65
Nervous system	9.10	0.33	2.45	0.97
Circulatory	12.40	0.67	3.66	1.26
Respiratory	28.00	0.76	0.58	1.66
Digestive	109.30	1.90	2.85	5.00
Lymphatic	26.20	0.02	0.26	3.01
Urinary	2.20	0.19	0.36	0.22
Other	361.80	0.67	12.28	28.61
Total disease	1,121.50	13.25	32.05	73.29
Injuries	99.90	1.79	1.12	4.56
Grand total	1,221.40	15.04	33.17	77.85

— No data.
N = c.70,400 annually.
Source: AMSR for 1905, p. 335.

Table A.24. *Health Indicators for European Troops Serving in India, 1909–13*

Disease	Rates per Thousand Mean Strength			
	Admitted	Died	Invalided/ Discharged	Constantly Sick
Enteric fever	3.70	0.62	0.04	0.80
Influenza	4.80	0.00	0.00	0.12
Beri-beri	0.20	0.01	0.01	0.02
Cholera	0.20	0.13	0.00	0.01
Dysentery	7.50	0.21	0.01	0.53
Kala azar	0.20	0.13	0.00	0.01
Malaria/blackwater	126.60	0.18	0.04	4.29
Septic diseases	46.40	0.11	0.03	2.17
Pneumonia	2.50	0.27	0.00	0.23
Tonsilitis	18.60	0.01	0.00	0.54
Rheumatic fever	4.80	0.00	0.07	0.41
Tuberculosis	1.40	0.24	0.96	0.42
Venereal disease	57.60	0.05	0.23	7.48
Diabetes	0.10	0.03	0.02	0.01
Carcinoma/Sarcoma	0.20	0.07	0.01	0.02
Nervous and mental	7.80	0.19	1.25	0.62
Diseases of the ear	12.30	0.03	0.72	0.67
Circulatory system	7.70	0.33	0.93	0.72
Respiratory system	13.30	0.10	0.14	0.63
Digestive system	62.70	0.80	0.14	2.87
Lymphatic system	0.20	0.01	0.00	0.01
Urinary system	2.20	0.12	0.11	0.19
Generative system	8.80	0.01	0.01	0.48
Locomotive system	19.20	0.01	0.31	0.99
Other diseases	112.70	0.12	0.59	4.43
Total diseases	521.70	3.78	5.62	28.67
Injuries/poisons	67.60	1.09	0.49	3.25
Grand total	589.30	4.87	6.11	31.92

N = c.71,000 annually.
Source: AMSR for 1914, pp. 144–57.

Table A.25. Causes of Death among French Troops Serving in France and in Algeria, 1862–6

Disease	Deaths per Thousand		Difference in Rates	Contribution (%)[c]	Percentage of Total Deaths from Disease	
	France[a]	Algeria[b]			France	Algeria
Typhoid fever	1.93	2.60	0.66	14.82	20.23	18.50
Other continued fevers	0.08	0.35	0.27	6.11	0.83	2.52
Intermittent fevers	0.22	2.69	2.47	55.12	2.25	19.13
Eruptive fevers	0.29	0.29	0.00	−0.01	3.02	2.05
Syphilis	0.02	0.01	−0.01	−0.28	0.24	0.07
Diseases of the Brain or spinal cord	0.40	0.27	−0.13	−2.86	4.19	1.94
Diseases of the circulatory system	0.23	0.23	0.00	0.06	2.36	1.62
Scurvy[d]	0.00	0.03	0.03	0.71	0.03	0.25
Bronchitis	0.43	0.38	−0.05	−1.05	4.51	2.74
Pneumonia/pleurisy	0.64	0.80	0.16	3.68	6.67	5.72
Phthisis of the lung	1.66	1.13	−0.52	−11.70	17.34	8.07
Diseases of the digestive system	1.14	2.68	1.54	34.32	11.91	19.06
Cholera	0.53	0.50	−0.02	−0.46	5.49	3.59
Other diseases	2.00	2.07	0.07	1.55	20.92	14.73
Total from disease	9.56	14.04	4.48	100.00	100.00	100.00
Action	0.01	0.08	0.07			
Accidents	0.26	0.37	0.11			
Suicides	0.18	0.33	0.15			
Total deaths	9.95	14.76	4.81			

[a] N = 266,000.
[b] N = 63,000.
[c] Percentage contribution of each disease to total relocation cost in deaths.
[d] French total appears to be zero only because of rounding.

Source: Statistique médicale, 1862–4, Tables E no. 1 and E no. 2 each year. For 1865 and 1866, Table F, no. 3. For 1862 through 1864, breakdown of deaths in hospitals alone was used as a sample of deaths in the unit as a whole. Accidental deaths are seriously underreported. In 1866, deaths from causes other than disease are established in proportion to those in the army as a whole.

Table A.26. *Causes of Death among French Troops Serving in France and in Algeria, 1872–6*

Disease	Deaths per Thousand		Difference in Rates	Contribution (%)[c]	Percentage of Total Deaths from Disease	
	France[a]	Algeria[b]			France	Algeria
Typhoid fever	3.40	3.50	0.10	2.86	37.28	27.68
Malaria	0.10	2.33	0.23	63.22	1.07	18.39
Smallpox	0.13	0.31	0.17	4.95	1.44	2.42
Heart disease	0.14	0.26	0.12	3.28	1.54	2.03
Respiratory disease	0.43	1.35	−0.08	−2.13	15.64	10.69
Tuberculosis	0.25	1.57	0.32	9.01	13.67	12.37
Diseases of the digestive system	0.66	1.38	0.72	20.31	7.26	10.90
Cholera	0.09	0.02	−0.07	−2.04	1.01	0.16
Diseases of liver and spleen	0.13	0.23	0.11	3.03	1.37	1.83
Diseases of the nervous system	0.43	0.50	0.06	1.82	4.76	3.94
Other disease	1.38	1.22	−0.17	−4.71	15.16	9.62
Total from Disease	9.13	12.65	3.53	100.00	100.00	100.00
Accidents and suicide	0.28	0.49	0.20			
Total deaths	9.41	13.14	3.73			

Note: French sample is all troops serving in France, 1872–4, those in Gouvernement de Paris only 1875–6. Algerian sample is all French troops serving in Algeria. These figures by cause of death disagree slightly with overall mortality figures reported elsewhere because of differences in mode of reporting. Disease classification was not identical for France and Algeria, 1872–4. It changed and was made uniform for both from 1875. Diseases listed separately as encephalitis, meningitis, and cerebrospinal meningitis are equated with diseases of the nervous system after 1875. Diarrhea, dysentery, gastritis, and gastroenteritis are equated with diseases of the digestive system after 1875.

[a] N = 65,847 in 1875.
[b] N = 40,830 in 1875.
[c] Percentage contribution of each disease of total relocation cost in deaths.

Source: Statistique médicale, Table D each year 1872–4, Table V 1875–6.

Table A.27. Causes of Death among French Troops Serving in France and in Algeria, 1882–6

Disease	Deaths per Thousand		Difference in Rates	Contribution (%)[a]	Percentage of Total Deaths from Disease	
	France	Algeria			France	Algeria
Typhoid fever	4.34	4.10	0.24	−15.45	53.66	42.63
Malaria	0.03	0.95	0.92	59.63	0.39	9.84
Smallpox	0.01	0.10	0.08	5.49	0.13	0.99
Heart disease	0.15	0.21	0.06	3.69	1.90	2.18
Respiratory diseases	0.95	0.75	−0.20	−13.32	11.78	7.77
Tuberculosis	0.81	0.69	−0.12	−7.56	9.97	7.17
Diseases of the digestive system	0.76	1.23	0.47	30.66	9.39	12.78
Cholera	0.09	0.21	0.12	7.88	1.07	2.16
Diseases of the nervous system	0.35	0.28	−0.08	−4.96	4.35	2.87
Other disease	0.60	1.12	0.52	33.95	7.36	11.60
Total from Disease	8.09	9.62	1.54	100.00	100.00	100.00
Traumatic lesions and surgery	0.20	0.77	0.57			
Total deaths	8.29	10.39	2.10			

Note: French sample consists of troops serving in the Gouvernement de Paris: N = 37,400 in 1883. Algerian sample consists of all troops serving in Algeria: N = 56,670 in 1883. These figures by cause of death disagree slightly with overall mortality figures reported elsewhere because of differences in mode of reporting.
[a] Percentage contribution of each disease to total relocation cost in deaths.
Source: Statistique médicale, Table V 1882, Table VI each year 1883–6.

Table A.28. Causes of Death among French Troops Serving in France and in Algeria, 1892–6

Disease	Deaths per Thousand		Difference in Rates	Contribution (%)[a]	Percentage of Total Deaths from Disease	
	France	Algeria			France	Algeria
Typhoid fever	0.98	3.66	2.68	63.88	22.80	43.05
Influenza	0.30	0.09	−0.21	−4.99	7.05	1.12
Malaria	0.00	0.75	0.75	17.82	0.00	8.78
Smallpox	0.00	0.02	0.02	0.50	0.00	0.25
Measles	0.14	0.03	−0.11	−2.66	3.30	0.37
Scarlet fever	0.28	0.02	−0.26	−6.28	6.59	0.24
Heart disease	0.07	0.13	0.06	1.46	1.63	1.55
Respiratory diseases	0.80	1.01	0.21	5.02	18.47	11.84
Tuberculosis	0.85	0.86	0.01	0.22	19.78	10.14
Diseases of the digestive system	0.28	0.71	0.43	10.21	6.43	8.29
Cholera	0.03	0.10	0.07	1.55	0.79	1.17
Diseases of nervous system	0.21	0.23	0.01	0.29	4.98	2.67
Other disease	0.35	0.90	0.54	12.98	8.18	10.54
Total from Disease	4.31	8.51	4.19	100.00	100.00	100.00
Accidents and suicides	0.11	0.20	0.09			
Total deaths	4.42	8.70	4.28			

Note: The French sample is troops serving in the Gouvernement de Paris: N = 57,000 in 1894. The Algerian sample is troops serving in Algeria: N = 45,150 in 1894. These figures by cause of death disagree slightly with overall mortality figures reported elsewhere because of differences in mode of reporting.
[a] Percentage contribution of each disease to total relocation cost in deaths.
Source: Statistiques médicale, 1892–6, annual series, Table VII.

Table A.29. Causes of Death among French Troops Serving in France and in Algeria, 1902–6

Disease	Deaths per Thousand		Difference in Rates	Contribution (%)[c]	Percentage of Total Deaths from Disease	
	France[a]	Algeria[b]			France	Algeria
Typhoid fever	0.59	2.74	2.15	70.85	16.77	41.79
Influenza	0.30	0.02	−0.29	−9.44	8.64	0.28
Malaria	0.01	0.58	0.57	18.78	0.27	8.84
Measles	0.09	0.03	−0.06	−1.99	2.54	0.44
Scarlet fever	0.13	0.03	−0.11	−3.49	3.74	0.39
Cerebrospinal meningitis	0.06	0.05	−0.01	−0.20	1.69	0.82
Dysentery	0.06	0.17	0.11	3.49	1.70	2.53
Tuberculosis	0.84	0.83	−0.01	−0.38	23.82	12.63
Diseases of the nervous system	0.12	0.16	0.04	1.35	3.46	2.49
Bronchopneumonia	0.31	0.27	−0.04	−1.18	8.68	4.12
Pneumonia	0.26	0.39	0.12	4.02	7.48	5.88
Other respiratory diseases	0.28	0.20	−0.07	−2.41	7.83	3.09
Diseases of the circulatory system	0.11	0.14	0.03	0.84	3.18	2.10
Diseases of the digestive system	0.26	0.41	0.14	4.74	7.52	6.23
Other diseases	0.31	0.55	0.24	7.95	8.75	8.38
Total disease	3.52	6.56	3.03	100.00	100.00	100.00
Accidents	0.19	1.02	0.83			
Suicides	0.13	0.37	0.23			
Other traumatic lesions	0.10	0.14	0.04			
Total deaths	4.17	8.09	3.92			

[a] French sample is all troops serving in the Gouvernement de Paris: N = 44,800 in 1904.
[b] Algerian sample is all troops serving in Algeria: N = 53,840 in 1904.
[c] Percentage contribution of each disease to total relocation cost in deaths.
Source: Statistiques médicales, 1892–96, annual series, Table VII.

Table A.30. Causes of Death among French Troops Serving in France and in Algeria, 1902–13

Disease	Deaths per Thousand		Difference in Rates	Contribution (%)[c]	Percentage of Total Deaths from Disease	
	France[a]	Algeria[b]			France	Algeria
Typhoid fever	0.27	1.50	1.23	65.40	9.08	31.12
Influenza	0.04	0.02	-0.02	-0.86	1.21	0.40
Malaria	0.00	0.34	0.34	18.30	0.00	7.16
Measles	0.19	0.03	-0.16	-8.43	6.43	0.62
Scarlet fever	0.14	0.02	-0.11	-6.02	4.67	0.48
Cerebrospinal meningitis	0.07	0.05	-0.02	-1.23	2.38	0.97
Dysentery	0.01	0.12	0.11	5.74	0.39	2.48
Tuberculosis	0.76	0.73	-0.03	-1.65	26.06	15.22
Diseases of the nervous system	0.12	0.15	0.03	1.68	4.08	3.14
Bronchopneumonia	0.25	0.25	0.01	0.41	8.42	5.29
Pneumonia	0.22	0.32	0.09	5.04	7.66	6.63
Other respiratory diseases	0.18	0.20	0.02	1.17	6.19	4.22
Diseases of the circulatory system	0.08	0.18	0.10	5.22	2.70	3.69
Diseases of the digestive system	0.18	0.38	0.20	10.40	6.22	7.85
Other diseases	0.42	0.52	0.09	4.83	14.50	10.72
Total disease	2.93	4.81	1.88	100.00	100.00	100.00
Accidents	0.17	0.71	0.54			
Suicides	0.16	0.39	0.24			
Other traumatic lesions	0.15	0.14	-0.01			
Total deaths	3.40	6.06	2.66			

[a] French sample is all troops serving in the Gouvernement de Paris: N = c.40,000.
[b] Algerian sample is all troops serving in Algeria: N = c.53,000.
[c] Percentage contribution of each disease to total relocation cost in deaths.
Source: Statistiques médicales, 1909–13, annual series, Table VII.

Table A.31. *Relocation Costs as Percentage Increase in Deaths: Great Britain to India, 1830–55*

Year	Deaths per Thousand United Kingdom	Madras	Cost	Deaths per Thousand Bombay	Cost	Deaths per Thousand Bengal	Cost
1830	9.50	32.66	243.79	24.84	161.47	61.90	551.58
1831	14.40	44.88	211.67	35.22	144.58	65.58	355.38
1832	15.60	35.86	129.87	24.33	55.96	68.30	337.82
1833	19.30	45.36	135.03	33.26	72.33	76.55	296.63
1834	13.40	35.70	166.42	35.33	163.66	91.43	582.28
1835	13.70	21.26	55.18	46.23	237.45	77.85	468.25
1836	14.00	23.83	70.21	31.46	124.71	59.40	324.29
1837	13.30	35.95	170.30	60.72	356.54	58.95	343.23
1838	13.80	21.22	53.77	41.48	200.58	82.75	499.64
1839	14.00	27.47	96.21	80.76	476.86	77.83	455.89
1840	10.70	32.70	205.61	64.02	498.32	70.88	562.38
1841	12.80	25.92	102.50	27.30	113.28	73.23	472.07
1842	13.20	33.04	150.30	54.18	310.45	72.00	445.45
1843	12.60	23.66	87.78	54.15	329.76	80.70	540.48
1844	10.30	26.00	152.43	66.53	545.92	74.88	626.94
1845	10.50	46.58	343.64	71.55	581.43	199.23	1797.39
1846	13.90	45.74	229.05	94.62	580.74	100.21	620.93
1847	16.73	37.25	122.66	25.02	49.54	63.24	278.03
1848	16.73	23.49	40.42	28.83	72.35	103.46	518.41
1849	16.73	31.71	89.55	46.83	179.95	88.83	430.93
1850	16.73	22.74	35.90	29.09	73.88	52.64	214.63
1851	16.73	21.14	26.38	33.60	100.83	49.74	197.29
1852	16.73	66.84	299.54	34.11	103.87	71.19	325.54
1853	16.73	46.76	179.49	19.22	14.90	56.68	250.74
1854		32.82		21.93		45.77	
1855		24.93		18.09		45.51	

Source: Data for 1830–47 are for Dragoon Guards and Dragoons, chosen because they did not include men recently returned from colonial service. Indian data from W. H. Sykes, "Vital Statistics of the East India Company's Armies in India, European and Native," JSSL, 10:113–15 (1847) to 1844. India, 1845–55, J. R. Martin, *The Influence of Tropical Climates in Producing the Eudemic Diseases of Europeans*, 2d ed. (London, 1861), p. 105. British 1830–6, PP. 1839, xvi [C.166], p. 4; 1836–47, PP. 1852–53, lix, p. 5.

Table A.32. *Relocation Costs: Great Britain to India, 1859–1914*

Year	Deaths per Thousand Great Britain	India	Cost	Year	Deaths per Thousand Great Britain	India	Cost
1859	7.94	45.35	471.16	1886	6.68	15.51	132.19
1860	9.95	36.77	269.55	1887	5.13	14.68	186.16
1861	9.24	45.93	397.55	1888	5.52	15.20	175.36
1862	8.72	28.11	222.36	1889	4.57	17.12	274.62
1863	8.86	25.08	183.07	1890	5.53	14.45	161.30
1864	9.99	21.10	111.21	1891	4.94	16.36	231.17
1865	8.86	24.24	173.59	1892	4.38	17.59	301.60
1866	9.62	20.11	109.04	1893	5.13	13.15	156.34
1867	9.40	30.95	229.26	1894	3.70	16.81	354.32
1868	9.34	20.11	115.31	1895	4.32	14.31	231.25
1869	9.51	18.20	91.38	1896	3.58	15.29	327.09
1870	9.48	22.86	141.14	1897	3.42	19.25	462.87
1871	8.62	18.73	117.29	1898	3.59	20.31	465.74
1872	7.95	25.30	218.24	1899	4.46	13.25	197.09
1873	8.26	16.25	96.73	1900	6.62	15.36	132.02
1874	8.79	14.22	61.77	1901	4.71	13.12	178.56
1875	9.36	18.52	97.86	1902	4.18	15.36	267.46
1876	8.43	16.10	90.98	1903	3.41	13.33	290.91
1877	7.20	13.75	90.97	1904	2.96	11.28	281.08
1878	6.53	22.30	241.50	1905	2.73	10.38	280.22
1879	7.55	25.88	242.78	1906	2.92	10.81	270.21
1880	6.83	24.65	260.91	1907	3.14	8.58	173.25
1881	7.45	17.19	130.74	1908	2.52	9.27	267.86
1882	6.94	12.82	84.73	1909	2.92	6.37	118.15
1883	6.28	12.03	91.56	1910	2.42	4.77	97.11
1884	5.33	13.03	144.47	1911	2.47	5.04	104.05
1885	6.68	15.18	127.25	1912	2.34	4.82	105.98
				1913	2.60	3.34	28.46
				1914	2.77	3.38	22.02

Source: AMSR, annual series. British sample is Dragoons and Dragoon Guards through 1860; all troops in the United Kingdom thereafter.

Table A.33. *Relocation Costs: Great Britain to the British West Indies, 1803–58*

Year	Deaths per Thousand	
	Windward	Jamaica
1803	117	195
1804	249	92
1805	277	167
1806	114	115
1807	128	87
1808	146	240
1809	99	112
1810	168	126
1811	146	137
1812	9	161
1813	73	140
1814	74	94
1815	96	126
1816	157	101
1817	162	68
1818	126	89
1819	83	294
1820	105	153
1821	109	116
1822	77	171
1823	49	65
1824	70	84
1825	76	307

Year	Deaths per Thousand			Relocation Cost	
	Great Britain	Windward	Jamaica	Windward	Jamaica
1830	14.4	65.00	97	451	574
1831	15.6	69.00	133	351	753
1832	19.3	64.00	111	342	475
1833	13.4	50.00	86	232	542
1834	13.7	43.00	93	273	579
1835	14.0	57.00	75	214	436
1836	13.3	77.00	61	307	359
1837	13.3	69.54	58	479	336
1838	13.8	69.54	55	423	299
1839	14.0	69.54	72	404	415
1840	10.7	69.54	94	397	779
1841	12.8	69.54	244[a]	550	1806
1842	13.2	69.54	33	443	151
1843	12.6	69.54	28	427	123
1844	10.3	69.54	37	452	260
1845	10.5	69.54	21	575	100
1846	13.9	69.54	22	562	58
1847	16.73	69.54	28	400	66
1848	16.73	69.54	44	316	161
1849	16.73	69.54	13	316	-21
1850	16.73	69.54	60[b]	316	259
1851	16.73	69.54	35	316	110
1852	16.73	69.54	14	316	-18

1826	68	80
1827	85	224
1828	81	74
1829	58	62
1853		50[c]
1854		14
1855		13
1856		113[d]
1857		14[e]
1858		3

[a] High barracks at Newcastle first used.

[b] Cholera epidemic.

[c] Two yellow fever cases in Newcastle and 20 others among military elsewhere on the island, but .not so stated in the military records.

[d] Yellow fever epidemic, including Newcastle.

[e] Six cases of yellow fever in Port Royal sent to Newcastle.

Source: British 1830–6, PP. 1839, xvi [C.166], p. 4; 1836–47, AMSR for 1853; later years, AMSR, annual series. Data for 1830–47 for Dragoon Guards and Dragoons, chosen because they do not include men recently returned from colonial service. West Indian Commands, PP. 1837–8, xii(136), pp. 5–6, 45; AMSR for 1869, pp. 81–4. AMSR for 1864, p. 6; for 1860, p. 22, for 1861, p. 10; for 1862, p. 11; (for 1863, p. 10; for 1874, p. 74–5. Jamaica Command data for 1838–58 are for 1838–9 and so on, identified by initial year. Notes and data from AMSR, 9:248–9 (1867); 1837 interpolated.

Table A.34. *Relocation Costs: Great Britain to the British West Indies, 1859–1914*

Year	Deaths per Thousand		Relocation Cost (%)	Year	Deaths per Thousand		Relocation Cost (%)
	Great Britain	West Indies			Great Britain	West Indies	
1859	7.94	20.0	148.74	1888	5.52	3.44	-37.68
1860	9.95	5.6	-43.92	1889	4.57	5.65	23.63
1861	9.24	13.0	35.82	1890	5.53	9.58	73.24
1862	8.72	13.0	50.23	1891	4.94	13.70	177.13
1863	8.86	9.0	1.58	1892	4.38	10.06	128.31
1864	9.99	16.0	56.16	1893	5.13	6.34	23.59
1865	8.86	21.0	136.91	1894	3.70	7.48	102.16
1866	9.62	27.0	180.04	1895	4.32	10.90	151.85
1867	9.40	33.0	254.26	1896	3.58	6.19	72.91
1868	9.34	27.0	193.79	1897	3.42	14.80	333.04
1869	9.51	5.7	-40.59	1898	3.59	7.19	100.28
1870	9.48	29.0	204.85	1899	4.46	7.07	58.52
1871	8.62	6.2	-27.96	1900	6.62	7.07	6.80
1872	7.95	8.9	11.82	1901	4.71	20.50	334.18
1873	8.26	13.0	54.96	1902	4.18	11.60	177.75
1874	8.79	17.0	92.26	1903	3.41	3.55	4.11
1875	9.36	8.8	-5.56	1904	2.96	3.32	12.16
1876	8.43	3.7	-56.35	1905	2.73	3.62	32.60
1877	7.20	16.0	120.56	1906	2.92	6.28	115.07
1878	6.53	13.0	105.21	1907	3.14	18.10	477.39
1879	7.55	10.0	36.03	1908	2.52	6.76	168.25
1880	6.83	8.7	26.09	1909	2.92	17.00	481.85
1881	7.45	61.0	722.95	1910	2.42	5.29	118.60
1882	6.94	10.0	46.40	1911	2.47	2.57	4.05
1883	6.28	14.0	129.94	1912	2.34	5.33	127.78
1884	5.33	11.0	112.57	1913	2.60	7.89	203.46
1885	6.68	7.8	16.32	1914	2.77	12.90	366.79
1886	6.68	15.0	120.06				
1887	5.13	12.0	126.12				

Source: Army Medical Service, *Reports*, Annual Series. Data for Windward and Leeward Command to 1874, then West Indies in general 1875–98; Jamaica alone, 1899 onward. Data missing for 1906 on account of earthquake, filled with annual average 1903–9, with 1906 omitted

Table A.35. *Relocation Costs: France to North Africa, 1831–53*

Year	Deaths per Thousand[a]		Relocation Cost (%)
	France	Algeria	
1831		58.77	
1832		92.88	
1833		94.33	
1834		66.68	
1835		79.19	
1836		71.55	
1837		112.14	
1838		50.10	
1839		71.48	
1840		156.16	
1841		108.36	
1842	24.60	78.87	220.60
1843	20.40	64.09	214.17
1844	15.60	56.85	264.44
1845	14.80	49.09	231.72
1846	17.60	68.22	287.64
1847	19.20	47.50	147.39
1848	24.30	56.64	133.09
1849	17.00		
1850	11.90		
1851	17.40		
1852	14.60		
1853	14.40		

[a] Excluding those killed in action.
Sources: France, 1845–53, Roudin, RMMM, 12(3rd ser.):377–8 (1864); Algeria, 1831–48, PP, 167, xv [Cd.1947], p.36.

Table A.36. *Relocation Costs: France to Algeria, 1859–1913*

Year	Deaths per Thousand[a] France	Algeria	Relocation Cost (%)	Year	Deaths per Thousand[a] France	Algeria	Relocation Cost (%)
1859		56.70		1887	6.55	11.09	69.31
1860		17.80		1888	6.09	11.54	89.49
1861		11.30		1889	5.39	11.07	84.39
1862	9.42	12.21	29.62	1890	5.81	11.94	105.51
1863	9.22	12.29	33.30	1891	6.77	12.50	84.64
1864	9.01	21.25	135.85	1892	5.59	9.09	62.61
1865	11.79	16.32	38.42	1893	5.23	13.45	157.17
1866	10.23	11.95	16.84	1894	5.29	13.30	151.42
1867	9.40	23.04	145.11	1895	6.08	12.27	101.81
1868	12.27	24.31	98.13	1896	5.57	9.49	70.38
1869	9.55	14.42	50.99	1897	4.57	9.87	115.97
1870	9.36	13.61	45.18	1898	4.41	9.03	104.76
1871	9.16	12.79	39.37	1899	4.72	9.78	107.20
1872	8.97	11.98	33.56	1900	4.85	11.53	137.73
1873	8.68	9.22	6.22	1901	4.51	11.10	146.12
1874	8.05	10.76	33.66	1902	4.24	8.30	95.75
1875	10.72	15.68	46.27	1903	3.78	9.53	152.12
1876	9.87	12.35	25.13	1904	3.21	7.56	135.51
1877	8.21	12.59	53.35	1905	3.14	6.20	97.45
1878	7.79	13.59	74.45	1906	3.53	5.98	69.41
1879	7.55	12.68	67.95	1907	3.92	6.15	56.89
1880	9.28	17.80	91.81	1908	4.04	7.91	95.79
1881	8.66	22.61	161.09	1909	3.75	5.53	47.47
1882	8.31	18.00	116.61	1910	3.01	5.72	90.03
1883	7.60	9.80	28.95	1911	3.44	6.25	81.69
1884	6.79	12.52	84.39	1912	2.53	5.39	113.04
1885	6.79	10.38	52.87	1913	2.52	3.62	43.65
1886	7.12	10.52	47.75				

Note: Data not reported separately for "interior" forces in 1874 through 1882, only for the entire army. The "interior" rates reported here are therefore adjusted according to the average difference between "interior" and "entire army" rates for 1872–3 and 1883–4.
[a] From all causes.
Source: Algeria 1859–62, PP, 1867, xv [Cd.19447], p. 7. Ministère de Guerre, *Statistique médicale de l'armée metropolitaine et de l'armée coloniale* (Annual Series). Calculations are based on *effectifs*, not those actually present. Data for 1870–1 filled by interpolation. Algerian data include Tunisia after 1898.

Table A.37. Relocation Costs: Netherlands to Netherlands East Indies, 1859–1913

Year	Deaths per Thousand		Relocation Cost (%)	Year	Deaths per Thousand		Relocation Cost (%)
	Netherlands	Netherlands Indies			Netherlands	Netherlands Indies	
1859	7.94	78.65	890.52	1887	5.73	16.57	189.32
1860	9.95	71.50	618.59	1888	5.93	23.29	292.98
1861	9.24	36.85	298.79	1889	4.01	23.80	492.83
1862	8.72	57.50	559.46	1890	3.79	19.32	409.66
1863	8.86	50.18	466.42	1891	4.35	20.94	380.78
1864	7.89	89.93	1040.13	1892	3.31	17.08	415.60
1865	8.17	78.62	862.17	1893	3.38	11.79	248.71
1866	14.55	54.40	273.86	1894	3.35	16.85	403.62
1867	8.45	46.33	448.21	1895	3.24	15.16	367.91
1868	7.15	81.25	1036.49	1896	3.52	18.34	420.90
1869	8.84	49.64	461.29	1897	3.80	17.10	349.93
1870	8.87	28.54	221.72	1898	3.36	10.97	226.47
1871	9.65	27.98	190.02	1899	2.92	8.30	184.19
1872	8.32	26.07	213.29	1900	3.21	8.71	171.22
1873	8.55	64.41	653.71	1901	3.50	8.38	139.39
1874	6.70	154.47	2207.05	1902	3.27	8.19	150.49
1875	6.35	97.23	1431.06	1903	2.78	7.96	186.28
1876	7.29	89.96	1134.82	1904	2.29	7.74	238.21
1877	5.43	67.27	1139.89	1905	2.61	7.58	190.34
1878	4.41	48.38	996.14	1906	2.39	6.63	177.43
1879	5.28	44.27	737.99	1907	3.14	5.80	84.77
1880	7.06	28.57	304.60	1908	2.52	5.08	101.45
1881	6.81	41.66	511.93	1909	2.92	6.09	108.46

Table A.37. (cont.)

Year	Deaths per Thousand		Relocation Cost (%)
	Netherlands	Netherlands Indies	
1882	5.79	37.86	554.32
1883	6.41	41.55	547.81
1884	5.40	24.68	356.73
1885	5.34	30.19	464.92
1886	6.19	31.80	413.92

Year	Deaths per Thousand		Relocation Cost (%)
	Netherlands	Netherlands Indies	
1910	2.42	6.88	184.14
1911	2.47	6.33	156.39
1912	2.34	6.25	167.05
1913	2.60	6.41	146.48

Source: For the Netherlands 1864–1907; Netherlands. Department van Oorlog, *Statistisch overzicht der bij het Neder landische leger in het yaar ... behandelden zieken* (Annual Series), with interpolations for 1898, 1900, and 1903. Data for British troops in Europe used as a surrogate for Dutch troops for the periods 1859–63 and 1908–13, AMSR, annual reports. For the Netherlands Indies 1859–94: Netherlands, *Koloniaal Verslag*, (Annual Series); for 1895–1900, Netherlands, Central Bureau voor de Statistiek, *Geneeskundig Tijdschrift voor Nederlandische Indie* (Annual Series), with interpolation for 1901–8.

Table A.38. *Causes of Death among British Troops Serving in the United Kingdom and Madras, 1837–46*

Disease	Deaths per Thousand		Difference in Rates	Contribution (%)	Percentage of all Deaths from Disease	
	United Kingdom	Madras			United Kingdom	Madras
Fevers	2.50	3.80	1.30	5.51	13.97	9.16
Eruptive fevers	0.40	0.20	−0.20	−0.85	2.23	0.48
Diseases of the lungs	10.20	2.90	−7.30	−30.93	56.98	6.99
Diseases of the liver	0.40	4.50	4.10	17.37	2.23	10.84
Diseases of the stomach and bowels	0.80	12.70	11.90	50.42	4.47	30.60
Epidemic cholera	0.00	8.30	8.30	35.17	0.00	20.00
Diseases of the brain	0.80	2.60	1.80	7.63	4.47	6.27
Dropsies	0.30	0.60	0.30	1.27	1.68	1.45
Other[a]	2.50	5.90	3.40	14.41	13.97	14.22
Total	17.90	41.50	23.60	100.00	100.00	100.00

Note: United Kingdom sample is infantry of the line. Madras sample is all European troops in the presidency.

[a] Includes other diseases, wounds, and injuries, but not killed in action.

Source: AMSR, 1860, pp. 134, 137. The U.K. data for the infantry of the line are used because they follow the same disease classification as the Madras figures. For a slightly more complex set of distinctions, see data for the footguards used in Table A.2 and in comparing mortality in Britain and the West Indies, Table A.45.

Table A.39. *Causes of Death among European Troops Serving in the United Kingdom and Madras, 1860–7*

Disease	Deaths per Thousand		Difference in Rates	Contribution (%)[a]	Percentage of all Deaths from Disease	
	United Kingdom	Madras			United Kingdom	Madras
Zymotic diseases						
Eruptive fevers	0.31	0.80	0.49	4.29	3.67	4.03
Paroxysmal fevers	0.00	0.70	0.70	6.11	0.00	3.52
Continued fevers	0.42	1.23	0.81	7.07	5.00	6.19
Dysentery/Diarrhea	0.23	3.07	2.84	24.75	2.78	15.46
Spasmodic cholera	0.00	2.76	2.76	24.08	0.00	13.90
Sore throat/influenza	0.04	0.00	-0.04	-0.34	0.46	0.00
Ophthalmia	0.00	0.00	0.00	0.00	0.00	0.00
Rheumatism	0.08	0.04	-0.04	-0.34	0.95	0.20
Enthetic diseases	0.11	0.36	0.25	2.18	1.31	1.81
Dietic diseases	0.07	0.17	0.10	0.87	0.83	0.86
Parasitic diseases	0.00	0.00	0.00	0.00	0.00	0.00
Constitutional diseases						
Diathetic	0.13	0.22	0.09	0.79	1.55	1.11
Tubercular	3.16	2.23	-0.93	-8.12	37.62	11.23
Local diseases						
Nervous system	0.72	1.54	0.82	7.16	8.57	7.75
Circulatory system	1.00	1.31	0.31	2.71	11.90	6.60
Respiratory system	1.32	0.63	-0.69	-6.02	15.71	3.17
Digestive system	0.54	3.96	3.42	29.84	6.43	19.94
Urinary system	0.16	0.17	0.01	0.09	1.90	0.86
Reproductive system	0.00	0.00	0.00	0.00	0.00	0.00
Locomotive system	0.02	0.03	0.01	0.09	0.24	0.15
Integumentary system	0.05	0.08	0.03	0.26	0.60	0.40

Other or not specified	0.04	0.56	0.52	4.54	0.48	2.82
Total disease	8.40	19.86	11.46	100.00	100.00	100.00
Accidents	0.61	1.85				
Homicide	0.02	0.00				
Suicide	0.30	0.30				
Punishment	0.01	0.00				
Grand total	9.34	22.01				

[a] Percentage contribution to total relocation cost.

Source: Tables A.3 and A.19.

Table A.40. Causes of Death among European Troops Serving in the United Kingdom and Madras, 1869–77

Disease	Deaths per Thousand		Difference in Rates	Contribution (%)ᵃ	Percentage of all Deaths from Disease	
	United Kingdom	Madras			United Kingdom	Madras
General diseases						
Febric group						
Eruptive fevers	0.24	0.08	−0.16	−1.60	3.11	0.45
Continued fevers	0.34	1.60	1.26	12.67	4.44	9.08
Paroxysmal fevers	0.00	0.35	0.35	3.52	0.00	1.99
Cholera	0.00	1.58	1.58	15.90	0.00	8.97
Constitutional group				0.00	0.00	0.00
Rheumatism	0.04	0.02	−0.02	−0.23	0.55	0.11
Syphilis	0.21	0.19	−0.02	−0.20	2.74	1.08
Scrofula, phthisis	2.55	1.63	−0.92	−9.23	33.17	9.25
Local diseases						
Nervous system/ear	0.57	1.99	1.42	14.29	7.42	11.29
Circulatory system	1.39	1.86	0.47	4.73	18.10	10.56
Respiratory system	1.32	0.51	−0.81	−8.15	17.19	2.89
Digestive system	0.55	6.74	6.19	62.27	7.16	38.25
Urinary/reproductive system	0.26	0.16	−0.10	−1.01	3.39	0.91
Locomotive system	0.05	0.03	−0.02	−0.20	0.65	0.17
Cellular tissue	0.03	0.02	−0.01	−0.10	0.39	0.11
Conditions						
Debility	0.01	0.06	0.05	0.50	0.13	0.34
Other or not specified	0.12	0.80	0.68	6.84	1.56	4.54
Total from disease	7.68	17.62	9.94	100.00	100.00	100.00
Injuries						
Battle						
Accidents	0.81	1.78	0.97			
Grand total	8.49	19.40	10.91			

ᵃ Percentage contribution to total relocation costs by disease.
Source: Tables A.4 and A.20.

Table A.41. *Causes of Death among European Troops Serving in Madras and the United Kingdom, 1879–84*

Disease	Deaths per Thousand		Difference in Rates	Contribution (%)[a]	Percentage of All Deaths from Disease	
	United Kingdom	Madras			United Kingdom	Madras
Febrile group						
Smallpox	0.01	0.05	0.04	0.80	0.17	0.45
Other eruptive fevers	0.05	0.00	-0.05	-1.00	0.83	0.00
Enteric fever	0.18	1.51	1.33	26.71	3.00	13.74
Other continued fevers	0.12	0.17	0.05	1.00	2.00	1.55
Paroxysmal fevers	0.01	0.28	0.27	5.42	0.17	2.55
Cholera	0.00	1.12	1.12	22.49	0.00	10.19
Constitutional group						
Rheumatism	0.07	0.02	-0.05	-1.00	1.16	0.18
Syphilis	0.02	0.05	0.03	0.60	0.33	0.45
Tubercular diseases	2.08	0.90	-1.18	-23.69	34.61	8.19
Local diseases						
Nervous system	0.46	1.32	0.86	17.27	7.65	12.01
Circulatory system	0.66	0.68	0.02	0.40	10.98	6.19
Respiratory system	1.30	0.41	-0.89	-17.87	21.63	3.73
Digestive system	0.49	3.23	2.74	55.02	8.15	29.39
Gonorrhea/urinary	0.15	0.24	0.09	1.81	2.50	2.18
Other	0.41	1.01	0.60	12.05	6.82	9.19
Total diseases	6.01	10.99	4.98	100.00	100.00	100.00
Injuries	0.72	1.44	0.72			
Grand total	6.73	12.43	5.70			

[a] Percentage contribution to total relocation cost.

Source: Tables A.5 and A.21.

Table A.42. *Causes of Death among European Troops Serving in India and the United Kingdom, 1886–94*

Disease	Deaths per Thousand		Difference in Rates	Contribution (%)[a]	Percentage of all Deaths from Disease	
	United Kingdom	India			United Kingdom	India
Other eruptive fevers	0.05	0.00	−0.05	−0.55	1.16	0.00
Enteric fever	0.27	5.11	4.84	53.72	6.26	38.36
Other continued fevers	0.01	0.04	0.03	0.33	0.23	0.30
Dysentery	0.02	0.70	0.68	7.55	0.46	5.26
Cholera	0.00	1.42	1.42	15.76	0.00	10.66
Malaria	0.01	0.74	0.73	8.10	0.23	5.56
Septic diseases	0.08	0.09	0.01	0.11	1.86	0.68
Rheumatism	0.05	0.07	0.02	0.22	1.16	0.53
Tuberculosis	0.93	0.83	−0.10	−1.11	21.58	6.23
Syphilis	0.05	0.10	0.05	0.55	1.16	0.75
Gonorrhea	0.00	0.00	0.00	0.00	0.00	0.00
Parasitic diseases	0.00	0.00	0.00	0.00	0.00	0.00
Alcoholism	0.04	0.07	0.03	0.33	0.93	0.53
Local diseases						
Eye	0.00	0.00	0.00	0.00	0.00	0.00
Nervous system	0.34	0.38	0.04	0.44	7.89	2.85
Circulatory	0.40	0.38	−0.02	−0.22	9.28	2.85
Respiratory	1.31	0.96	−0.35	−3.88	30.39	7.21
Digestive	0.35	1.82	1.47	16.32	8.12	13.66
Lymphatic	0.01	0.03	0.02	0.22	0.23	0.23
Urinary	0.16	0.16	0.00	0.00	3.71	1.20
Generative	0.01	0.02	0.01	0.11	0.23	0.15
Locomotive	0.03	0.03	0.00	0.00	0.70	0.23
Connective Tissue	0.01	0.01	0.00	0.00	0.23	0.08
Skin	0.00	0.00	0.00	0.00	0.00	0.00
Other disease	0.18	0.36	0.18	2.00	4.18	2.70
Total disease	4.31	13.32	9.01	100.00	100.00	100.00
Injuries/poisons	0.74	2.34	1.60			
Grand total	5.05	15.66	10.61			

[a] Percentage of total relocation costs.
Source: Tables A.6 and A.22.

Table A.43. *Causes of Death among European Troops Serving in the United Kingdom and India, 1895–1904*

Disease	Deaths per Thousand		Difference in Rates	Contribution (%)[a]	Percentage of All Deaths from Disease	
	United Kingdom	India			United Kingdom	Madras
Smallpox	0.01	0.06	0.05	0.51	0.28	0.45
Other eruptive fevers	0.06	0.02	−0.04	−0.41	1.70	0.15
Influenza	0.04	0.02	−0.02	−0.21	1.14	0.15
Diphtheria	0.02	0.00	−0.02	−0.21	0.57	0.00
Enteric fever	0.21	5.62	5.41	55.60	5.97	42.42
Other continued fevers	0.02	0.03	0.01	0.10	0.57	0.23
Dysentery	0.02	0.79	0.77	7.91	0.57	5.96
Cholera	0.00	0.55	0.55	5.65	0.00	4.15
Malaria	0.02	0.62	0.60	6.17	0.57	4.68
Septic diseases	0.05	0.11	0.06	0.62	1.42	0.83
Tuberculosis	0.59	0.77	0.18	1.85	16.76	5.81
Syphilis	—	—	—	—	—	—
Gonorrhea	0.00	0.00	0.00	0.00	0.00	0.00
Parasitic diseases	0.00	0.00	0.00	0.00	0.00	0.00
Alcoholism	0.06	0.09	0.03	0.31	1.70	0.68
Rheumatism/rheumatic fever	0.06	0.03	−0.03	−0.31	1.70	0.23
Local diseases						
Eye	0.00	0.00	0.00	0.00	0.00	0.00
Nervous system	0.26	0.33	0.07	0.72	7.39	2.49
Circulatory	0.41	0.67	0.26	2.67	11.65	5.06
Respiratory	0.99	0.76	−0.23	−2.36	28.13	5.74
Digestive	0.30	1.90	1.60	16.44	8.52	14.34
Lymphatic	0.00	0.02	0.02	0.21	0.00	0.15
Urinary	0.11	0.19	0.08	0.82	3.13	1.43
Other	0.30	0.67	0.37	3.80	8.52	5.06
Total disease	3.52	13.25	9.73	100.00	100.00	100.00
Injuries	0.68	1.79	1.11			
Grand total	4.20	15.04	10.84			

— No data.
[a] Percentage of total relocation costs, by disease.
Source: Tables A.1 and A.23.

Table A.44. Causes of Death among European Troops Serving in the United Kingdom and India, 1909–13

Disease	Deaths per Thousand		Difference in Rates	Contribution (%)[a]	Percentage of all Deaths from Disease	
	United Kingdom	India			United Kingdom	India
Enteric fever	0.06	0.62	0.56	30.60	3.08	16.40
Influenza	0.01	0.00	-0.01	-0.55	0.51	0.00
Beri-beri	0.00	0.01	0.01	0.55	0.00	0.26
Cholera	0.00	0.13	0.13	7.10	0.00	3.44
Dysentery	0.00	0.21	0.21	11.48	0.00	5.56
Kala azar	0.00	0.13	0.13	7.10	0.00	3.44
Malaria	0.00	0.18	0.18	9.84	0.00	4.76
Septic diseases	0.08	0.11	0.03	1.64	4.10	2.91
Pneumonia	0.29	0.27	-0.02	-1.09	14.87	7.14
Tonsilitis	0.00	0.01	0.01	0.55	0.00	0.26
Rheumatic fever	0.02	0.00	-0.02	-1.09	1.03	0.00
Tuberculosis	0.25	0.24	-0.01	-0.55	12.82	6.35
Venereal disease	0.01	0.05	0.04	2.19	0.51	1.32
Diabetes	0.02	0.03	0.01	0.55	1.03	0.79
Carcinoma/sarcoma	0.06	0.07	0.01	0.55	3.08	1.85
Nervous and mental	0.17	0.19	0.02	1.09	8.72	5.03
Diseases of the ear	0.02	0.03	0.01	0.55	1.03	0.79
Circulatory system	0.29	0.33	0.04	2.19	14.87	8.73
Respiratory system	0.12	0.10	-0.02	-1.09	6.15	2.65
Digestive system	0.28	0.80	0.52	28.42	14.36	21.16
Lymphatic system	0.00	0.01	0.01	0.55	0.00	0.26
Urinary system	0.12	0.12	0.00	0.00	6.15	3.17
Generative system	0.00	0.01	0.01	0.55	0.00	0.26
Locomotive system	0.01	0.01	0.00	0.00	0.51	0.26
Other diseases	0.14	0.12	-0.02	-1.09	7.18	3.17
Total disease	1.95	3.78	1.83	100.00	100.00	100.00
Injuries/poisons	0.60	1.09	0.49			
Grand total	2.55	4.87	2.32			

[a] Percentage contribution to total relocation costs.
Source: AMSR for 1914, pp. 144–57. Tables A.8 and A.24.

Table A.45. *Causes of Death among European Troops Serving in the United Kingdom and the Windward and Leeward Command, 1837–46*

	Deaths per Thousand		Difference in Rates	Contribution (%)[a]	Percentage of all Deaths from Disease	
Disease	United Kingdom	Windward/Leeward Command			United Kingdom	Windward/Leeward Command
Zymotic diseases						
Miasmatic diseases						
Eruptive fevers	0.32	0.03	−0.29	−0.59	1.61	0.04
Intermittent fevers	0.00	34.66	34.66	70.08	0.00	50.01
Continued fevers	2.44	5.24	2.80	5.66	12.29	7.56
Dysentery/Diarrhea	0.02	13.65	13.63	27.56	0.10	19.69
Cholera	0.07	0.00	−0.07	−0.14	0.35	0.00
Ophthalmia	0.00	0.17	0.17	0.34	0.00	0.25
Rheumatism	0.00	0.06	0.06	0.12	0.00	0.09
Enthetic diseases	0.02	0.06	0.04	0.08	0.10	0.09
Dietic diseases	0.02	0.00	−0.02	−0.04	0.10	0.00
Parasitic disease	0.00	0.00	0.00	0.00	0.00	0.00
Constitutional diseases						
Diathetic	0.09	0.73	0.64	1.29	0.45	1.05
Tubercular	12.58	5.22	−7.36	−14.88	63.38	7.53
Local diseases						
Nervous system	0.59	3.88	3.29	6.65	2.97	5.60
Circulatory system	0.62	0.14	−0.48	−0.97	3.12	0.20
Respiratory system	1.62	3.33	1.71	3.46	8.16	4.80
Digestive system	0.64	1.65	1.01	2.04	3.22	2.38
Urinary system	0.04	0.01	−0.03	0.06	0.20	0.01
Reproductive system	0.00		0.00	0.00	0.00	0.00
Integumentary system	0.04	0.26	0.22	0.44	0.20	0.38

Table A.45. (cont.)

Disease	Deaths per Thousand		Difference in Rates	Contribution (%)[a]	Percentage of all Deaths from Disease	
	United Kingdom	Windward/Leeward Command			United Kingdom	Windward/Leeward Command
Other or not specified	0.74	0.22	−0.52	−1.05	3.73	0.32
Total from disease	19.85	69.31	49.46	100.00	100.00	100.00
Accidents	0.58	0.23				
Punishment	0.00	0.00				
Grand total	20.43	69.54				

[a] Percentage contribution to total relocation cost.
Source: Tables A.2 and A.10.

Table A.46. *Causes of Death among European Troops Serving in the United Kingdom and the British West Indies Commands, 1859–67*

	Deaths per Thousand		Difference in Rates	Contribution (%)[a]	Percentage of all Deaths from Disease	
Disease	United Kingdom	British West Indies			United Kingdom	British West Indies
Zymotic diseases						
Miasmatic diseases						
Eruptive fevers	0.31	0.00	−0.31	−4.15	3.69	0.00
Paroxysmal fevers	0.00	3.21	3.21	42.97	0.00	20.23
Continued fevers	0.42	1.54	1.12	14.99	5.00	9.70
Yellow fever	0.00	3.43	3.43	45.92	0.00	21.61
Dysentery/diarrhea	0.23	0.29	0.06	0.80	2.74	1.83
Sore throat/influenza	0.04	0.05	0.01	0.13	0.48	0.32
Ophthalmia	0.00	0.00	0.00	0.00	0.00	0.00
Rheumatism	0.08	0.06	−0.02	−0.27	0.95	0.38
Enthetic diseases	0.11	0.00	−0.11	−1.47	1.31	0.00
Dietic diseases	0.07	0.50	0.43	5.76	0.83	3.15
Parasitic diseases	0.00	0.00	0.00	0.00	0.00	0.00
Constitutional diseases						
Diathetic	0.13	0.06	−0.07	−0.94	1.55	0.38
Tubercular	3.16	1.62	−1.54	−20.62	37.62	10.21
Local diseases						
Nervous system	0.72	1.74	1.02	13.65	8.57	10.96
Circulatory system	1.00	1.25	0.25	3.35	11.90	7.88
Respiratory system	1.32	0.44	−0.88	−11.78	15.71	2.77
Digestive system	0.54	0.99	0.45	6.02	6.43	6.24
Urinary system	0.16	0.06	−0.10	−1.34	1.90	0.38
Reproductive system	0.00	0.00	0.00	0.00	0.00	0.00

Table A.46. (cont.)

Disease	Deaths per Thousand				Percentage of all Deaths from Disease	
	United Kingdom	British West Indies	Difference in Rates	Contribution (%)[a]	United Kingdom	British West Indies
Locomotive system	0.02	0.06	0.04	0.54	0.24	0.38
Integumentary system	0.05	0.00	−0.05	−0.67	0.60	0.00
Other or not specified	0.04	0.55	0.51	6.83	0.48	3.47
Total disease	8.40	15.87	7.47	100.00	100.00	100.00
Accidents	0.61	1.00				
Homicide	0.02	0.00				
Suicide	0.30	0.30				
Punishment	0.01	0.00				
Grand total	9.34	17.17				

[a] Percentage contribution to total relocation cost.
Source: AMSR, 9:70–1, 82–3. The British West Indies figure represents an average of the data for the Windward and Leeward Command plus the Jamaica Command, weighted according to their relative strengths in 1868. See also Tables A.3 and A.11.

Table A.47. Causes of Death among European Troops Serving in the United Kingdom and the British West Indies, 1869–77

	Deaths per Thousand				Percentage of all Deaths from Disease	
Disease	United Kingdom	British West Indies	Difference in Rates	Contribution (%)[a]	United Kingdom	British West Indies
General diseases						
Febrile group						
Eruptive fevers	0.24	0.00	−0.24	−10.30	3.11	0.00
Continued fevers	0.34	1.76	1.42	61.16	4.44	17.60
Yellow fever	0.00	2.20	2.20	94.83	0.00	22.00
Paroxysmal fevers	0.00	0.97	0.97	41.81	0.00	9.70
Constitutional group						
Rheumatism	0.04	0.00	−0.04	−1.83	0.55	0.00
Syphilis	0.21	0.00	−0.21	−9.05	2.74	0.00
Scrofula, phthisis	2.55	1.76	−0.79	−33.94	33.17	17.60
Local diseases						
Nervous system	0.57	0.97	0.40	17.24	7.42	9.70
Ear/eye/nose/circulatory	1.39	0.97	−0.42	−18.10	18.10	9.70
Respiratory system	1.32	0.27	−1.05	−45.26	17.19	2.70
Digestive system	0.55	0.70	0.15	6.47	7.16	7.00
Urinary/reproductive system	0.26	0.09	−0.17	−7.33	3.39	0.90
Locomotive system	0.05	0.00	−0.05	−2.16	0.65	0.00
Cellular tissue	0.03	0.00	−0.03	−1.29	0.39	0.00
Conditions						
Debility	0.01	0.17	0.16	6.90	0.13	1.70
Other or not specified	0.12	0.14	0.02	0.86	1.56	1.40
Total from disease	7.68	10.00	2.32	100.00	100.00	100.00
Injuries						
Battle			0.00			
Accidents	0.81	1.27	0.46			
Grand total	8.49	11.27	2.78			

[a] Percentage of total relocation cost, by disease.
Source: Tables A.4 and A.12.

Table A.48. Causes of Death among European Troops Serving in the United Kingdom and the British West Indies, 1879–84

	Deaths per Thousand		Difference in Rates	Contribution (%)[a]	Percentage of all Deaths from Disease	
Disease	United Kingdom	British West Indies			United Kingdom	British West Indies
Febrile group						
Smallpox	0.01	0.00	−0.01	−0.08	0.17	0.00
Other eruptive fevers	0.05	0.00	−0.05	−0.42	0.83	0.00
Enteric fever	0.18	1.32	1.14	9.56	3.00	7.36
Other continued fevers	0.12	0.00	−0.12	−1.01	2.00	0.00
Yellow fever	0.00	8.12	8.12	68.12	0.00	45.29
Paroxysmal fevers	0.01	3.02	3.01	25.25	0.17	16.84
Constitutional group						
Rheumatism	0.07	0.00	−0.07	−0.59	1.16	0.00
Syphilis	0.02	0.00	−0.02	−0.17	0.33	0.00
Tubercular diseases	2.08	0.94	−1.14	−9.56	34.61	5.24
Local diseases						
Nervous system	0.46	0.57	0.11	0.92	7.65	3.18
Circulatory system	0.66	0.75	0.09	0.76	10.98	4.18
Respiratory system	1.30	1.13	−0.17	−1.43	21.63	6.30
Digestive system	0.49	1.51	1.02	8.56	8.15	8.42
Gonorrhea/urinary	0.15	0.19	0.04	0.34	2.50	1.06
Other	0.41	0.38	−0.03	−0.25	6.82	2.12
Total diseases	6.01	17.93	11.92	100.00	100.00	100.00
Injuries	0.72	1.51				
Grand total	6.73	19.44				

[a] Percentage of total relocation cost, by disease.
Source: Tables A.5 and A.13.

Table A.49. Causes of Death among European Troops Serving in the United Kingdom and the British West Indies, 1886–94

Disease	Deaths per Thousand		Difference in Rates	Contribution (%)[a]	Percentage of all Deaths from Disease	
	United Kingdom	British West Indies			United Kingdom	British West Indies
Other eruptive fevers	0.05	0.00	-0.05	-1.38	1.16	0.00
Enteric fever	0.27	2.81	2.54	69.97	6.26	35.39
Other continued fevers	0.01	0.19	0.18	4.96	0.23	2.39
Dysentery	0.02	0.49	0.47	12.95	0.46	6.17
Yellow fever	0.00	0.68	0.68	18.73	0.00	8.56
Malaria	0.01	0.97	0.96	26.45	0.23	12.22
Septic diseases	0.08	0.00	-0.08	-2.20	1.86	0.00
Rheumatism	0.05	0.10	0.05	1.38	1.16	1.26
Tuberculosis	0.93	0.19	-0.74	-20.39	21.58	2.39
Syphilis	0.05	0.19	0.14	3.86	1.16	2.39
Gonorrhea	0.00	0.00	0.00	0.00	0.00	0.00
Parasitic diseases	0.00	0.00	0.00	0.00	0.00	0.00
Alcoholism	0.04	0.00	-0.04	-1.10	0.93	0.00
Local diseases						
Eye	0.00	0.00	0.00	0.00	0.00	0.00
Nervous system	0.34	0.39	0.05	1.38	7.89	4.91
Circulatory	0.40	0.49	0.09	2.48	9.28	6.17
Respiratory	1.31	0.68	-0.63	-17.36	30.39	8.56
Digestive	0.35	0.29	-0.06	-1.65	8.12	3.65
Lymphatic	0.01	0.00	-0.01	-0.28	0.23	0.00
Urinary	0.16	0.29	0.13	3.58	3.71	3.65
Generative	0.01	0.00	-0.01	-0.28	0.23	0.00
Locomotive	0.03	0.10	0.07	1.93	0.70	1.26
Connective tissue	0.01	0.00	-0.01	-0.28	0.23	0.00
Skin	0.00	0.00	0.00	0.00	0.00	0.00

Table A.49. (cont.)

Disease	Deaths per Thousand		Difference in Rates	Contribution (%)[a]	Percentage of all Deaths from Disease	
	United Kingdom	British West Indies			United Kingdom	British West Indies
Other disease	0.18	0.08	−0.10	−2.75	4.18	1.01
Total disease	4.31	7.94	3.63	100.00	100.00	100.00
Injuries/poisons	0.74	1.08	0.34			
Grand total	5.05	9.02	3.97			

[a] Percentage of total relocation costs, by disease.
Source: Tables A.7 and A.14.

Table A.50. Causes of Death among European Troops Serving in the United Kingdom and the British West Indies, 1895–1904

Disease	Deaths per Thousand		Difference in Rates	Contribution (%)[a]	Percentage of all Deaths from Disease	
	United Kingdom	British West Indies			United Kingdom	British West Indies
Other eruptive fevers	0.06	0.00	−0.06	−1.54	1.70	0.00
Influenza	0.04	0.00	−0.04	−1.02	1.14	0.00
Diphtheria	0.02	0.07	0.05	1.20	0.57	0.90
Enteric fever	0.21	0.88	0.67	17.04	5.97	11.79
Other continued fevers	0.02	0.00	−0.02	−0.51	0.57	0.00
Dysentery	0.02	0.14	0.12	3.13	0.17	1.91
Yellow fever	0.00	1.52	1.52	38.90	0.00	20.46
Malaria	0.02	1.48	1.46	37.40	0.57	19.94
Septic diseases	0.05	0.00	−0.05	−1.28	1.42	0.00
Tuberculosis	0.59	0.71	0.12	3.19	16.76	9.62
Gonorrhea	0.00	0.00	0.00	0.00	0.00	0.00
Parasitic diseases	0.00	0.00	0.00	0.00	0.00	
Alcoholism	0.06	0.21	0.15	3.96	1.70	0.00
Rheumatism	0.06	0.07	0.01	0.17	1.70	0.90
Local diseases						
Eye	0.00	0.00	0.00	0.00	0.00	0.00
Nervous system	0.26	0.14	−0.12	−3.02	7.39	1.91
Circulatory	0.41	0.43	0.02	0.49	11.65	5.78
Respiratory	0.99	0.28	−0.71	−18.15	28.13	3.79
Digestive	0.30	0.50	0.20	5.20	8.52	6.77
Lymphatic	0.00	0.00	0.00	0.00	0.00	0.00
Urinary	0.11	0.29	0.18	4.61	3.13	3.90

Table A.50. (*cont.*)

Disease	Deaths per Thousand		Difference in Rates	Contribution (%)[a]	Percentage of all Deaths from Disease	
	United Kingdom	British West Indies			United Kingdom	British West Indies
Other	0.30	0.70	0.40	10.25	8.52	9.43
Total disease	3.52	7.42	3.90	100.00	100.00	100.00
Injuries	0.68	2.32	1.64			
Grand total	4.20	9.75	5.55			

[a] Percentage of total relocation costs, by disease.

Source: AMSR for 1905, pp. 274–5, 302–3, 306–7. Tables A.8 and A.15. West Indian data are the average of separate reports for the Barbados and Jamaican Commands, weighted in proportion of troops in each as of 1900.

Table A.51. Causes of Death among European Troops Serving in the United Kingdom and Jamaica, 1909–13

Disease	Deaths per Thousand		Difference in Rates	Contribution (%)[a]	Percentage of all Deaths from Disease	
	United Kingdom	Jamaica			United Kingdom	Jamaica
Cerebrospinal fever	0.01	0.52	0.51	9.64	0.51	7.18
Enteric fever	0.06	1.03	0.97	18.34	3.08	14.23
Influenza	0.01	0.00	-0.01	-0.19	0.51	0.00
Dysentery	0.00	0.00	0.00	0.00	0.00	0.00
Malaria	0.00	1.52	1.52	28.73	0.00	20.99
Septic diseases	0.08	0.00	-0.08	-1.51	4.10	0.00
Pneumonia	0.29	0.52	0.23	4.35	14.87	7.18
Tonsilitis	0.00	0.00	0.00	0.00	0.00	0.00
Rheumatic fever	0.02	0.00	-0.02	-0.38	1.03	0.00
Tuberculosis	0.25	0.52	0.27	5.10	12.82	7.18
Venereal disease	0.01	0.52	0.51	9.64	0.51	7.18
Diabetes	0.02	0.52	0.50	9.45	1.03	7.18
Carcinoma/sarcoma	0.06	0.52	0.46	8.70	3.08	7.18
Nervous and mental	0.16	0.00	-0.16	-3.02	8.21	0.00
Diseases of the ear	0.02	0.00	-0.02	-0.38	1.03	0.00
Circulatory system	0.29	1.03	0.74	13.99	14.87	14.23
Respiratory system	0.12	0.00	-0.12	-2.27	6.15	0.00
Digestive system	0.28	0.52	0.24	4.54	14.36	7.18
Urinary system	0.12	0.00	-0.12	-2.27	6.15	0.00
Generative system	0.00	0.00	0.00	0.00	0.00	0.00
Locomotive system	0.01	0.00	-0.01	-0.19	0.51	0.00
Other diseases	0.14	0.02	-0.12	-2.27	7.18	0.28
Total disease	1.95	7.24	5.29	100.00	100.00	100.00
Injuries/poisons	0.60	0.52				
Grand total	2.55	7.76				

[a] Percentage of total relocation costs, by disease.
Source: Tables A.9 and A.16.

Table A.52. *Admissions and Deaths of Female Dependents, Officers, and Other Ranks in India, 1899–1913*

	Admissions per Hundred Thousand			Deaths per Thousand		
Year	Female Dependents[a]	Officers	ORs	Female Dependents	Officers	ORs
1899	6.70	7.68	11.49	14.55	13.63	13.25
1900	8.02	8.13	11.43	17.54	14.61	14.62
1901	7.15	8.31	11.04	12.83	11.12	12.38
1902	8.00	8.18	10.78	14.87	16.05	14.68
1903	7.59	8.11	10.36	14.18	13.39	12.78
1904	6.97	7.77	8.97	12.42	8.73	10.81
1905	6.47	6.89	8.34	10.96	9.08	10.06
1906	7.58	7.27	8.71	12.24	17.54	10.43
1907	6.58	6.33	7.56	6.58	7.71	8.18
1908	7.20	6.47	8.36	13.53	7.87	9.09
1909	5.97	6.39	7.17	7.67	9.58	6.25
1910	5.05	5.73	5.77	6.28	7.19	4.66
1911	4.96	5.82	5.25	7.30	8.10	4.89
1912	5.11	5.80	5.48	9.16	4.39	4.62
1913	5.27	5.46	5.81	6.31	2.09	3.26

[a] Number of Women in 1913 was 4,123.
Source: AMSR, 49:103–4 (1908); 55:57 (1913).

BIBLIOGRAPHY

The sources for this study fall into two categories. First are the annual and other reports from various army medical authorities. These are the basis for the statistics that appear in the appendix tables, and are further refined in text tables and discussions. The second principal source is the literature on tropical and military medicine, supplemented by later, secondary works on the history of medicine and on military medicine in particular. Those works are listed in the general bibliography.

Statistical Sources

Anon. "Report of a Committee of the Statistical Society of London, Appointed to Collect and Inquire into Vital Statistics, upon Sickness and Mortality among European and Native Troops ... in ... Madras .... JSSL, 3:113–43, 4:137–55 (1840–1).

"Statistiques coloniale. Mortalité des troupes." RC, 10(2d ser.):473–81 (1853).

Internationale militärärtzliche Commission für Einheitliche Militäsrs Sanitäts-Statistik zu Budapest im September 1894. Budapest, 1894.

"International Medico-Military Statistics." JAMA, 26:293– (1896).

"La mortalité des troupes en France, en Algérie, et aux colonies." *Revue scientifique*, 10(4th ser.):269–76 (1898).

Benoitson de Chateauneuf. "Essai sur la mortalité de l'infantrie française." AHPML, 10:239–316 (1833).

Bryden, James L. *Annual Reports of the European Army of the Bengal Presidency from 1858–1868, and of the Native Army Each Year Since Its Reorganization in 1861, and of the Jails for Each Year since 1859*. Calcutta, 1871.

Chenu, Jean-Charles. *Statistique médico-chirurgicale de la campagne d'Italie en 1859 et 1860*, 2 vols. Paris, 1870.

France, Ministère des colonies. *Statistiques médicale des troupes coloniales en France et aux colonies pendant l'année....* Paris, 1903–13.

France, Ministère de Guerre. *Statistiques médicale de l'armée metropolitaine et de l'armée coloniale*. Paris, annual series, 1862–1914.

Statistiques médicale: I. Donnée statistique relative à la guerre 1914–18. II. Statistique du Maroc de 1907 à 1919. III. Pandémie de grippe du 1er mai 1918 au 30 avril 1919. Paris, 1922.

Ministère du la marine. *Statistiques médicales de la marine*. Annual Series.

Germany, Reichsgesundheitsamt. *Arbeiten aus den Kaiserlichen Gesundheitsamt*. Annual Series, 1884+.

Kolonialamt. *Medizinal-Berichte über die Deutschen Schutzgebeiten 1903/04–1911/12*.

Great Britain, Army Medical Service. *Reports* (1859–1914).

Royal Commission on the Sanitary State of the Army in India. *Report of the Commissioners Appointed to Inquire into the Sanitary State of the Army in India....* 2 vols. London, 1863.

Parliamentary Sessional Papers, 1837–8, xl (138). *Statistical Report of Sickness, Invaliding, and Mortality among Troops in the West Indies.*

1839, xvi [C.166]. *Statistical Reports of the Sickness, Mortality, and Invaliding among Troops in the United Kingdom, Mediterranean, and British North America.* By Major Alexander M. Tulloch.

1840, xxx [C.228]. *Statistical Reports on Sickness, Mortality, and Invaliding among Troops in Western Africa, St. Helena, Cape of Good Hope, and Mauritius.*

1842, xxvii [C.358]. *Statistical Reports on the Sickness, Mortality, and Invaliding among Her Majesty's Troops serving in Ceylon, the Tenasserim Provinces, and the Burmese Empire.* By Major Alex M. Tulloch.

1849, xxxiii (436). *Statistical Reports on the Health of the Navy 1837–43. Part I. South Atlantic Station, North American and West Indian Stations, Mediterranean Station.*

1852–3. lix, *Statistical Reports on the Sickness, Mortality, and Invaliding among the Troops in the United Kingdom, the Mediterranean, and British America.*

Kozlovski, N. "Statistical Data Concerning the Losses of the Russian Army from Sickness and Wounds in the War against Japan, 1904–05." JRAMC, 18:330–46 (1912).

Lawson, Thomas. *Statistical Report on the Sickness and Mortality in the Army of the United States.* 3 vols. Washington, D.C., 1840–60.

Lemos Junior, Maximiano. "A mortalidade do exercito portuguez." RMMP, 1:137–42 (1886–7).

Marshall, Henry. "Mortality of the French Infantry." *British Annals of Medicine, Pharmacy, Vital Statistics, and General Science*, 1:585–7 (1837).

Netherlands, Central Bureau voor de Statistiek. *Jaarcifers voor het Koninkrijk der Nederlanden: Koloniën.* The Hague, Annual Series, 1884+.

Supplément à la statistique medicale de l'armée Indo-néerlandaise pendant l'année ... comme contribution à la statistique médicale militaire internationale. The Hague, 1912–17.

Statistisch Overzicht der Behandelde Zieken van het Nerderlanissch-Indisch Lager. Batavia, Annual Series, 1905–18.

Department van Kolonien. *Kolonial Verslag.* Annual Series, 1848+.

Department van Oorlog. *Geneeskundig Dienst der Landmacht. Statistisch overzicht der bij het Nederlandische leger in het yaar ... behandelde zieken.* The Hague, Annual Series.

Pollock, C. E., "Losses in the Russo-Japanese War, 1904–05." JRAMC, 17:50–4 (1911).

Portugal, Ministerio das obras publicas. *Annuario estatistico de Portugal.*

Spain, Ministerio de la Guerra. *Resumen de la estadistica sanitaria del ejercito española.* Madrid, 1884+.

Statistical Society of London. "Report of the Committee of the Statistical Society of London, Appointed to Enquire into Vital Statistics, upon the Sickness and Mortality among the European and Native Troops Serving in Madras Presidency, from the year 1793 to 1838." JSSL, 3:113–43 (1840).

Sykes, W. H. "Vital Statistics of the East India Company's Armies in India, European and Native." JSSL, 10:100–15 (1847).

U.S. Army, Surgeon General. *Report of the Surgeon General of the Army to the Secretary of War for the Fiscal Year Ending ....* Annual Series, Washington, D.C.

General Bibliography

Acherknecht, Erwin H. "Anticontagionism between 1821 and 1867." BHM, 22:562–93 (1948).

"Broussais or a Forgotten Medical Revolution." BHM, 27:320–43 (1957).

History and Geography of the Most Important Diseases. New York, 1965.

Adams, Catherine F. *Nutritive Value of American Foods.* Washington, D.C., 1975.

Ageron, Charles Robert. *Les algériens musulmans et la France, 1871–1914.* Paris, 1968.

Allen, S. Glen. "Enteric Fever in Ambala, 1880–1905." JRAMC, 8:123–40 (1907).

Alvernhe. "État sanitaire des troupes coloniales françaises." AMPM, 47:58–72 (1906).

American Society of Civil Engineers. *Pure and Wholesome: A Collection of Papers on Water and Waste Treatment at the Turn of the Century.* New York, 1982.

Anderson, J. B. "Malaria in India." JRAMC, 14:50–60 (1910).

Annesley, James. *Sketches of the Most Prevalent Diseases of India.* 2d ed. London, 1931.

Annett, H. E., J. Everett Dutton, and J. H. Elliott. *Report of the Malaria Expedition to Nigeria of the Liverepool School of Tropical Medicine and Medical Parasitology.* London, 1902.

Anon. "On Sickness and Mortality among Soldiers' Wives." AMSR, 9:155–65 (1865).

"Estadistica sanitaria del ejécito de Cuba: gráfica comparativa del estado sanitario del segundo cuatrimestre de los años 1896 y 1897," *Medicina militar española*, 3:118–21 (1897).

"Mortality of French and British Naval Expeditions." *British Medical Journal* (1898):991.

Hints and Suggestions for Travelling on the West Coast of Africa. (London, 1901).

"The Sterilisation of Drinking Water for Troops in the Field." JRAMC, 4:349–52(1905).

"Chronique. France. Statistique médicale des Troupes Coloniales en France et aux Colonies pour l'année 1910." RTC, 12:763–8 (1913).

"On Sickness and Mortality among Soldiers' Wives." AMSR, 9:155–65 (1865).

Armand, Adolphe. *L'algérie médicale: topographie, climatologie, pathogénie, pathologie, prophylaxie, hygiène, acclimatement et colonisation.* (Paris, 1854).

Souvenirs d'un médecin militaire: France, Afrique, Italie, Turquie, Crimée. Paris, 1858.

Médecine et hygiène des pays chauds; et spécialment de l'Algérie et des colonies. . . . Paris, 1859.

Traité de climatologie générale du globe: études médicales sur tous les climats. Paris, 1873.

Arnould, Jules. *Nouveaux eléments d'hygiène* (1881).

Arnould, Jules, E. and H. Surmont. *Nouveaux éléments d'hygiène.* 3d ed. (1895).

Ashburn, P. M. *The Ranks of Death: A Medical History of the Conquest of America.* New York, 1947.

Aufderheide, Arthur C., J. Lawrence Angel, Jennifer O. Kelley, Alain C. Outlaw, Merry O. Outlaw, George Rapp, Jr., and others. "Lead in Bone III. Prediction of Social Correlates from Skeletal Lead Content in Four Colonial American Populations . . ." *American Journal of Physical Anthropology*, 66:353–61 (1985).

Azan, Paul. *L'armée d'Afrique de 1830 à 1852.* Paris, 1936.

Badoul. "Note sur le traitement sénégalais de la fièvre jaune." AMN, 74:139–40 (1900).

Badour. "Souvenirs de l'éxpedition de 1881 en basse Tunisie (colonne de Tébassa). *Gasette d'hôpital*, 40:180–, 180–, 876– (1887).

Baeza Gonzales, Federico. *Contribución a la história medicoquirurgica de la ultima campaña de Cuba.* Valencia, 1899.

Baills, J. J. "Deux cas d'empoisonnement par le sulfate de quinine." AMPH, 6:320–4 (1885).

Baker, M. N. *The Quest for Pure Water: The History of Water Purification from the Earliest Records to the Twentieth Century.* New York, 1948.

Balck, J. A., and A. Harpur Napier. "Notes on the Treatment of Cholera." JRAMC, 12:192–7 (1909).

Balfour, Edward. *Observations on the Means of Preserving the Health of Troops by Selecting Healthy Localities for their Cantonments.* London, 1845.

Remarks on the Causes for Which Native Soldiers of the Madras Army Were Discharged the Service in the Five Years from 1842–3 to 1846–7. Madras, 1850.

Balfour, T. Graham. "Comparison of the Sickness, Mortality, and Prevailing Diseases among Seamen and Soldiers, as Shown by the Naval and Military Statistical Reports." JSSL, 8:77–86 (1845).

"Summary of the Reports on the Health of the Army Published Previous to 1859." AMSR, 2:131–41 (1860).

Ballhatchet, Kenneth. *Race, Sex, and Class under the Raj: Imperial Attitudes and Policies and Their Critics, 1793–1905.* London, 1980.

Barclay. "Report to the Assistant Quarter-Master-General, Mysore Division, on the Causes of Enteric Fever at Bangalore." AMSR, 13:208–11 (1871).

Barnier, Jean-Baptiste. "Note sur l'épidemie de choléra qui a sévi dans l'île de Nossi-Bé." AMN, 16:190–8 (1871).

Barwise, Sydney. *The Purification of Sewage*. London, 1899.

Baudens, J. B. L. *Rélation de l'expédition de Constantine*. Paris, 1838.

Rélation historique de l'expédition de Tagdempt. Paris, 1841.

Baudens, Lucien. *Sur la guerre de Crimée*. 2d ed. Paris, 1858.

Beckerling, Joan Letitia. *The Medical History of the Anglo-Boer War: A Bibliography*. Cape Town, 1967.

Benson, Bryan. "Mortality Variation in the North of England." 2 vols. Ph.D. diss., Johns Hopkins, 1981.

Bérenger-Féraud, Laurent Jean Baptiste. "Le Sénégal 1817–1874." RC, 41:28–45 (1875).

De la fièvre bilieux mélanique des pays chauds. Paris, 1874.

Traité clinique des maladies des européens au Sénégal. 2 vols. Paris, 1875–8.

De la fièvre dite bilieuse inflammatoire aux Antilles et dans l'Amérique tropicale. Paris, 1878.

Berger, Charles, and Henri Rey. *Répertoire bibliographique des travaux des médecins and des pharmaciens de la marine française, 1698–1873*. Paris, 1974.

Bertillon. "Acclimatement." *Dictionaire encyclopédique des sciences médicales*. Paris, 1861, I, 270–328.

Bett, Walter R. *The History and Conquest of Common Diseases*. Norman, Okla., 1954.

Beveridge, W. W. O. "Some Essential Factors in the Construction of Field Service and Expeditionary Rations." JRAMC, 23:377–96 (1914).

Billet, A. "La fièvre typhoïde dans la garnison de Constantine en 1899." AMPH, 37:94–145 (1901).

Birch, Edward A. "The Influence of Warm Climates on the Constitution." In *Hygiene and Disease in Warm Climates*, ed. A. Davidson. London, 1893, pp. 1–24.

Birt, C., and H. R. Bateman. "Kala-Azar." JRAMC, 7:341–7 (1906).

Bishop, W. J., and Sue Goldie. *A Bio-Bibliography of Florence Nightingale*. London, 1962.

Blackham, Robert J. "A Soldier's Head-Dress." JRAMC, 21:670–5.

"The Goux System and Its Applications to India." JRAMC, 6:662–75 (1906).

"The Treatment of Dysentery." JRAMC, 10:436–45 (1908).

"Micro-organisms of Dysentery." JRAMC, 11:582–92 (1908).

"The Sanitary Organization of the Imperial and Indian Armies, with Sanitary Lessons from the Oriental Campaign." JRAMC, 19:231–51 (1912).

Blanco, Richard L. *Wellington's Surgeon General: Sir James McGrigor*. Durham, N. C., 1974.

Blane, Gilbert. "Statements of the Health of the British Navy from the Year 1779 to the Year 1814, with Proposals for Its Further Improvement." *Medico-Chirurgical Transactions*, 6:490–573 (1815).

Bonnafy, M. "Statistique Médicale de la Cochinchine (1861–1888)" AMN, 67:161–96 (1897).

"Les moyens d'assurer la salubrité de l'eau au point de vue de l'hygiène coloniale." *Transactions, Twelfth* ICHD, 10:667–78 (Paris, 1900).

Bonnette. "Epuration de l'eau potable en campagne." AMPM, 42:271–4 (1903).

Borius, Alfred. "Topographie médicale du Sénégal." AMN, 33:114–, 270–, 321–, 416–; 34:278–, 330–, 340–; 35:114–, 280–, 473–; 36:117–, 321–; 37:140–, 230–, 297–, 367–, 456– (1879–82).

Boudin, Jean Chrisitan Marc François Joseph. *Traité des fièvres intermettentes remittentes et continue, des pays chauds et des régions marécaseusses, suivi des recherches sur l'emplois des préparations arsénales*. Paris 1812.

Essai de géographie médicale ou étude sur les lois qui préside à la distribution géographique des maladies, ainsi qu'à leurs rapports topographiques entre elles. Lois de coincidence et d'antagonisme. Paris, 1843.

Statistique de l'état sanitaire des armées de terre et de mer. Paris, 1846.

"Étude sur la mortalité et l'acclimatement de la population françaises en Algérie." AHPML, 37(2):358–91 (1847).

Hygiène militaire comparée et statistique médicale des armées de terre et de mer. Paris, 1848.

"Histoire statistique de la colonisation et de la population en Algérie." AHPML, 50:281–314 (1852).

Traité de géographie et de statistique médicale et des maladies endémiques. 2 vols. Paris, 1857.

"Essai de pathologie ethnique; de l'influence de la race sur la fréquence, la forme, et la gravité des maladies." AHPML, 16:5–50, 17:64–103 (1861–2).

"Examen de deux questions de géographie médicale." RMMM, 7(3d ser.):97–108 (1862).

"Statistique médicale de l'armée anglaise." RMMM, 12 (3d ser.):369–89; 13:1–22 (1864–5).

Bourdas. "Fièvre jaune et moustiques. AMPM, 40:171–(1902).

Boyd, Mark F. *Malariology: A Comprehensive Survey of All Aspects of This Group of Diseases from a Global Standpoint.* 2 vols. Philadelphia and London, 1949.

Brault, Jules. *Hygiène et prophylaxie des maladies dans les pays chauds. L'Afrique française.* Paris, 1900.

Brereton, J. M. *The British Soldier: A Social History from 1661 to the Present Day.* London: Bodley Head. 1986.

Brice and Bottet. *Le corps de santé militaire en France: son évolution, ses campaigns 1708–1882.* Paris, 1907.

Brignon, René. *Contribution de la France à l'étude des maladies coloniales.* Lyon, 1942.

Brockway, Lucille H. *Science and Colonial Expansion: The Role of the British Royal Botanic Society.* New York, 1979.

Brooke, Gilbert E. *Tropical Medicine, Hygiene, and Parasitology: A Handbook for Practitioners and Students.* London, 1908.

Bruce, Charles. "Some Imperial Aspects of the Study of Tropical Medicine." JRAMC, 11:164–9 (1908).

Bruce, David. "Analysis of the Results of Professor Wright's Method of Anti-Typhoid Inoculation." JRAMC, 4:244–55 (1905).

Bruce-Chwatt, Leonard Jan. *Essential Malariology.* London, 1980.

Bruce-Chwatt, Leonard J., and Joan M. Bruce-Chwatt. "Malaria and Yellow Fever," in *Health in Tropical Africa during the Colonial Period,* ed. Sabben-Clare, E. E., David J. Bardley, and Kenneth Kirkwood. Oxford, 1980; pp. 43–62.

Bruce-Chwatt, Leonard Jan, and Julian de Zulueta. *The Rise and Fall of Malaria in Europe – A Historical-Epidemiological Study.* Oxford, 1980.

Bryden, James L. *Age and Length of Service as Affecting the Sickness and Mortality of Europeans....* Calcutta, 1874.

Bryson, Alexander. "On the Prophylactic Influence of Quinine," MTG, 8(n.s.):6–7 (January 7, 1854).

Burge, Wylie D., and Paul B. Marsh. "Infectious Hazards of Landspreading Sewage Waste." *Journal of Environmental Quality,* 7:1–9 (1978).

Burnet, Macfarlane, and David O. White. *Natural History of Infectious Disease.* 4th ed. Cambridge, 1972.

Burnett, James. *Plenty and Want: A Social History of Diet in England from 1815 to the Present.* London, 1966.

Burot, Fernand, and Maximilien Albert Legrand. *Les troupes colonialiaux. Statistiques de la mortalité. Maladies du soldat aux pays chauds. Hygiène du soldat sous les tropiques.* 3 vols. Paris, 1897–98.

Burot, Fernand, and Maximilien-Albert Legrand. "Maladies de marins, épidémies nautiques." RC, 130:17–81 (1897).

Burot, Fernand, and M. Vincent. "Les altitudes dans les pays paludéens et la zone toride." AHPML, 1 Dec. 1896.

228 **Bibliography**

Caille, H. A. *Considerations sanitaires sur les expéditions coloniales*. Bordeaux, Thesis no. 64, 1904.

Calmette. "Stérilisation des eaux par l'ozone." *Annales de l'institut Pasteur*, 13:344 (April 1899).

Camail. "Morbidité et mortalité des troupes aux colonies (Tonkin, Cochinchine, Magadascar, Sénégal, Guyane)." AHMC, 4:284–94 (1901).

Cambay, Charles. *Traité des maladies des pays chauds, et specialment de l'Algérie*. Paris, 1847.

Cantile, Neil. *A History of the Army Medical Department*. 2 vols. London and Edinburgh, 1974.

Carbonnel, Pierre François Auguste Thomas. *De la mortalité actuelle au Sénégal et particulièrement à Saint-Louis*. Paris, Thesis no. 10, 1873.

Carlson, Dennis G. "African Fever, Prophylactic Quinine, and Statistical Analysis: Factors in the European Penetration of a Hostile West African Environment." BHM, 51:386–96 (1977).

Carpenter, Kenneth J. *The History of Scurvy and Vitamin C*. New York, 1986.

Cassedy, James H. *American Medicine and Statistical Thinking, 1800–1860*. Cambridge, 1984.

Medicine and American Growth 1800–1860. Madison, Wisc., 1986.

Castellani, Aldo, and Albert J. Chalmers. *Manual of Tropical Medicine*. London, 1910.

Cell, John W. "Anglo-Indian Medical Theory and the Origins of Segregation in West Africa." AHR, 91:307–35 (1986).

Chandra, R. K., and P. M. Newberne. *Nutrition, Immunity, and Infection: Mechanisms of Interactions*. New York, 1977.

Chaudoye. "Le paludisme à Touggourt en 1902." AMPM, 42:14–38 (1903).

"La fièvre typhoïde dans la garnison et dans la ville de T'bessa de 1890 à 1906." AMPM, 50:169–(1909).

Chenu, Jean-Charles. *De mortalité dans l'armée et les moyens d'économiser la vie humaine, extraits des statistiques médico-chirugicales des campagnes de Crimée en 1854 et d'Italie en 1859*. Paris, 1878.

Chevalier, A. "Sur la necessité de proscrire les vases de plomb...." AHPML, 50:314–36 (1853).

Christie, James. "Notes on the Cholera Epidemics in East Africa." *Transactions of the Epidemiological Society of London*, 3:265–87 (1870).

Cholera Epidemics in East Africa. London, 1876.

Christophers, S. R., and J. W. W. Stephens. "Segregation of Europeans." *Reports of the Malaria Commission of the Royal Society*, 3:21–5 (1900).

Cockburn, Aiden. *The Evolution and Eradication of Infectious Diseases*. Baltimore, Md., 1963.

Cohen, William B. "Health and Colonialism in French Africa." In *Études africaine offertes à Henri Bruinschwig*, ed. Jan Vansina and others. Paris, 1982.

"Malaria and French Imperialism," JAH, 24:23–36 (1983).

Coleman, William. *Yellow Fever in the North: The Methods of Early Epidemiology*. Madison, 1987.

Coley, Noel G. "Physicians and the Chemical Analysis of Mineral Waters in Eighteenth-Century England." MH, 26:123–44 (1982).

Colin, Léon. *Traité des fièvres intermittendes*. Paris, 1870.

Colnat, A. *Epidémiologie et histoire*. Paris, 1937.

Condamy. "Habitations coloniales." RTC, 6(1):18–55 (1906).

Cornish, W. R. *A Record of the Progress of Cholera in 1870, and Resumé of the Records of Former Epidemic Invasions of the Madras Presidency*. Madras, 1871.

Corre, Armand. "De l'influence de la race dans les maladies infectieuses." GHMC, no. 37:580–3, 598–601 (1869).

Traité clinique des maladies des pays chauds. Paris, 1887.

Coudray, F. E. C. "Notes épidemiologiques du passé: La peste à l'armée d'Orient de la 1re république." AMPM, 85:389–403 (1926).

Courtet and Delaborde. "L'épidemie cholérique du Djérid (Sud-Tunisen) en 1893," AMPM, 25:15–34 (1895).

Coustan, M. "Aperçu topographique et climatologique dans ses rapports avec l'étiologie des principales maladies observées à la colonne expéditionaire du sud de la Tunisie." AMPM, 1:9–35 (1883).

Covell, G. "Malaria and War." Journal of the United Service Institute of India, 73:298 (1943).

Cronjé, Gillian. "Tuberculosis and Mortality Decline in England and Wales, 1851–1910." In Urban Disease and Mortality in Nineteenth-century England, ed. Robert Woods and John Woodward. London and New York, 1984, pp. 79–101.

Crosby, Alfred W. Ecological Imperialism: The Biological Expansion of Europe, 900–1900. New York, 1986.

Cullen, Michael J. The Statistical Movement in Early Victorian Britain. New York, 1975.

Cullimore, D. H. The Book of Climates: Acclimatization; Climatic Disease; Health Resorts and Mineral Springs; Sea Sickness; and Sea Bathing. 2d ed. London, 1891.

Curtin, Philip D. "The White Man's Grave: Image and Reality, 1780–1850." Journal of British Studies, 1:94–110 (1961).

The Image of Africa. Madison, Wisc., 1964.

"Epidemiology and the Slave Trade." Political Science Quarterly, 83:191–216 (1968).

"African health at Home and Abroad." Social Science History, 10:369–98 (1986).

Czernicki. "La fière typhoïde aux colonnes d'opération du sud-Oranais en 1881," AMPM, 3:401–7 (1884).

"La fièvre typhoïde au corps d'occupation de Tunisie en 1881." AMPM, 2:397–416 (1882).

Dabry de Thiersant, P. "L'armée coloniale de l'Inde néerlandaise." RC, 84 (4th ser.):5–64 (1885).

Daniels, C. W. Tropical Medicine and Hygiene. 3 parts. London, 1913.

Danziger, Raphael. Abd al-Qadir and the Algerians: Resistance to the French and Internal Consolidation. New York and London, 1977.

Dashwood, R. L. The Health of British Troops in India and other Foreign Stations. London, 1897.

Davidson. "Medico-Topographical and Statistical Report of the Convalescent Depot at Wellington, India, for the Year 1870." AMSR, 12:474–85 (1870).

Davidson, Andrew (ed.). Hygiene and Diseases of Warm Climates. Edinburgh, 1893.

Davies, A. M. "Report on Bacterial Cultivations from Drinking Water." AMSR, 29:307–66 (1887).

"Enteric Fever on Campaigns – Its Prevalence and causation." Seventh Transactions ICHD, 8:84–96. London, 1891.

"Review of the Progress of Hygiene, 1906." JRAMC, 8:398–422 (1907).

"Review of the Progress of Hygiene in 1907." JRAMC. 10:542–6, 647–67 (1908).

De Chaumont, F. "Amount of Fresh Air Required to Reduce the Normal Standard of Carbonic Acid in Air Vitiated by Respiration." Lancet, 1866 (2):230–1 (Sept. 1, 1866).

"On Ventilation and Cubic Space." Edinburgh Medical Journal, 1867 (1) 1024–34 (May 1867).

"Report on Hygiene for Part of 1875." AMSR, 17:206–12 (1875).

"Report on the Progress of Hygiene for the Year 1876 and Part of 1877." AMSR, 18:205–23 (1876).

"Report on the Progress of Hygiene for the Year 1877 and Part of 1878." AMSR, 19:165–97 (1877).

"Report on the Progress of Hygiene for the Year 1878 and Part of 1879." AMSR, 20:187–222 (1878).

"Report on the Progress of Hygiene for the Close of the Year 1879 and Part of 1880." AMSR, 21:209–37 (1879).

"Report on the Progress of Hygiene for the Close of the Year 1880." AMSR, 22:251–61 (1880).

Dechambre, A. "Tahiti." DESM, 15(3d ser.):554–81 (1885).

Delmas, L. "Rélation médico-chirurgicale de la campagne du Sud-Oranais en 1881–82." AMPM, 10:81–, 187–(1887).

Delmont, Jean. "Paludisme et variations climatiques saisonnière en savanne soudanienne d'Afrique de l'Ouest." Cahiers d'études africaines, 22:117–34 (1983).

Demontes, Victor. Le peuple algérien: essai de démographie algériene. Alger, 1906.

Desgenettes, Renée Nicholas Dufirche. Histoire médicale de l'armée d'Orient. 3d ed. London, 1835.

Devaux. "Suite aux quelques conseils de médicine pratique à l'usage des officiers en campagne." RTC, 3(2):175–82 (1904).

Deveau. "Une épidemie de malaria sans moustiques." RTC, 2:87–8 (1902).

Diaz-Briquets, Sergio. The Health Revolution in Cuba. Austin, Tex., 1983.

Dixon, Cyrill William. Smallpox. London, 1962.

Dowling, H. F. Fighting Infection: Conquests of the Twentieth Century. Cambridge, Mass., 1977.

Drevon. "Morbidité et mortalité du personnel militaire de la Guadeloupe pendant l'année 1897." AHMC, 1:361–8 (1898).

Du Bois Saint-Servin. "Le diagnostique bacteriologique du paludisme." AMN, 65:335–46 (1896).

Duchesne, Charles. "Rapport fait au ministre de la guerre le 25 avril 1896." Journal Officiel, 1896, pp. 5105–14, 5131–40, 5158–69 (September 12–14, 1896).

Dufour, Georges. "Compte rendu de la statistique médicale de l'armée espagnole pour l'année 1895." AMN, 71:224–31 (1899).

Duncan, Andrew. "Remarks on Some Recent theories on the Action of Heat in the Tropics." JRAMC, 11:71–6 (1908).

Duran-Reynals, Marie L. The Fever-Bark Tree: The Pageant of Quinine. Garden City, N.Y., 1946.

Durand, François Auguste. Traité dogmatique et pratique des fièvres intermittentes appuyé sur les travaux des médecins militaires en Algérie. Paris, 1862.

Dutroulau, Auguste Frédéric. Traité des maladies des Européens dans les pays chauds. 2d ed. Paris, 1868.

Edmonds, T. R. "On the Mortality and Sickness of Soldiers Engaged in War." Lancet, 1837–8(2):143–8.

"On the Mortality and Diseases of Europeans and Natives in the East Indies." Lancet, 1837–8(2):433–600.

Ellis, Robert S. Report on the Station, Barracks, and Hospitals of Bangalore. Madras, 1865.

Evans, Richard J. Death in Hamburg: Society and Politics in the Cholera Years 1830–1910. Oxford, 1987.

Evatt, G. J. H. "The Sanitary Care of the Soldier by His Officer." JRAMC, 18:189–23 (1912).

Ewarth, Joseph. A Digest of the Vital Statistics of the European and Native Armies of India. London, 1859.

Eyler, John M. "Mortality Statistics and Victorian Health Policy: Program and Criticism." BHM, 50:335–55 (1976).

Fabre, P. "Morbidité et mortalité comparées pour 1000 hommes, en Cochinchine, dans l'Inde anglaise et dans les Indes néerlandaises." Janus, 2:96 (1897).

Fahey, G. "Rations on Active Service." JRAMC, 19:714–29 (1912).

Fair, G. M., J. C. Geyer, and D. A. Okun. Water and Wastewater Engineering. New York, 1966.

Feacham, Richard, Michael McGarry, and Duncan Mara. Water, Wastes and Health in Hot Climates. London, 1977.

Felsenfeld, Oscar. The Epidemiology of Tropical Diseases. Springfield, Ill., 1966.

Firth, R. H. "Report of the Progress of Hygiene from the Year 1900–01." AMSR, 42:369–98 (1900).

"Report of the Progress of Hygiene from the Year 1901–02." AMSR, 43:345–68 (1901).

"The Griffith Water Steriliser." JRAMC, 7:218–25 (1906).

"Hygiene and Preventive Medicine during 1905." JRAMC, 6:251–90 (1906).

"On the Application of Heat for the Purification of Water, with Troops in the Field." JRAMC, 11:570–81 (1908).

"Fifty Years of Sanitary Effort." JRAMC, 21:654–9 (1913).

Firth, R. H., James Lane Notter, and Robert Hammill. *The Theory and Practice of Hygiene.* 3d ed. London, 1908.

FitzSimons, Neal, and others. *Pure and Wholesome: A Collection of Papers on Water and Waste Treatment at the Turn of the Century.* New York, 1982.

Foley, Antoine Edouard, and Martin. *De l'acclimatement et de la colonisation en Algerie.* Paris, 1847.

Fosnagrive, Jean Baptiste. *Traité d'hygiène navale.* 2d ed. Paris, 1877.

France, Armée, État major, Service historique. *Guide bibliographique sommaire d'histoire militaire et coloniale françaises.* Paris, 1979.

Frankland, Percy, and Grace Frankland. *Micro-Organisms in Water: Their Significance, Identification, and Removal, together with an Account of the Bateriological Methods Employed in Their Investigation.* London, 1894.

Freeman, Ernest Carrick. *The Sanitation of British Troops in India.* London, 1899.

Freer, E. L. "Enteric Fever and Dysentery in South Africa." BMJ, 1903 2:776–77.

Frison. "Contribution à l'histoire de la fièvre typhoïde en Algérie; relation d'une épidémie de fièvre typhoïde qui a régné à Ténès, pendant l'été de 1866." RMMM, 18(3d ser.):433–58 (1867).

Froment. "De l'épuration chimique des eaux en campagne par le procédé Georges Lambert." AMPM, 62:400–4.

Gallagher, Nancy Elizabeth. *Medicine and Power in Tunisia, 1780–1900.* Cambridge, 1983.

Garnet. "De l'épuration chimique de l'eau en campagne et en garnison, par le procédé Laurent. AMPM, 57:360–(1911).

Garnier, Marcel, Valery Dalamare, Jean Delamare, and Jacques Delamare. *Dictionaire des termes techniques de médecine.* Rev. ed. Paris, 1978.

Gärtner, August. *Leitfaden der Hygiene.* Berlin, 1896. French translation, *Précis d'hygiène publique et privée.* Bruxelles, 1896.

Geggus, David. *Slavery, War, and Revolution: The British Occupation of Saint Domingue 1793–1798.* Oxford, 1982.

Gentil, Pierre. *Les troupes du Sénégal de 1816 à 1890.* Dakar, 1978.

Gestin, Robert Héristel. *L'influence des climats chauds sur l'Européen.* Paris, Thesis no. 182, 1857.

Gilbert, Nicolas Pierre. *Histoire médicale de l'armée française à Saint-Domingue, en l'an dix: ou mémoire sur la fièvre jaune, avec un aperçu de topographie médicaler de cette colonie.* Paris, 1803.

Girault, L. *Contribution à l'étude du rôle du service santé militaire: Conquête d'Algérie 1830–47.* Paris, 1937.

Glitzky, A. *Enteric Fevers: Causing Organisms and Hosts' Reactions.* Basel and New York, 1971.

Gordon, Charles Alexander. *Army Hygiene.* London, 1866.

Experiences of an Army Surgeon in India. London, 1872.

A Lecture on Some Points of Comparison between the French and British Soldier. London, 1872.

Gordon, Charles Alexander, and Kehoe. "On Tropical Fevers." MTG, 8(n.s.), January 14, 1854, p. 31.

Gore, A. A. *The Story of Our Services under the Crown: A Historical Sketch of the Army Medical Staff.* London, 1849.

Goubert, Jean Pierre. *La conquête de l'eau: l'avènement de la santé à l'âge industriel.* Paris, 1986.

232   Bibliography

Granjux. "Etiologie de la fièvre jaune typhoïde dans l'armée d'Afrique." RHPS, 23:245–58 (1910).

Grant, Allen Ewing, and Henry King. *The Indian Manual of Hygiene: Being King's Madras Manual of Hygiene, Revised, Rearranged, and in Great Part Rewritten.* Madras, 1894.

Great Britain, Army Medical Department. "Index to Appendices of the Reports 1859 to 1896." AMSR, 39:540–99 (1897).

Great Britain, Parliamentary Sessional Papers, 1843, xlviii [C.472], *Papers Relating to the Expedition to the River Niger.*

1843, xxi (83). *Niger Expedition – Mortality.*

1857–8, xviii [C.2318], *Report of the Commissioners Appointed to Enquire into the Sanitary Condition of the Army.*

1857–8, xxviii, *Medical and Surgical History of the British Army which Served in Turkey and the Crimea during the War against Russia in the Years 1854–5–6.*

1857–8, xxxii, 347. *First Report of the Commissioners Appointed to Enquire into the Utilization of Sewage.*

1861, xxxiii, 463. *Second Report of the Commissioners Appointed to Enquire into the Utilization of Sewage.*

1862, xiv, 321 and 439. *Report on the Best Means of Utilizing Sewage of Cities and Towns.*

1863, xix [C.3184]. *Report of Commissioners Appointed to Enquire into the Sanitary Condition of the Army in India.*

1865, xxvii, 303. *Third Report of the Commissioners Appointed to Enquire into the Utilization of Sewage.*

1865, xxxviii (467). *Reports of the Barrack and Hospital Improvement Commission. Report of Dr. Leith of the Bombay Army.*

1865–6, li, 183. *Report of the Sanitary Commission for Madras for the year 1866.*

1867, xv [Cd.1947]. *Report of the Causes of Reduced Mortality in the French Army Serving in Algeria.*

1874, xlvii (195). *Bombay Army (Medical Reports).*

1875, xliii (48). *Abstract of Medical Returns for All India and for Each Presidency, from 1861 to 1873.*

Greig, E. D. W. "The Recent Work of Koch in East Africa." JRAMC, 6:110–12 (1906).

Grellois, M. "Étude hygiènique sur les eaux potables." RMMM, 2(3d ser.):120–212 (1859).

Griffith, P. G. "Heat as a Means of Purifying Water." JRAMC, 7:116–231 (1906).

Gros, Henri. "Encore le climat tropical." RGI, 22:205–8, 230–2 (1896).

"Statistiques médicales de l'armée des Index néelandaises (Orientales) pour 1894." AMN, 65:392–398 (1896).

Gunter, F. E. "Notes on the Health of Europeans and Natives in Peking." JRAMC, 6:24–30, 151–60 (1906).

Guy, William Augustus. *Public Health, A Popular Introduction to Sanitary Science: Being a History of the Prevalent and Fatal Diseases of the English Population from the Earliest Times to the End of the Eighteenth century.* 2 vols. London, 1870–4.

Guyon, J. L. G. "Histoire médicale et chirurgicale de l'expédition dirigée contre Constantine en 1837." RMMM, 44:235–303 (1838).

H. W. S. "Beri-Beri." JRAMC, 19:257–9 (1912).

Halliday, Andrew. *A Letter to the Right Honourable, the Secretary of War, on Sickness and Mortality in the West Indies, Being a Review of Captain Tulloch's Statistical Report.* London, 1839.

Hamet. "Malaria and Military Medicine during the Conquest of Algeria." MS, 25:24–33 (1932).

Handler, Jerome, Arthur C. Aufderheide, Robert S. Corruccini, Elizabeth M. Brandon, and Lorentz E. Wittmers, Jr. "Lead Contact and Poisoning in Barbados Slaves: Historical, Chemical, and Biological Evidence." *Social Science History*, 10:399–425 (1986).

Hanley, Susan B. "Urban Sanitation in Preindustrial Japan." JIH, 18:1–26 (1987).

Harding, N. E. "The Value of Koch's Treatment of Malaria." JRAMC, 11:263–76 (1908).

Hardy, Anne. "Water and the Search for Public Health in London in the Eighteenth and Nineteenth Centuries." MH, 28:250–82 (1984).

Harrison, Gordon. *Mosquitos, Malaria, and Man.* New York, 1978.

Harrison, W. S. "Our Present Position with Regard to Enteric Fever in India." JRAMC, 3:452–5 (1904).

Haspel, Auguste. *Maladies de l'Algérie; des causes, de la symptomatologie, de la nature et du traitement des maladies endémo-épidémique de la province d'Oran.* 2 vols. Paris, 1850–2.

Helye, Alphonse Méderic. *De la maladie en Algérie et dans les pays chauds.* Paris, 1864.

Henderson, D. A. "Smallpox." In *Epidemiology and Community Health in Warm Countries,* ed. Robert Cruickshank, H. B. L. Russell, and Kenneth L. Standard. Edinburgh, 1976, pp. 164–6.

Hercouët. *Étude sur les maladies des européens aux îles Tahiti.* Paris, Thesis no. 433, 1880.

Hirsch, A. *Handbook of Geographical and Historical Pathology.* 3 vols. London, 1883–6. Translated by C. Creighton.

Hodge, William Barwick. "On Mortality Arising from Military Operations." JSSL, 19:219–71 (1856).

Hoeppli, R. J. C. *Parasites and Parasitic Infections in Early Medicine and Science.* Singapore, 1959.

Parasitic Disease in Africa and the Western Hemisphere: Early Documentation and Transmission by the Slave Trade. Basel, 1969.

Hoffman, Elizabeth. *The Sources of Mortality Changes in Italy since Unification.* New York, 1981.

Hoile, Edmond. "Report of the Epidemic of Yellow Fever at Barbados in 1881." AMSR: 22:331–9 (1881).

Holmes, Frederick Lawrence. *Lavoisier and the Chemistry of Life: An Exploration of Scientific Creativity.* Madison, Wisc., 1985.

Hopkins, Donald. *Princes and Peasants: Smallpox in History.* Chicago, 1983.

Horrocks, W. H. "Report on the Progress of Hygiene for the Year 1900." AMSR, 41:349–72 (1899).

Horton, James Africanus Beale. *Physical and Medical Climate and Meteorology of the West Coast of Africa with Valuable Hints to Europeans for the Preservation of Health in the Tropics.* London, 1867.

Houdaille, Jacques. "La mortalité (hors combat) des militaires français à la fin du XVIIIe et au debut du XIXe siècle." *Population,* numéro special, 481–97 (1977).

Huas, Pierre Camioe Victor. *Considerations sur l'hygiène des troupes en campagne dans les pays intertropicaux.* Bordeaux, Thesis no. 17, 1886.

Huddleston, W. E. "An Analysis of Our Present Position with regard to the Prevention and Cure of Malarial Infections." JRAMC, 21:320–38 (1913).

Hudson, Robert P. *Disease and Its Control: The Shaping of Modern Thought.* Westport, 1983.

Huisman, L., and W. E. Wood. *Slow Sand Filtration.* Geneva, 1974.

India, Madras Presidency. *Proceedings of the Sanitary Commission for Madras.* Madras, Annual Series, 1864–77.

India. Presidencies. *Report on the Extent and Nature of the Sanitary Establishments for European Troops in the Bengal, Madras, and Bombay Presidencies.* Calcutta, 1861.

Jackson, Robert. *A Treatise on the Fevers of Jamaica, with Some Observations on the Intermitting Fever of America, and with an Appendix, Containing Some Hints on the Means of Preserving the Health of Soldiers in the Tropics.* London, 1791.

A Systematic View of the Formation, Discipline, and Economy of Armies. London, 1804.

A System for Arrangement and Discipline for the Medical Department of Armies. London, 1805.

Jacquot, Félix, and Topin. *De la colonisation et de l'acclimatement en Algérie.* Paris, 1849.

Jannetta, Ann Bowman. *Epidemics and Mortality in Early Modern Japan*. Princeton, 1987.

Jarco, Saul. "Lavernan's Discovery in the Retrospect of a Century." BHM, 58:215–24 (1984).

Johnson, H., R. J. O'Flaherty, and Lt.-Col. Gain. "Report of the Commission Appointed to Assemble to Investigate the Origin, Progress, and Results of the Epidemic of Yellow Fever in the Island of Jamaica in 1866 and 1867." AMSR, 9:224–48 (1867).

Journal of Interdisciplinary History. "The Relationship of Nutrition, Disease, and Social Conditions: A Geographical Presentation." JIH, 14:503 (1983).

Jousset, A. "De l'acclimatement et de l'acclimatation." AMN, 40:5–, 81–, 161–, 273–, 321–, 422–; 40:79–, 97–, 273–, 387–(1883–4).

Kelsch, Achille Louis Félix and Paul Louis Keiner. *Traité des maladies des pays chauds, région prétropicale*. Paris, 1889.

Keogh, Alfred. "The Results of Sanitation on the Efficiency of Armies in Peace and War." JRAMC, 12:357–785 (1909).

Kérandel. "Dysenterie bacillaire (distribution géographique et bactériologie)." AHMC, 17:762–78 (1914).

Kermorgant, A. "Maladies épidémiques et contagieuses qui ont régné dans les colonies françaises au cours de l'année 1900," AHMC, 5:277–305 (1902).

"Aperçu sur maladies vénériennes." AHMC, 6:428–60 (1903).

"Maladies épidémiques et contagieuses qui ont régné dans les colonies françaises en 1901." AHMC 6:60–5–635 (1903).

"Maladies épidémiques et contagieuses qui ont régné dans les colonies françaises en 1902." AHMC, 7:385–416 (1904).

"Maladies épidémiques et contagieuses qui ont régné dans les colonies françaises en 1904." AHMC, 90:349–57 (1906).

"La tuberculose dans les colonies françaises et plus particulièrement chez les indigènes." AHMC, 9:220–41 (1906).

"Prophylaxie du paudisme." AHMC, 9:18–46 (1906).

"Maladies épidémiques et contagieuses qui ont régné dans les colonies françaises en 1905." AHMC, 10:285–333 (1907).

"Maladies épidémiques et contagieuses qui ont régné dans les colonies françaises en 1906," AHMC, 11:334–80 (1908).

Kermorgant, Alexandre Marie, and Gustave Reynaud. "Précautions hygièniques à prendre pour les expéditions et les explorations au pays chauds." AHMC 3:305–414 (1900).

King, Anthony D. *Colonial Urban Development: Culture, Social Power and Environment*. London, 1976.

The Bungalow: Production of a Global Culture. London, 1984.

King, Henry. *The Madras Manual of Hygiene*. Madras, 1875.

Kiple, Kenneth F. and Virginia H. "Black Yellow Fever Immunities, Innate and Acquired as Revealed in the American South." SSH, 1:419–36 (1977).

Another Dimension of the Black Diaspora: Diet, Disease, and Racism. Cambridge, 1981.

Kiple, Kenneth F. "Deficiency Disease in the Caribbean." JIH, 11:197–215 (1980).

The Caribbean Slave: A Biological History. Cambridge, 1984.

"Cholera and Race in the Caribbean." *Journal of Latin American Studies*, 17:157–77 (1984).

Klein, Richard. "The 'Fever Bark' Tree." *Natural History*, 85:10–19 (1976).

Knox, E. Blake. "Some Medical Notes on War." JRAMC, 4:440–6, 580–6, 616–22, 703–14 (1905); 5:230–9, 616–22 (1906), 7:703–14 (1907).

Kolb, Edmond. *Étude sur l'hygiène de l'Algérie*. Montpellier, 1859.

Lalande, M. E. "Nouveau procédé de dosage de la quinine dans les quinquinas." AMN, 32:134–8 (1879).

Lambert, Gabriel. "De la purification des eaux de boisson et nouveau procédé chimique de purification totale et rapide des eaux destinèes à l'alimentation." AHMC, 9:266–

97 (1906).

"L'épuration chimiqu`. des eaux de boisson par les permanganates & les coagulants insoluable." RTC, 11(1):655–67 (1911).

"Sur un nouveau procédé pour l'épuration des eaux de boisson – coagulation des oxydes de manganèse par entraînement." AHMC, 15:103–29 (1912).

Lambert, Sylvester M. *The Population of Pacific Peoples*. Honolulu, 1934.

Largeau, G. "Étude statistique sur la mortalité des marins et soldats français dans les colonies." *Journal des sociétés scientifiques*, no. 7, pp. 59–60 (13 Fev. 1889).

Laudan, Rachel. *From Mineralogy to Geology: The Foundations of a Science, 1650–1830.* Chicago, 1987.

Laveran, Alphonse. "Antagonisme." DESM, lère ser., v. 5, pp. 229–45 (Paris, 1867).

Traité des maladies et épidémies des armées. Paris, 1875.

Nature parasitaire des accidents du l'impaludisme; description d'un pouve aud parasite trouvé dans le sang des malades atteints de fièvre palustre. Paris, 1881.

Traité des fièvres palustres. Paris, 1884.

Du paludisme et de son hémotozaire. Paris, 1891.

Prophylaxie du paludisme. Paris, 1908.

Laveran, Louis. "Recherches statistiques sur les causes de la mortalité de l'armée, servant à l'intérieur." AHPML, 13(2d ser.): 233–91 (1860).

"Algérie." DESM, 2(2d ser.):748–78 (1869).

"Cholera." DESM, 16(1st ser.):758–887 (1874).

Lawson, Robert. "Observations on the Outbreak of Yellow Fever among the Troops at Newcastle, Jamaica, in the Latter Part of 1856." *British and Foreign Medical and Chirurgical Review*, 59:445–480 (1859).

Layet, Alexandre. *La santé des européens entre les tropiques. Leçons d'hygiène et de médecine sanitaire coloniales.* Paris, 1906.

Le Dantec, Aristide. "Phagédénisme des pays chauds, son identité avec la purriture d'hôpital, pathogénie, symptomes, traitement." AMN, 71:133–45 (1899).

Précis de pathologie exotique (maladies des pays chauds et des pays froids). 3d ed. Paris, 1911.

Lecrain, Émile. *Introduction à l'étude des fièvres des pays chauds (région prétropicale): la fièvre intermittente; la quinine; les pyrexies & cachexies des pays chauds.* Paris, 1899.

Legrand, A. *L'hygiène des troupes européens aux colonies et dans les expéditions coloniales.* Paris, 1895.

Leishman, W. B. "The Progress of Anti-Typhoid Inoculation in the Army." JRAMC, 8:463–71 (1907).

Lelean, P. S. "Quinine as a Malarial Prophylactic." JRAMC, 17:463–80 (1911).

"Bacteriological Examination of Waters in the Field." JRAMC, 23:292–319 (1914).

Leriche, Marc. "Notes sur l'évolution démographique de Tahiti, jusqu'en 1918." *Bulletin de la société d'études océanien*, 16:741–61 (1977).

Leveugle, J. *Contribution à l'êtude de l'influence des sejours en pays tropicaux sur la mortalité.* Paris, 1949.

Lévy, Claude. *Emancipation, Sugar, and Federalism: Barbados and the West Indies, 1833–76.* Gainesville, Fla., 1980.

Levy, Michel. *Traité d'hygiène publique et privé.* 4th ed. Paris, 1862.

Rapport sur les progrès de l'hygiène militaire. Paris, 1868.

Lillianfeld, Abraham M. *Foundations of Epidemiology.* New York, 1976.

Limagne, E. *Manuel de service sanitaire: receuil des règlements et instructions sur la police sanitaire en France et en Algérie.* 2d ed. Paris, 1858.

Lind, James. *Essay on the Diseases Incidental to Europeans in Hot Countries.* 6th ed. London, 1808. (Originally published 1768)

Livi-Bacci, M. "The Nutrition-Mortality Link in Past Times: A Comment." JIH, 14:192– (1983).

Livingstone, David N. "Human Acclimatization: Perspectives on a Contested Field of Inquiry in Science, Medicine, and Geography." *History of Science*, 25:359–94 (1987).

Luckin, Bill. "Evaluating the Sanitary Revolution: Typhus and Typhoid in London, 1851–1900." In *Urban Disease and Mortality in Nineteenth-century England*, ed. Robert Woods and John Woodward. London and New York, 1984, pp. 102–19.

Lyle, A. A. "Some Remarks on 'Beri-Beri', A Disease Largely Prevalent in the Straits Settlements, with a Few Notes of Cases, & c." AMSR, 37:379–84 (1885).

M., C. H. "Sterilization of Water by Means of Ultra-Violet Rays." JRAMC, 18:235–9 (1912).

M., W. G. "The Influence of Rice on Beri-Beri." JRAMC, 12:583–4 (1909).

"Supervision of Water Supplies in the French Army," JRAMC, 11:317–18 (1908).

McCulloch, T. "The Field Service Filter Water Cart." JRAMC, 6:449–54 (1906).

"Malaria Fever amongst British Troops." JRAMC, 3:79–86 (1904).

Macdonald, George. *The Epidemiology and Control of Malaria*. London, 1957.

McGill, H. S. "Water Supply and Sanitation of Camps in India." JRAMC, 3:512–22 (1904).

McGrew, Roderick E. "The First Cholera Epidemic and Social History." BHM, 34:61–2 (1960).

Russia and the Cholera, 1823–32. Madison, Wisc., 1965.

Encyclopedia of Medical History. London, 1985.

MacGrigor, James. "Sketch of the Medical History of the British Armies in the Peninsula of Spain and Portugal during the Late Campaigns." *Medico-Chirurgical Transactions*, 6:381–489 (1815).

McKeown, Thomas. *The Modern Rise of Population*. New York, 1976.

"Fertility, Mortality and the Causes of Death: An Examination of Issues Related to the Modern Rise of Population." PS, 32:535–42 (1978).

"Food, Infection, and Population." JIH, 14:227 (1983).

Macnamara, C. "On Cholera." *Indian Medical Gazette*, 3:246–9, 267–70; 4:4–9, 26–30, 39a–30d. (1868–9).

McNeill, John R. "The Ecological Basis of Warfare in the Caribbean, 1700–1804" in *Adapting to Conditions: War and Society in the Eighteenth Century*, ed. Maarten Utlee, Tuscaloosa, Aa., 1986, pp. 16–42.

McNeill, William H. *Plagues and Peoples*. New York, 1976.

Macpherson, W. G. "Some Practical Points in the Prevention of Disease in Panama and Cuba." JRAMC, 11:277–97 (1908).

Madras (Presidency). *Report on the Medical Topography of the Nizam's Military Cantonments and Army*. Madras, 1852.

Maillot, François Clément. "Recherches sur les fièvres intermittentes du nord de l'Afrique." RMMM, 38(1st ser.):150–86 (1835).

Traité des fièvres ou irritations cérebro-spinales intermittentes. Paris, 1836.

"État sanitaire de la garnison de Bône, de 1832 à 1881." *Gazettes des hôpitaux*, 57:266–8, 275–6 (20 and 22 March 1884).

"Mon dernier mot sur la fièvre d'Algérie." *Lancette française*, 57:895–9 (30 Sept. 1884).

Mangin, F. M. "Causation and Prevention of the Spread of Yellow Fever." JRAMC, 7:369–71 (1906).

Manson, Patrick. *Tropical Diseases: A Manual of the Diseases of Warm Climates*. 4th ed. London, 1907.

Manson-Bahr, Philip Heinrich. *History of the School of Tropical Medicine in London, 1899–1949*. London, 1956.

"The March of Tropical Medicine during the Last Fifty Years (Footprints on the Sands of Time)." *Transactions of the Royal Society of Tropical Medicine and Hygiene*, 56:483–99 (1958).

Manson-Bahr, Philip, and A. Alcock. *Life and Work of Sir Patrick Manson*. London, 1927.

Marchoux. "Au sujet de la transmission du paludisme par les moustiques." AHMC, 2:22–6 (1899).

Marit, Jean Joseph. *Hygiène de l'Algérie. Exposeé des moyens de conserver la santé et de se preserver des maladies dans les pays chauds et spécialement en Algérie.* Paris, 1862.

Maroix. "Notice sur l'armée des Indes nérlandaises." RTC 6(2):542–71, 631–52 (1907).

Martin, Alfred Etienne Victor. *Manual d'hygiène à l'usage des Européens qui viennent d'ètablir en Algérie.* Alger, 1847.

Martin, James Ranald. *Practical Observations on the Disorders and Diseases of European Invalids on Their Return from Tropical Climates.* London, 1850.

The Influence of Tropical Climates in Producing the Acute Endemic Diseases of Europeans. 2d ed. London, 1861.

Marvaud. "La fièvre typhoïde au corps d'occupation en Tunisle." AMPM:3:273–83 (1884).

Maurel, E. "De la mortalité dans l'armée coloniale." *Bulletin de la société de géographie de Toulouse,* 17:246–9 (1898).

Mayne, C. B. *How Far Past Legislation Proved Effective in Securing the Health of British Troops in India, with Suggestions as to Future Legislation on This Important Subject.* London, 1897.

Melville, C. H. "The Place of Sanitation as a Factor in Strategy." JRAMC, 11:64–9 (1908).

Miller, Louis H., S. H. Mason, D. F. Clyde, and M. H. McGinniss. "The Resistance Factor to Plasmodium Vivax in Blacks: The Duffy-Blood-Group Genotype, FyaFyb." *New England Journal of Medicine,* 295:302–4 (1976).

Molinier, M. "Quelques remarques sur les filtres Chamberland en usage dans la colonne expéditionaire du Dahomey (1892)." AMN, 62:460–6 (1894).

Moore, William James. *A Manual of the Diseases of India.* London, 1861.

Health in the Tropics; or, Sanitary Art Applied to Europeans in India. London, 1862.

The Constitutional Requirements for Tropical Climates; and Observations on the Sequel of Diseases Contracted in India. London, 1890.

"Sanitary Progress in India." Seventh Transactions, ICHD, 11:15–89 (London, 1891).

Moore, William James, and John Henry Tull. *A Manual of Family Medicine and Hygiene for India.* 7th ed. London, 1903.

Morache, George Auguste. *Traité d'hygiène militaire.* 2d ed. Paris, 1886.

Moreau de Jonnès, Alexandre. *Essai sur l'hygiène militaire des Antilles.* Paris, 1817.

"Observations pour servir à l'histoire de la fièvre jaune des Antilles suivies de tables de la mortalité des troupes européenes dans les Indes-Occidentale." *Bulletin de la société médicale d'émulation,* 6:237–47 (1817).

Morel, Auguste Désiré. "Statistique générale de la morbidité et de la mortalité dans les établissements hospitaliers françaises en 1902." AHMC, 8:135–45 (1905).

Morin. "L'essai des eaux en campagne." RMMMM, 9(3d ser.): 310–16 (1863).

Nasmith, G. G., and R. R. Graham. "Simple Method of Purifying Almost Any Infected Water for Drinking Purposes." JRAMC, 17:50–4 (1911).

Navarre, Pierre. *Manuel d'hygiène coloniale.* Paris, 1895.

Nelson, T. "Medical Results of the Recent Chinese Wars." *British and Foreign Medico-Chirurgical Review,* 63:203–19 (1863).

Nesfield, V.B. "The Chemical Sterilization of Water for Military Purposes." JRAMC, 18:513–22 (1912).

"The Rapid Chemical Sterilization of Water." JRAMC, 24:146–54 (1915).

"The Chemical Sterilization of Water for Military Purposes." JRAMC, 12:513–22 (1919).

Nicolas, Adolphe C. A. M. *Hygiène industrielle et coloniale. Chantiers et terassements en pays palunéen.* Paris, 1889.

Nicolas, Adolphe C. A. M. (ed.). *Guide hygiènique et médicale du voyageur dans l'Afrique centrale.* Paris, 1885. (Originally published 1881)

Manuel d'hygiène coloniale. Rédigé par une commission de la société (Paris, 1894).

Noel. "La mortalité des troupes en France, en Algérie et aux colonies." *Bulletin médicale d'Algérie,* 12:797–802 (1898).

Notter, J. Lane. "Report on the Progress of Hygiene for the Year 1888." AMSR, 39:285–336 (1887).

"Report on the Progress of Hygiene for the Year 1890." AMSR, 31:321–41 (1889).

"Enteric Fever in the European Army in India: Its Etiology and Prevention." *Seventh Transactions*, ICHD, 10:210–15 (London, 1891).

"Report on the Progress of Hygiene for the Year 1892." AMSR, 33:339–49 (1891).

"Report on the Progress of Hygiene for the Year 1893." AMSR, 33:281–300 (1892).

"Military Hygiene." In *A Treatise on Hygiene and Public Health*, ed. Thomas Stevenson and Shirley F. Murray. London, 1893, 2:599–670.

"The Hygiene of the Tropics." In *Hygiene and Diseases of Warm Climates*, ed. Andrew Davidson. London, 1893, pp. 25–75.

"Report on the Progress of Hygiene for the Year 1895." AMSR, 34:307–14 (1894).

"Report on the Progress of Hygiene for the Year 1896." AMSR, 37:279–90 (1895).

"Report on the Progress of Hygiene for the Year 1897." AMSR, 38:323–41 (1896).

"Report on the Progress of Hygiene for the Year 1898." AMSR, 39:351–71 (1897).

"Report on the Progress of Hygiene for the Year 1899." AMSR, 40:389–410 (1898).

Spread and Distribution of Infectious Diseases; Spread of Typhoid Fever, Dysentery, and Allied Diseases among Large Communities, with Special Reference to Miltary Life in Tropical and Sub-Tropical Countries. London and Manchester, 1904.

Notter, J. Lane, and R. H. Firth. *The Theory and Practice of Hygiene*. London, 1896.

Noury. "De la cinchonidine comme succédant de la quinine." AMN, 30:449–55 (1879).

Nouschi, André. *Enquête su le niveau de vie des populations rurales constantinoises*. Paris, 1961.

Nuttall, G. H. F. *The Rôle of Insects, Arachnids, and Myriapods as Carrieres in the Spread of Bacterial and Parasitic Diseases of Man and Animals: A Critical and Historical Study*. Baltimore, Md., 1899.

O'Reilly, Patrick, and Edouard Reitman. *Bibliographie de Tahiti et de la Polynésie française*. Paris, 1967.

Ogilvie, W. H. "Sunstroke – A Heresy." JRAMC, 19:444–6 (1912).

Oldham, Charles Frederick. *What is Malaria? And Why It Is Most Intense in Hot Climates*. London, 1871.

Ouanès, Mahmoud. "Le paludisme et la lutte antipaludique en Tunisie (1945–80.)" *Revue tunisienne de science et education*, nos. 11–12:91–122 (1982).

Ouy-Vernazobres, Charles. "L'abandon de l'Algérie et les médecins militaires." *Pro Medico* (1930).

P., C. E. "Water Sterilizers and Ice Machines with Troops in Morocco." JRAMC, 22:380–1 (1914).

Palmer, Roy. *The Water Closet: A New History*. Newton Abbott, 1973.

Parkes, Edmund Alexander. *Remarks on the Dysentery and Hepatitis of India*. London, 1846.

"Review of the Progress of Hygiene during the Year 1861," AMSR for 1860, 2:343–67.

"Review of the Progress of Hygiene during the Year 1862." AMSR for 1861, 3:308–34.

"Report on Hygiene for 1863." AMSR for 1862, 3:335–54.

"Report on Hygiene for 1866." AMSR, 7:333–54 (1865).

"On Relative Power of Certain So-Called Disinfectants in Preventing the Putrefaction of Human Sewage." AMSR, 318–(1866).

"Report on Hygiene for 1867." AMSR, 8:296–317 (1866).

"Report on Hygiene for 1868." AMSR, 9:250–64 (1867).

"Report on Hygiene for 1869." AMSR, 10:219–241 (1868).

"Report on Hygiene for 1870." AMSR, 11:205–28 (1869).

"Report on Hygiene for 1871." AMSR for 1870, 12:226–59.

"Report on Hygiene for the Year 1872." AMSR, 13:174–201 (1871).

"Report on Hygiene for the Year 1873." AMSR, 15:220–56 (1872).

"Report on Hygiene for the Year 1874 and Part of 1875." AMSR, 15:181–205 (1873).

"Report on Hygiene for the Year 1875." AMSR, 15:181–205 (1873).

On Personal Care of Health. London, 1897.

Patterson, K. David. *Pandemic Influenza, 1700–1900: A Study in Historical Epidemiology*. Totowa, N.J., 1986.

Paynter, Joshua. "Report upon the Sanitary Condition of French Troops Serving in Algeria." AMSR, 7:437–51 (1865).

Pellarin, A. *Hygiène des pays chauds: Contagion du choléra demontrée par l'épidémie de la Guadaloupe. Conditions hygièniques de l'émigration dans les pays chauds et de la colonisation de ces pays* ... Paris, 1872.

Pelling, Margaret. *Cholera, Fever and English Medicine.* London, 1978.

Pembrey, M. S. "Heat-Stroke." JRAMC, 21:156–64 (1913).

"Heat Stroke. Further Observations on an Analysis of Fifty Cases." JRAMC, 22:629–38 (1914).

Pepper, Edouard. *De la malaria.* Paris, 1891.

Perier, M. J. De l'acclimatement en Algerie. AHPML, 33:301–38, 34:24–41 (1845).

Perier, S.A.N. "Biographie du Dr. Boudin, suivie d'un index bibliographique de ses ouvrages." RMMM, 19(3d ser.), 249–67, 350–63 (1867).

Pickford, John. "Water Treatment in Developing Countries" in *Water, Wastes, and Health in Hot Climates*, Richard Feachem, Michael McGarry, and Duncan Mara. London, 1977.

Pinchard. "Filtre destiné à la purification de l'eau." RMMMM, 18(3d ser.):504–7 (1867).

Pinot Bey, J. B. "L'eau d'alimentation des villes du Caire et d'Alexandrie." AHPML, 33(3d ser):487–96 (1895).

Plouzané, Edouard François. *Contribution à l'étude de 'hygiène pratique des troupes européenes dans les pays intertropicaux: Haut Sénégal et Haut Niger.* (Bordeaux, Thesis no., 89, 1887).

Población y Fernandez, Antonio. *História médica de la guerra de Africa.* Madrid, 1866.

Poggio, H. "De la aclimatación en Canarias de las tropas destinadas al Ultramar." RGCMSM, 4:257–, 289–, 353–, 385–429, 460–, 517–, 554–, 591– (1867).

Pollitzer, R. *Cholera.* Geneva, 1959.

Pollock, C. E. "The Effect of the Sun in the Tropics on Animals and Man." JRAMC, 17:50–4 (1911).

"Indian Field Service Ration." JRAMC, 19:647–8 (1912).

"Medical Arrangements of the French Expeditionary Force to Fez, Morocco." JRAMC, 19:507–8 (1912).

"Water Sterilizers and Ice Machines with the Troops in Morocco." JRAMC, 21:380–1 (1913).

Porter, R. "Bacterial Treatment of Sewage." JRAMC, 6:194–200 (1906).

Porter, Theodore M. *The Rise of Statistical Thinking, 1820–1900.* Princeton, 1986.

Portugal, Ministério de Guerra. *Estatistica geral do servicio de exercito.* Lisboa, Annual Series.

Portugal, Ministério de Marinha e Ultramar. *Archivos Médico-coloniães.*

Pottier. "Épuration de l'eau potable en campagne." AHMC, 5:599–605 (1902).

Poynter, F. N. L. "Evolution of Military Medicine" in *A Guide to the Sources of British Military History*, ed. Robin Higham. Berkeley, 1971, pp. 591–605.

Prat. *Contribution à la géographie médicale de l'île de Tahiti.* Toulon, 1869.

Preston, S. H., and E. van de Walle. "Urban French Mortality in the Nineteenth Century." *Population Studies*, 32:275– (1978).

Preston, Samuel H., Nathan Keyfitz, and Robert Schoen. *Causes of Death.* New York and London, 1972.

Pringle, John. *Observations on the Diseases of the Army*, 7th ed. London, 1775.

Proust, A. "Mesures hygièniques prescrites dans l'Inde par le gouvernement anglais." AGM, 1894:468–73.

Prudhomme, Emile. "Le quinine à Madagascar." RM, 4:128–43 (1902).

Quill, Richard H. "Enteric Fever: Is It Invariably a Water-Borne Disease?" JRAMC, 7:232–35 (1906).

Rançon, Laurent Ferdinand André Moyse Paoul. *De la dysenterie endémique des pays chauds, notamment au Sénégal* (Bordeaux, thesis no. 14, 1886).

Razzell, P. E. "An Interpretation of the Modern Rise of Population – A Critique." PS,

28:5–(1973).

Régniard. "La première expédition de Constatine." AMPH, 10:316–7 (1887).

Régnier. "Résumé de la statistique médicale des troupes stationées aux colonies pendant l'anée 1905." AHMC, 10:393–8 (1907).

Reiux, J. "Paludisme." in Anon., *L'oeuvre du service de santé militaire en Algérie, 1830–1930.* Paris, 1931.

Reuss, L. "Prophylaxie du paludisme." AHPML, 34(3d ser.):400–11 (1895).

Rey-Goldzeiguer, Annie. *Le royaume arabe: La politique algérienne de Napoléon III, 1861–70.* Alger, 1977.

Reynaud, Gustave A. "Hygiène coloniale." AMN, 53:123–47, 212–6 (1890).

L'armée coloniale au point de vue de l'hygiène pratique. Paris, 1892.

Considerations sanitaires sur l'expédition de Madagascar et quelques autres expéditions coloniales, françaises et anglaises. Paris, 1898.

"Compte rendu sommaire du XIe congrès international d'hygiène et de démographie tenu à Bruxelles du 2 au 8 septembre 1903." AHMC, 7:445–9 (1904).

Hygiène coloniale. 2 vols. Paris, 1903.

"Sur les sanatoriums dans les pays chauds." ICHD 10:678–86 (1910).

Ricoux, René, *Contribution à l'étude de l'acclimatement des français en Algérie.* Paris, 1874.

La population européenne en Algérie (1873–1881): étude statistique. Alger, 1883.

Rieux, J., and Paul Hormous. "Note sur le paludisme dans le Maroc occidental." AMPM, 62:1–32 (1913).

Riley, James C. *The Eighteenth-Century Campaign to Avoid Disease.* London, 1986.

"Insects and European Mortality Decline." AHR, 91:833–58 (1986).

Roberts, George W. *Population of Jamaica: An Analysis of Its Structure and Growth.* Cambridge, 1957.

Rosen, George. *A History of Public Health.* New York, 1958.

Rosenberg, Charles E. *The Cholera Years: The United States in 1832, 1849, and 1866.* Chicago, 1962.

"The Therapeutic Revolution: Medicine, Meaning and Social Change in Nineteenth-Century America." PBM, Summer 1977, pp. 485–506.

"Florence Nightingale on Contagion: The Hospital as a Moral Universe." In *Healing and History: Essays for George Rosen,* ed. C. E. Rosenberg. London and New York, 1979, pp. 116–36.

"Disease and Social Order in America: Perceptions and Expectations." *The Millbank Quarterly,* 64:34–55 (1986).

Ross, H. C. "A Rapid Means of Sterilising Water for Troops by Using 'Thermite' as Fuel." JRAMC, 6:145–9 (1906).

Ross, Ronald. *Memoires.* London, 1923.

"Prevention of Malaria in British Possessions, Egypt, and Parts of America." RAMC, 10;155–70, 263–80 (1908).

Roth, Wilhelm August, and Rudolph Lex. *Handbuch der Militär-Gesundheitspflege.* 3 vols. Berlin, 1872–7.

Rouget, J. F. A. "Étiologie de la tuberculose pulmonaire dans l'armée." MPM, 38:1–26, 169–83 (1901).

Rozier-Joly, A. "Considerations générale sur les constitutions médicales des pays marécageux." *Gazette médicale de l'Algérie,* 4:33–, 51–, 101–(1859); 5:4–, 42–, 62–, 157–, 178–(1860); 6:2–(1861); 7:45–, 80–, 147–(1862); 8:47–, 65–, 78–, 91–(1863).

Russell, M. W. "Recent Tendencies in the Development of Army Medical Services." JRAMC, 4:178–86 (1905).

"Sir James McGrigor." JRAMC, 12:117–48 (1909).

Russell, Paul F. *Man's Mastery of Malaria.* London, 1955.

Ryan, M. R. "A Brief Survey of the Effects of High Temperature on the Body, with Special Reference to the Nature, Prevention, and Treatment of Heat Stroke." AMSR, 37:396–411 (1885).

Sadoul, Louis. *Hygiène et médecine coloniale: guide pratique à usage des postes militaires déprouvu de médecin.* Paris, 1895.

Sari, Djilali. "Le désastre démographique de 1867 en Algérie." *Revue d'histoire megrebine,* 8:55–9 (1981).

Le désastre démographique. Alger, 1982.

Saxena, Krishnan M. *The Military System of India.* New Delhi, 1974.

Schneider. "Prophylaxie de la fièvre typhoïde dans l'armée française." *Seventh ICHD,* 8:101–3 (London, 1891).

Schoutetten, L. *Rélation médico-cirurgicale succinct de la campagne de Kabylie en 1857, et spécialement des faits qui se rapportent au 2e bataillon du 70e régiment de ligne.* Metz, 1858.

Schrimshaw, Nevin S., Carl E. Taylor, and John E. Gordon. *Interactions of Nutrition and Infection.* Geneva, 1968.

Scott. "Remarks on the Outbreak of Cholera at Secunderabad." AMSR, 13:212–13 (1871).

Scott, Henry Harold. *A History of Tropical Medicine.* 2 vols. London, 1939.

Sérèz. "Considérations hygiènique et sanitaires sur Tahiti." AMN, 57:280–4 (1892).

"Morbidité et mortalité en Annam et Tonkin pendant l'année 1897." AHMC, 2:182–212 (1899).

Sheridan, Richard B. *Doctors and Slaves: A Medical and Demographic History of Slavery in the British West Indies, 1680–1834.* Cambridge, 1985.

Shrimpton, C. *Relation médico-chirurgicale de l'expédition du Bou Thaled de Constantine.* Constantine, 1846.

Sigfried, André. *Routes of Contagion.* New York, 1965. Translated by Jean Henderson and Mercedes Claraso.

Simpson, R. J. S. "The Solar Element in Heat Stroke, in Its Physical Relations." JRAMC, 11:541–9 (1908).

"Tuberculosis in the British Army and Its Prevention." JRAMC, 12:18–27 (1909).

"Humidity and Heat-Stroke." JRAMC, 23:1–11 (1914).

Simpson, W. J. R. *The Principles of Hygiene as Applied to Tropical and Sub-Tropical Climates.* London, 1908.

Simpson, W. J. "Water Supplies." JTM, 6:132–8, 1723–74, 192–4 (1903).

Sistach. "De l'emploi des préparations arsenicales dans le traitement des fièvres intermittentes." RMMM, 5(3d ser.): 1–42, 97–114 (1861).

Skelton, D. S. "Some Observations on Blackwater Fever." JRAMC, 10:602–15 (1908).

Smart. "On the Distribution of Asiatic Cholera in Africa." *Transactions of the Epidemiological Society of London,* 3:336–55 (1866–76).

Smith, C. E. Gordon. "Changing Patterns of Disease in the Tropics." *British Medical Bulletin,* 28:3–9 (1972).

Smith, Dale C. "Quinine and Fever: The Development of the Effective Dosage." JHM, 30:343–67 (1974).

Snow, John. *On the Mode of Communication of Cholera.* 2d ed., London, 1855.

Solente, Lucy. "Histoire de l'évolution des méningites cérébro-spinales aiguës." *Revue médicale,* 55:18–29 (1983).

Squire, J. Edward. "Camp Fevers: Their Origin and Spread." *Seventh ICHD,* 8:97–110 (London, 1891).

Stephens, James William Watson. *Blackwater Fever: A Historical Survey and Summary Observations Made over a Century.* Liverpool, 1937.

Stephens, J. W. W., and S. R. Christophers. *The Practical Study of Malaria and Other Blood Parasites.* London, 1903.

Stevenson, Thomas, and Shirley F. Murphy. *A Treatise on Hygiene and Public Health.* 3 vols. London, 1892–4. (Originally published 1890–2)

Stokvis. "Le colonization et l'hygiène tropicale." *Revue de géographie internationale,* 22:115–18, 138–9, 161–4 (1896).

Stone, Mary M. "The Plumbing Paradox." *Winterthur Portfolia,* 14:292, 284 (1979).

Stott, H. "A Contribution to the Study of the Aetiology of Berri-Berri." JRAMC, 17:231–

44 (1911).

Strauss, W. Patrick. *Americans in Polynesia 1783–1842*. East Lansing, Mich., 1963.

Strickland, G. Thomas. *Hunter's Tropical Medicine*, 6th ed., Philadelphia, 1984.

Sullivan. *Endemic Diseases of Tropical Climates*. London, 1877.

Sutherland, J., J. Paynter, C. B. Ewart, and R. S. Ellis. "Report on the Causes of Reduced Mortality in the French Army Serving in Algeria." PP, 1867, xv [Cd.19447].

Tarr, Joel A. "From City to Farm: Urban Wastes and the American Farmer." *Agricultural History*, 49:598–612 (1975).

"Water and Wastes: A Retrospective Assessment of Wastewater Technology in the United States, 1800–1932." *Technology and Culture*, 25:226–63 (1984).

Tarr, Joel A., James McCurley, and Terry F. Yosie. "The Development and Impact of Urban Wastewater Technology: Changing Concepts of Water Quality Control, 1850–1930." In *Population and Reform in American Cities, 1870–1930*, ed. Marton V. Melosi. Austin, Tex., 1980, pp. 59–82.

Taylor, Norman. *Quinine: The Story of Cinchona*. New York, 1943.

Temkin, Osei. *The Double Face of Janus*. Baltimore, Md., 1977.

Tesnière. "Notes recueillies pendant la campagne d'Alger pour servir à l'histoire médico-chirurgicale de l'expédition d'Afrique." RMMM, 31:70–109 (1831).

Thévenot, Jean Pierre Ferdinand. *Traité des maladies des Européens dans les pays chauds, et specialement au Sénégal, ou essai statistique, médicale et hygiènique sur le sol, le climat et les maladies de cette partie de l'Afrique*. Paris, 1840.

Thomas, Félix. "Européens et zone tropicale." AMN, 29:16–61 (1878).

Thompson, H. N. "The Prophylactic Use of Quinine." JRAMC, 21:587–89 (1913).

Thomson, Arthur S. "On the Doctrine of Acclimatization." *Madras Quarterly Medical Review*, 2:69–72 (1840).

Thomson, T. R. H. "On the Value of Quinine in African Remittant Fever." *Lancet*, 1846(1), 244–5.

Thornton, J. H. *Memoires of Seven Campaigns. A Record of Thirty-Five Years' Service in the Indian Medical Department in India, China, Egypt, and the Sudan (1856–1891)*. Westminster, 1895.

Thresh, J. C. *The Examination of Water and Water Supplies*. 2d ed., London, 1913.

Tostivint and Remlinger. "Sur la prédesposition de la race arabe à la pneumonie." AMPM, 38:107–25 (1901).

"Sur la situation favorisée de l'Algérie et privilégiée de la Tunisie vis-à-vis de la tuberculose – Fréquence plus grande de la maladie chez les arabes que chez les européens." AMPM, 38:272–306 (1901).

Treherne, F. H. "Quinine in Malarial Fever." JRAMC, 9:276–81 (1907).

Treherne, F. H., and J. J. H. Nelson. "Sterilization of Infected Water in Camp and on the March in India." JRAMC, 21:443–51 (1913).

Treille, George Félix. *De l'acclimation des européens dans les pays chauds*. Paris, 1888.

Principles d'hygiène coloniale. Paris, 1899.

"Malaria sans moustiques?" *Janus*, 8:505–6 (1903).

Trotter, J. Lane. "The Hygiene of the Tropics." In *Hygiene and Disease in Warm Climates*, ed. A. D. Davidson. pp. 25–71.

Tulloch, Alexander. "Comparison of the Sickness, Mortality and Prevailing Diseases among Seamen and Soldiers. As Shown by the Naval and Military Statistical Reports." JSSL, 4:1–16 (1841).

Turin, Yvonne. *Affrontements culturels dans l'Algérie coloniale: Écoles, médecines, réligion, 1830–1880*. Paris, 1971.

Turner, J. A. *Sanitation in India*. Bombay, 1914.

Vaillard. "L'épuration de l'eau potable en campagne." AMPM, 40:1–37 (1902).

Vallin, E. "L'enseignement de la médecine et de l'hygiéne coloniales." RHPS, 23:481–91 (1901).

Vallin, Kelsch, Raillet, Blanchard, and Laveran. "Instruction pour le prophylaxie du paludisme." AMPM, 39:160–7 (1901).

Vedder, Edward B. *Beriberi*. London, 1913.

Védrenne. "Climatologie générale de la Grande Kabylie et topographie, physique et médicale de Tizi-Ouzou." RMMM, 2(3d ser.):213–78 (1858).

Verdon. "La fièvre intermittant à Ourgla." AMPM, 6:289–(1885).

Vidal. "Contribution à l'étude de l'immunité de la race arabe à l'égard de la fièvre typhoïde." AMPM, 42:438–43 (1903).

Villedary, Paul Edward. *Guide sanitaire des troupes et du colon aux colonies. Hygiène coloniale, prophylaxie et traitement des principals maladies des pays chauds.* Paris, 1893.

Vincent, H. "Sur l'immunité de la race arabe à l'égard de la fièvre typhoîde." AMPM, 37:145–52 (1901).

Vincent, L. "Prophylaxie de la fièvre jaune." RTC, 3(1):29–38 (1904).

Vincent, L., and F. Burot. "Les altitudes dans les pays paludéens de la zone torride." AHPML, 5(3d ser.):500–25 (1896).

Vincent, M. A., and V. Collardot. *Le choléra d'après les neuf epidémies qui ont règné à Alger, depuis 1835 jusqu'en 1865.* Paris, 1867.

Viry. *Principes d'hygiène militaire.* Paris, 1896.

Vital, Auguste Edmond. *Correspondence de A. Vital avec I. Urbain (1845–74).* Alger, 1958. (Reprinted edited by A. Nouschi)

Waksman, Selman A. *The Conquest of Tuberculosis.* Berkeley, 1966.

Walker, N. Dunbar. "Water-Bottles and Mess-Tins." JRAMC, 19:419–443 (1912).

Wallace, J. *Sanitary Engineering in India.* Bombay, 1893.

Wanhill, C. F. "Water Supply in the Field," JRAMC, 17:157–64 (1911).

"Factors Which May Influence the Production of 'Heat-Stroke' among Troops on the March or on Service." JRAMC, 22:661–4 (1914).

Webb, A. L. A. "Notes on some Experiments Made to Determine the Rate of Absorbability and Intensity of Action of Quinine Given Hyperdermically and by Mouth as Shown by the Minimum-Lethal-Dose Method." JRAMC, 20:280–5 (1912).

Welch, S. G., I. A. McGregor, and K. Williams. "The Duffy Blood Group and Malaria Prevalence in Gambian West Africans." *Transactions of the Royal Society of Tropical Medicine and Hygiene*, 71:295–6 (1977).

Wellcome Insititute for the History of Medicine, London. *Subject Catalogue of the History of Medicine and Related Sciences.* Munich, Kraus International, 1980.

Wintle, A. T. "The Dietary of Troops." *Transactions of the Seventh ICHD*, 8:144–50 (London, 1891).

Wohl, Anthony S. *Endangered Lives: Public Health in Victorian Britain* (Cambridge, Mass., 1983).

Wood, Evelyn. "Tactics and Health in the Army, 1848–1908," JRAMC, 12–8–17 (1909).

Woodhull, Alfred Alexander. *Observations upon the Medical Department of the British Army.* St. Louis, Mo., 1894.

Woods, Robert. The Effects of Population Redistribution on the Level of Mortality in Nineteenth-Century England and Wales. *Journal of Economic History*, 45:645–51 (1985).

Woods, Robert, and John Woodward (eds.). *Urban Disease and Mortality in Nineteenth-Century England.* New York, 1984.

Woods, Robert, and P. R. Andrew Hinde. "Mortality in Victorian England: Models and Patterns." JIH, 18:27–54 (1987).

Worboys, Michael. "Science and British Colonial Imperialism, 1895–1940." Unpublished Ph.D. Diss., University of Sussex, 1979.

World Health Organization (WHO). *International Standards for Drinking Water.* 3d ed. Geneva, 1971.

Wrigley, E. Anthony, and Roger S. Schofield. *The Population History of England, 1541–*

1871. Cambridge, Mass., 1981.

Wylie, John Capie. *The Wastes of Civilization.* London, 1959.

Yabé, Tatsusaburo. "Disparition du Kakké (Béribéri) dans la marine japonais." AMN, 73:58–551 (1900).

Yeo, Isaac Burney. *Food in Health and Disease.* London, 1889.

Zuckerman, Arie, J., and C. R. Howard, *Hepatitis Viruses in Man.* New York, 1979.

INDEX